Infections Affecting Pregnancy and Childbirth

JUDY BOTHAMLEY

RN, RM, ADM PGCEA, MA

Senior Lecturer in Midwifery
University of West London

and

MAUREEN BOYLE

RN, RM, ADM PGCEA, MSc

Senior Lecturer in Midwifery
University of West London

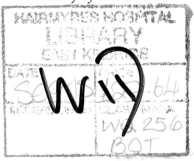
Radcliffe Publishing
London • New York

Radcliffe Publishing Ltd
St Mark's House
Shepherdess Walk
London N1 7BQ
United Kingdom

www.radcliffehealth.com

British Library Cataloguing in Publication Data

A catalogue record for this book is available from the British Library.

ISBN-13: 978 190936 835 4

The paper used for the text pages of this book is FSC® certified. FSC (The Forest Stewardship Council®) is an international network to promote responsible management of the world's forests.

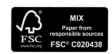

Typeset by Darkriver Design, Auckland, New Zealand
Printed and bound by Hobbs the Printers, Totton, Hants, UK

Contents

About the authors

Judy Bothamley, RN, RM, ADM PGCEA, MA, is a senior lecturer in midwifery at the University of West London. Following nurse training in her native country of Australia she qualified as a midwife in the UK in 1983, and she has had a varied clinical and teaching career. She has worked on a tertiary referral high-risk labour ward and as the lead midwife in the antenatal clinic and antenatal/postnatal ward and has always felt that women with complications of pregnancy deserve supportive and knowledgeable midwifery care. Her teaching interests include physiology and pathophysiology, high dependency care, emergencies and complications of pregnancy. She has published articles on a range of subjects including the experience of fathers, tuberculosis in pregnancy, cardiac disease and the challenge of obesity. She has collaborated with her colleague Maureen Boyle on a number of projects including as co-author for *Medical Conditions Affecting Pregnancy and Childbirth* (Radcliffe Publishing 2009).

Maureen Boyle, RN, RM, ADM PGCEA, MSc, is a senior lecturer in midwifery at the University of West London. After working as a nurse in Canada, she qualified as a midwife in the UK in 1985, and has practised since then at St Mary's Hospital in Paddington, London. She has specialised in the support of women experiencing complications in pregnancy and delivery, using this to underpin the development of a continuing personal and professional development module for experienced midwives, *High Dependency Care for Midwives*. She has published widely, including editing *Emergencies Around Childbirth: A Handbook for Midwives* first and second editions (Radcliffe Publishing 2002, 2011), *Wound Healing in Midwifery* (Radcliffe Publishing 2006) and, together with Judy Bothamley, *Medical Conditions Affecting Pregnancy and Childbirth* (Radcliffe Publishing 2009).

List of abbreviations

AAP	American Academy of Pediatrics
ABC	Airway, Breathing and Circulation
ABG	arterial blood gas
ABM	Academy of Breastfeeding Medicine
ACA	acrodermatitis chronica atrophicans
ACOG	American College of Obstetricians and Gynecologists
AIDS	acquired immune deficiency syndrome
ALT	alanine aminotransferase
ANTT	aseptic non-touch technique
APH	antepartum haemorrhage
ARM	artificial rupture of membranes
ART	antiretroviral therapy
AST	aspartate aminotransferase
BASHH	British Association for Sexual Health and HIV
BCG	bacillus Calmette–Guérin
BIA	British Infection Association
BLT	British Liver Trust
BV	bacterial vaginosis
CDC	Centers for Disease Control and Prevention (United States)
CEMD	Confidential Enquiries into Maternal Deaths
CHIVA	Children's HIV Association
CMACE	Centre for Maternal and Child Enquiries
CMV	cytomegalovirus
CNS	central nervous system
CO_2	carbon dioxide
CRP	C-reactive protein
CRS	congenital rubella syndrome

CS	caesarean section
CTG	cardiotocography
CVP	central venous pressure
DH	Department of Health
DNA	deoxyribonucleic acid
DTaP/IPV	diphtheria, tetanus, five-component acellular pertussis and inactivated polio antigens vaccine
DTaP/IPV/Hib	diphtheria, tetanus, acellular pertussis, inactivated polio and *Haemophilus influenzae* type b vaccine
DTPa	diphtheria, tetanus and acellular pertussis vaccine
ELISA	enzyme-linked immunosorbent assay (a technique for detecting antigens and antibodies)
EMDC	European Mode of Delivery Collaboration
EOGBS	early-onset group B streptococcus
FBC	full blood count
FCU	first-catch urine
fFN	fetal fibronectin
GAS	group A beta-haemolytic streptococcus
GBS	group B streptococcus
GBSS	group B Strep Support
GP	general practitioner
GUM	genitourinary medicine
HAART	highly active antiretroviral therapy
HAV	hepatitis A virus
HBcAg	hepatitis B core antigen
HBeAg	hepatitis B envelope antigen
HBIG	hepatitis B immunoglobulin
HBsAg	hepatitis B surface antigen
HBV	hepatitis B virus
HCC	hepatocellular carcinoma
HCV	hepatitis C virus
HDV	hepatitis D (delta) virus
HEV	hepatitis E virus
HICPAC	Hospital Infection Control Practices Advisory Committee
HIV	human immunodeficiency virus
HNIG	human normal immunoglobulin
HPA	Health Protection Agency (UK) – now defunct
HPV	human papilloma virus
HSE	Health and Safety Executive
HSV	herpes simplex virus

ICNARC	Intensive Care and National Audit Research Centre
ICU	intensive care unit (or ITU: intensive therapy unit)
IgA	immunoglobulin A
IgG	immunoglobulin G
IgM	immunoglobulin M
IP HIV Group	International Perinatal HIV Group
IPTp	intermittent preventive treatment in pregnancy
ITNs	insecticide-treated mosquito nets
IUGR	intrauterine growth restriction
IV	intravenous (into a vein)
JCVI	Joint Committee on Vaccination and Immunisation
LFTs	liver function tests
LOGBS	late-onset group B streptococcus
M, C & S	microscopy, culture and sensitivity
MDR TB	multi-drug-resistant tuberculosis
MDT	multidisciplinary team
MEOWS	modified early obstetric warning system
MMR vaccination	measles, mumps, rubella vaccination
MRSA	methicillin-resistant *Staphylococcus aureus*
MSM	men who have sex with men
MSU	midstream specimen of urine
NaTHNaC	National Travel Health Network and Centre
NCSP	National Chlamydia Screening Programme
NHS	National Health Service (UK)
NHS IDPSP	NHS Infectious Diseases in Pregnancy Screening Programme
NICE	National Institute for Health and Care Excellence (UK)
NMC	Nursing and Midwifery Council
PaCO$_2$	partial pressure of carbon dioxide
PCR	polymerase chain reaction
PEP	post-exposure prophylaxis
PHE	Public Health England
PID	pelvic inflammatory disease
PROM	prolonged rupture of membranes
RANZCOG	Royal Australian and New Zealand College of Obstetricians and Gynaecologists
RBCs	red blood cells
RCM	Royal College of Midwives
RCN	Royal College of Nursing
RCOG	Royal College of Obstetricians and Gynaecologists (UK)
RCP	Royal College of Physicians

RNA	ribonucleic acid
SaO$_2$	oxygen saturation
SIGN	Scottish Intercollegiate Guidelines Network
SIRS	systemic inflammatory response syndrome
SSPE	subacute sclerosing panencephalitis
STI	sexually transmitted infection
TOP	termination of pregnancy
U&E	urea and electrolytes
UK	United Kingdom
UK NSC	UK National Screening Committee
US DHHS	US Department of Health and Human Services
UTI	urinary tract infection
VZIG	varicella zoster immunoglobulin
VZV	varicella zoster virus
WBCs	white blood cells
WHO	World Health Organization

Introduction

The Confidential Enquiries into Maternal Deaths in the United Kingdom report for 2006–08, *Saving Mothers' Lives*, highlighted an alarming rise in the number of maternal deaths attributed to sepsis (CMACE 2011). This launched the issue of infection-related illness once again into the forefront of the care of mothers and babies. Alongside concerns about the impact of sepsis, questions have been raised about why this increase has occurred and what is the effect of infective illness in pregnancy generally. At the same time there has been growing concern about antimicrobial resistance, which means that the drugs used to fight a range of infectious diseases are becoming less effective (DH 2013). The World Health Organization (2014) considers antimicrobial resistance an increasingly serious threat to global public health. It has identified tuberculosis, malaria and the human immunodeficiency virus (HIV) as particularly problematic, but it also cites the risk of the high proportions of antibiotic resistance in bacteria that cause common infections (e.g. urinary tract infections, pneumonia, bloodstream infections) in all regions of the world.

It is therefore timely to consider the role midwives have in preventing, identifying, referring and managing infection-related illness. This book aims to provide midwives with accessible information about a range of infections that affect pregnancy and childbirth. The field of infectious diseases moves quickly, with new techniques of diagnosis and treatment being developed and the emergence of newly identified infections. This book brings together policy guidelines from a range of specialist areas including Public Health England; the British Association for Sexual Health and HIV; the UK National Screening Committee; the Royal College of Obstetricians and Gynaecologists; and epic3: national evidence-based guidelines for preventing healthcare-associated infection. While every effort has been made to keep abreast of changes, readers are advised to access up-to-date resources and contemporary clinical guidance when directing care. Each chapter in this book therefore provides a list of useful Internet-based resources.

Why are pregnant and postnatal women vulnerable to infections?

Pregnant women, in the same way as the general population, can be exposed to the pathogenic organisms that cause infection. However, some features of pregnancy, labour and the postnatal period mean that susceptibility to those infective agents is altered. Some aspects are protective; pregnant women are usually healthy and young and they usually adopt healthy lifestyle choices such as giving up smoking and improving their nutrition. Other aspects of pregnancy make women more vulnerable to infection, including the relative suppression of the immune response that protects the fetus from rejection (*see* section 'Changes to immunity in pregnancy' in Chapter 1).

The normal physiological adaptations of pregnancy mean that some infections can be more severe in pregnant women. Influenza and chickenpox are more likely to be complicated by the development of pneumonia, for example, and there is an increased risk of infections of the urinary tract. Interventions related to labour and delivery, including urinary catheterisation, cannulation and surgical procedures, allow entry to infection. The postnatal period, in particular, is a vulnerable time for infection, with the potential for development of sepsis, as the delivery of the placenta leaves an exposed area on the lining of the uterus and the opportunity for infective agents to enter the bloodstream. Nutritional demands and lack of sleep may contribute to the vulnerability of the immune system at this time.

The changing profile of pregnant women and susceptibility to infection

Women from poor socio-economic groups, those from minority ethnic groups and those born outside of the UK are more likely to suffer from an infective illness. A multitude of reasons may contribute to this profile. Travel and immigration mean that some infections (HIV, hepatitis, tuberculosis, malaria) that are more prevalent in other countries are now seen in UK settings (*see* Chapters 7, 8, 9 and 13). Women from outside the UK may not have had the advantage of relevant vaccinations. Vulnerable women, including those who don't speak English, will have more difficulty accessing services and getting treatment early. Poor nutrition, increased stress and overcrowded living conditions will make them more susceptible to the spread of infection. Midwives who understand the transmission and management of infections are well placed to offer effective, non-judgemental care and support for women affected by an infectious disease.

The numbers of women with coexisting medical complications such as diabetes, obesity, anaemia and sickle-cell disease are increasing, and these women are more likely to suffer from the effects of an infectious illness.

Infections that may affect the fetus or newborn

Another area of concern for midwives and mothers alike regarding infections is the potential for mother-to-child transmission. Most viruses and many bacteria are able to cross the placenta, although few do. Midwives will be familiar with the antenatal screening programme for HIV, which aims to both identify women with HIV in order to prevent HIV infection in the newborn and improve the health of the mother.

Women come into contact with common childhood illnesses through their own children and some of these infections can harm the fetus (*see* Chapter 11). Midwives are well placed to recognise the features of these illnesses and ensure prompt referral for diagnosis and management. Midwives also have a role in providing information about vaccination programmes that will help prevent morbidity associated with these infections. Recent outbreaks of whooping cough (*see* Chapter 10) and measles were reminders of the importance of vaccination and parents require clear information to support their decision-making.

Infection is a significant cause of preterm labour. Ascending genital tract infection is a known cause of preterm rupture of the membranes. In addition, many infectious diseases cause a high temperature and this may lead to preterm labour with increased morbidity for the newborn.

Food-borne and vector-transmitted infections (*see* Chapters 12 and 13) are another area of infections that may affect the fetus, and midwives need to provide information to women regarding both the transmission of these infections and how to prevent them.

What is the role of the midwife in addressing the problems associated with infectious diseases in pregnancy?
A key component of midwifery care is to *prevent* the spread of infective illness. The essential tenets of prevention centre on handwashing and aseptic technique along-side education regarding transmission. In theory these are the same basic principles of infection control that have been known for years and yet strict adherence and acknowledgement of the importance of these factors needs persistent emphasis (*see* Chapter 14).

Pregnancy brings women into contact with health professionals including mid-wives and provides the opportunity for *screening*. Under the direction of the UK National Screening Committee, all pregnant women are offered screening for hepatitis B, HIV, syphilis and susceptibility for rubella at booking. These are just a few of the conditions discussed in this book. Suitability for universal screening is assessed according to availability of an appropriate test and that for the condition diagnosed there is suitable treatment available with proven benefit. Issues around screening and approaches to identifying those at risk are discussed within each chapter of this book.

A challenging aspect of screening for infectious diseases involves the midwife identifying those at risk of a particular infection. The midwife requires knowledge of factors that might make a woman more vulnerable to infection as well as *recognising* the signs and symptoms of infective illness in the woman or those around her. The midwife may be responsible for the collection of samples to aid diagnosis and the follow-up of results. Timely and appropriate *referral* by the midwife to medical care is likely to significantly improve the outcome for mother and baby.

When a woman is diagnosed with an infectious condition, midwives will be responsible for supporting the woman through what may be a period of great concern for her health and that of her baby. Many infectious conditions carry stigma and can lead the woman to feel isolated and vulnerable. Sympathetic, confidential and respectful care by the midwife that provides ongoing support and education is essential to restore dignity and a sense of well-being alongside physical recovery.

REFERENCES

Centre for Maternal and Child Enquiries (CMACE) (2011) Saving mothers' lives: reviewing maternal deaths to make motherhood safer: 2006–2008. The Eighth Report of the Confidential Enquiries into Maternal Deaths in the United Kingdom. *Br J Obstet Gynaecol.* **118**(Suppl. 1): 1–203.

Department of Health (DH) (2013) *UK Five Year Antimicrobial Resistance Strategy 2013 to 2018* [online]. London: DH. Available at: www.gov.uk/government/uploads/system/uploads/attachment_data/file/244058/20130902_UK_5_year_AMR_strategy.pdf (accessed 11 June 2014).

World Health Organization (2014) *Antimicrobial Resistance: global report on surveillance 2014* [online]. Geneva: WHO. Available at: http://apps.who.int/iris/bitstream/10665/112642/1/9789241564748_eng.pdf?ua=1 (accessed 11 June 2014).

CHAPTER 1

Infectious organisms and the immune system

> → **Infectious organisms**
> → **Defence against infection: the immune system**
> → **Support of the immune system in pregnancy**

INFECTIOUS ORGANISMS

CLASSIFICATION OF INFECTIOUS ORGANISMS

There are five main classes of pathogens that cause infectious disease. These are *viruses*, *bacteria*, *fungi*, *protozoa* and *worms* (also known as helminths). Table 1.1 gives an overview of their size, their structure and the typical diseases they cause. In addition to these pathogens, there are *prions*, which are not organisms but are proteins that cause infection. A sixth class of organisms are insects that inhabit the skin, known collectively as *ectoparasites*.

Viruses

Viruses are the most commonly occurring pathogen with more than 1550 species having been identified (Murray *et al.* 2005). The simplest virus consists of a core of nucleic acid surrounded by a protein coat known as a capsid. Viruses contain either RNA or DNA, which contain the genetic code of the virus and serve as a blueprint for many more viruses. Viruses can only multiply inside a host cell. Entry to the cell is gained by attachment to molecules on the surface of the host cell. In order to multiply, a virus enters the body's cell where it 'taps into' the DNA of the host cell and directs it to make more copies of the virus. Once the virus has reproduced itself thousands of times inside the cell, particles can be released by budding out of the cell, or burst out causing the cell to rupture, and each viral particle attempts to infect another cell (Wilson 2006). This injures or kills the host cell and when enough cells are injured or

TABLE 1.1 Major classes of infectious organisms

Class	Visibility	Structure	Typical organisms and diseases
Prions	Electron microscope	Protein	Variant Creutzfeldt–Jakob disease
Viruses	Electron microscope	Nucleic acid (DNA or RNA) wrapped in a coat of protein	Common cold Influenza Measles, rubella, parvovirus Hepatitis Human immunodeficiency virus Cytomegalovirus Human papilloma virus Herpes Dengue fever
Bacteria	Light microscope	Single-cell organisms with a cell wall but lacking a nucleus (prokaryotic)	Staphylococci Group A and B streptococci Gonorrhoea Listeria Syphilis Tetanus Tuberculosis Chlamydia Whooping cough Lyme disease
Protozoa	Light microscope	Single cell with nucleus (eukaryotic)	Malaria Trichomoniasis Toxoplasmosis Chagas' disease
Fungi	Light microscope Naked eye (some)	Single or multicellular	Candidiasis (thrush)
Worms	Naked eye	Multicellular	Threadworms Roundworms (nematodes) Hookworms Tapeworms
Insects	Naked eye	Multicellular – inhabit skin only	Head and body lice, scabies

destroyed, recognisable illness such as influenza, the common cold or herpes occurs (Stanberry 2006). Some viruses insert all or part of their nucleic acid into the host cell's DNA, where it may code that cell for unlimited cell division. This may cause malignancy and is possibly the mechanism by which human papilloma virus causes cervical cancer.

Because viruses are hidden inside the cells they are difficult to eliminate. T-lymphocytes (*see* section 'Adaptive immunity' later in this chapter) detect and destroy cells that are infected by viruses by recognising certain receptor molecules on the infected cells' surfaces. These receptor molecules are a combination of host cell receptors and virus particles.

Many viruses, however, cause no harm and are dealt with effectively by the immune system, which kills the virus-infected cell. Carrier status is when viruses survive in cells without damaging them. The person suffers no illness but can be infectious to others. Women may be 'carriers' of a virus after recovery from the acute phase of the initial infection (e.g. hepatitis B). A virus can also become dormant or latent (e.g. herpes) and become reactivated in the future, possibly when the immune system is stressed, causing another symptomatic infection.

Bacteria

Bacteria are single-cell organisms, the majority of which live independently. Bacteria inhabit the environment (air, food, water), and although many of these don't cause disease, some can cause life-threatening illness. Bacteria are known as prokaryotes; that is, they have a single chromosome but don't have a defined nucleus. The cell wall structure of bacteria is complex and determines its classification. A rapid staining method using a simple iodine/crystal violet-based technique, the Gram stain, distinguishes the two main types of bacteria.

1. In *Gram-positive* bacteria the purple stain gets trapped in the peptidoglycan layer (a thick, mesh-like structure) that surrounds the cell.
2. *Gram-negative* bacteria have a thin peptidoglycan layer and an overlaying membrane that doesn't stain (Murray *et al.* 2005).

Some bacteria lack a cell wall and survive only inside host cells – for example, chlamydia. Mycobacterium, such as *Mycobacterium tuberculosis*, have a waxy outer layer and are known as acid-fast bacilli. Outside the cell wall bacteria may have *capsules* to protect them, *flagella* to enable movement or *pili* to aid attachment to mucosal surfaces. Further classification is determined according to size, shape (spheres (cocci), rods (bacilli), spirals (spirilla)) and arrangement (single cell, chains (strep), clusters (staph)).

Thousands of different bacteria inhabit the body. Many are 'good' bacteria forming the normal flora of the skin and gut and provide benefit to the human host. Intestinal flora, for example, are essential for vitamin synthesis. Antibiotics, although highly successful in treating bacterial infections, may alter this normal flora, which can be dangerous, allowing more harmful organisms such as *Clostridium difficile* to establish themselves.

Some dangerous bacterial diseases are due to the harmful effect of bacterial toxins (tetanus, diphtheria and cholera are examples) (Playfair & Bancroft 2004). Exotoxins are secreted by organisms, while endotoxins are an integral part of the cell wall of the bacteria. Some toxins act as superantigens, causing activation of T-cells and an inflammatory cytokine response. This can result in toxic shock syndrome, a widespread physiological reaction causing fever, shock, gastrointestinal disturbance and a rash (Gillespie & Bamford 2012).

Protozoa

Protozoa are single-cell eukaryotic organisms. The immune system finds it difficult to control these pathogens and it is also difficult to design drugs to combat them.

Malaria is commonly caused by the protozoan *Plasmodium falciparum*, which is transmitted by the bite of a particular mosquito (*see* Chapter 13). Another protozoan condition of significance in maternity care is toxoplasmosis, which is acquired from food and from water contaminated with cat faeces. Up to 50% of the human population harbour toxoplasmosis but don't have any symptoms. The protozoan survives in the form of cysts that can be reactivated if the host becomes immunocompromised. An active infection in the mother can pass to the fetus via the placenta, damaging the fetus (Playfair & Bancroft 2004) (*see* Chapter 12). *Trichomonas vaginalis* is a sexually transmitted protozoan of the vagina and urethra (*see* Chapter 5).

Fungi

Fungi come in an enormous range of shapes and sizes but only a very few are medically important. The yeast *Candidia albicans* is a normal commensal of the gut and moist skin sites. However, it can overgrow in the mouth, vagina and other sites, causing considerable irritation (*see* Chapter 5). Long-term antibiotic treatment that disturbs the normal flora may allow this yeast to flourish (Playfair & Bancroft 2004).

Worms (helminths)

Worms are more commonly a cause of disease in tropical countries. Examples include roundworms, hookworms, tapeworms and flukes. The presence of intestinal worms will result in poor uptake of nutrients by the host and is a common cause of iron-deficiency anaemia. Threadworms (also known as pinworms) are common in the UK, especially in those under 10 years of age. As their name implies, threadworms look like tiny pieces of white thread and may be seen around the anus or in the stool. A distinguishing feature indicating their presence is itchiness around the anus, usually worse at night.

Insects

Ectoparasites is the name given to insects that live on the outside of the body and that are of medical importance (Playfair *et al.* 1998). These cause itchiness and rashes.

Head lice are common among school-age children and therefore may be seen in pregnant women. Table 1.2 lists some of the more common ectoparasites.

TABLE 1.2 Common ectoparasites

Example of ectoparasite	Name
Mites	*Sarcoptes scabiei (scabies)*
Lice	*Pediculus* spp (head lice, body lice, pubic lice)
Bugs	*Cimex* spp (bedbug)

THE RELATIONSHIP BETWEEN PATHOGENS AND DISEASE

The relationship between pathogens and disease is not a simple case of cause and effect but, rather, a complex interaction between opportunity, the tenacity of the organism and the susceptibility of the host. Figure 1.1 shows the chain of infection with recommendations on how the cycle of infection can be broken. *See* Chapter 14 for further detail on methods of infection control, particularly within hospital settings.

An individual can be *colonised* with a microorganism, and when this does not cause any clinical symptoms, it is not considered to be an infection. Some women are colonised by group B streptococcus in the vagina and this usually does not cause harm to the mother, although it may cause an infection if passed to the infant (*see* Chapter 6). Pathogenic organisms are usually only able to establish themselves under certain circumstances. Infection is the detrimental colonisation of microorganisms that causes ill health, although the actual symptoms of an infectious disease are sometimes caused by the immune system itself rather than the pathogen (Playfair & Bancroft 2004).

Most organisms don't cause a particular distinct disease, although some do (e.g. *Treponema pallidum* causes syphilis). More often the location in the body of an organism determines the nature of the disease (e.g. *Staphylococcus aureus* may be responsible for wound infection, pneumonia and/or food poisoning). In addition, one disease can be caused by any number of different organisms making it difficult to identify a possible cause to treat (Murray *et al.* 2005). Maternal sepsis, for example, can be caused by a range of pathogens.

Sources of infection

Much human disease derives from the person's own 'normal flora' that finds its way into the wrong place. This is known as *endogenous* infection. For example, *S. aureus*, normally found in the nose, may cause wound infection if it gets into a surgical wound. Surgery and intravenous cannulation allow normal skin flora (*Staphylococcus epidermidis*) to penetrate beneath the skin. *Escherichia coli*, which is a normal inhabitant of the gut, can cause symptoms of infection if transferred to the vagina. Women

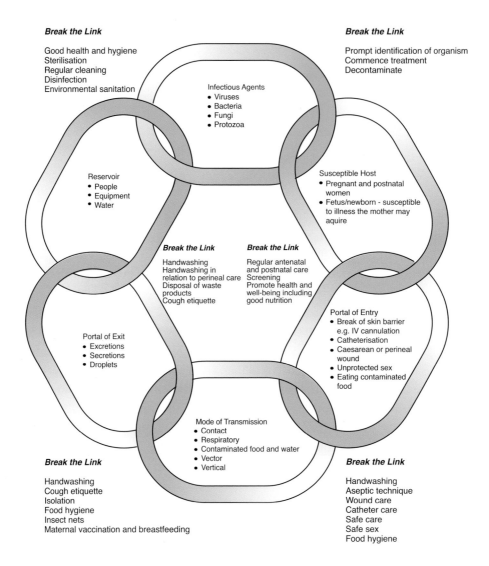

Break the Link

Good health and hygiene
Sterilisation
Regular cleaning
Disinfection
Environmental sanitation

Infectious Agents
- Viruses
- Bacteria
- Fungi
- Protozoa

Break the Link

Prompt identification of organism
Commence treatment
Decontaminate

Reservoir
- People
- Equipment
- Water

Susceptible Host
- Pregnant and postnatal women
- Fetus/newborn - susceptible to illness the mother may aquire

Break the Link

Handwashing
Handwashing in relation to perineal care
Disposal of waste products
Cough etiquette

Break the Link

Regular antenatal and postnatal care
Screening
Promote health and well-being including good nutrition

Portal of Entry
- Break of skin barrier e.g. IV cannulation
- Catheterisation
- Caesarean or perineal wound
- Unprotected sex
- Eating contaminated food

Portal of Exit
- Excretions
- Secretions
- Droplets

Mode of Transmission
- Contact
- Respiratory
- Contaminated food and water
- Vector
- Vertical

Break the Link

Handwashing
Cough etiquette
Isolation
Food hygiene
Insect nets
Maternal vaccination and breastfeeding

Break the Link

Handwashing
Aseptic technique
Wound care
Catheter care
Safe care
Safe sex
Food hygiene

FIGURE 1.1 Breaking the chain of infection

who have conditions that lower their natural immunity (such as HIV) are prone to infection from organisms normally held in check by the body's defences. Latent tuberculosis, for example, can become active in individuals with HIV.

Exogenous infections are those a person 'catches' from external sources such as inhaling the cold virus after someone coughs or sneezes, or through sexual contact. This makes other people, such as partners, close family members and, in particular, young children, a significant source of infection for pregnant women. Ingestion of contaminated food and water is another significant cause of infection (*see* Chapter 12).

ROUTES OF TRANSMISSION

The more efficient the transmission of an organism, the more rapidly it will spread disease through a population. Influenza, for example, is spread very efficiently via respiratory droplets and through contact with contaminated surfaces. Understanding routes of transmission provides a platform to control the spread of infection. Table 1.3 gives an overview of the principle routes of transmission and Figure 1.2 illustrates routes of mother-to-child transmission.

TABLE 1.3 Principle routes of transmission

Routes of transmission	Explanation	Examples
Direct contact	Touching, kissing, skin contact	Chickenpox Cold virus Glandular fever Oral herpes type 1
Respiratory route There are two classes of respiratory transmission: 1. droplet nuclei, where particles travel less than a metre 2. airborne transmission, when particles remain airborne and can travel more than a metre	Coughs, sneezes, laughing and talking	Cold virus Influenza Pulmonary tuberculosis Whooping cough Chickenpox Measles Mumps Rubella
Sexual contact	Sexual intercourse permits organisms with poor survival ability outside the body to be transmitted through direct contact of mucosal surfaces and via secretions (sperm, vaginal fluid, saliva) Transmission of HIV is enhanced where genital ulceration caused by other sexually transmitted diseases exists	Syphilis Gonorrhoea HIV Human papilloma virus Herpes 1 and 2 Hepatitis B
Indirect contact	Via objects (also known as fromites): tissues, bedding, drinking cups, toys, money	Influenza
Via blood and blood products	Blood transfusion Sharing of needles	Hepatitis HIV
Mother-to-child transmission (also known as vertical transmission)	Via the placenta	Rubella HIV Cytomegalovirus

(continued)

Routes of transmission	Explanation	Examples
Mother-to-child transmission (also known as vertical transmission)	During the birth	Chlamydia Gonorrhoea HIV Active herpes
	In breast milk	HIV Cytomegalovirus
Faecal–oral and other contaminated food and water	Food and water may contain microorganisms that will infect the gastrointestinal tract; this may occur when hands are not washed before preparing and eating food Poor storage of food, inadequate cooking or lack of pasteurisation	Hepatitis A Salmonella Listeria Toxoplasmosis
Iatrogenic	Transmission due to medical procedures and interventions	Infection following catheterisation, cannulation, surgery
Vector-borne transmission	A vector is an organism that does not cause a disease but acts as a vehicle to transmit the pathogen from one host to the next; an example is the mosquito that transmits malaria	Malaria (mosquito) Lyme disease (ticks) Chagas' disease (tritomine bug) Dengue (mosquito)

(Playfair & Bancroft 2004, Gillespie & Bamford 2012, Brankston *et al.* 2007)

Maternal infection passes to fetus via the placental barrier

Rubella, CMV, Parvovirus B19, Herpes simplex, HIV, Varicella, Listeria, Syphilis, Toxoplasmosis

During birth
Passage through infected birth canal
Colonisation of ascending infection after rupture of membranes
Exposure to maternal blood

CMV, Herpes, HIV, *E. coli*, Group B strep, Chlamydia, Gonorrhoea, Listeria

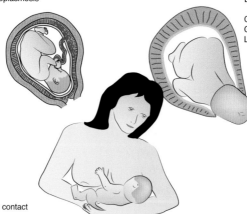

Postnatal
Close oral/respiratory contact
Breastfeeding
Faecal/oral spread via milk, blood, respiratory droplet

CMV, Hepatitis B, Varicella, HIV, Herpes

FIGURE 1.2 Mother-to-child transmission

DEFENCE AGAINST INFECTION: THE IMMUNE SYSTEM

OVERVIEW

The immune system involves a remarkable array of cells, proteins and chemicals that provide constant surveillance for any signs of invading pathogens or foreign particles. The immune system can be thought of as a complex war strategy. Some of the elements of that strategy include:

- alerting the rest of the army (complement)
- cooperation and communication (cytokines)
- short- and long-term strategy and defence: innate (short term) and adaptive (long-term immunity)
- avoidance of 'friendly fire' (T regulatory cells and avoidance of autoimmune diseases).

It uses:

- external defences, which aim to simply keep pathogens out
- innate (or inbuilt) immunity, which is a set of phagocytic cells, enzymes and proteins that attack invading microorganisms; the hallmark of innate immunity is inflammation
- adaptive immunity, which utilises a specialised set of cells that includes B- and T-lymphocytes; these cells identify the pathogens, mark them for disposal and importantly retain memory so that future attacks can be dealt with efficiently.

TABLE 1.4 Components of innate and adaptive immunity

	Innate immunity	**Adaptive immunity**
External defences	Skin, normal bacterial flora, lysozymes, pH, mucous membranes	Antibodies in mucosal membranes
Cellular elements	Phagocytes: neutrophils, macrophages (from monocytes), eosinophils Basophils (mature to mast cells) Natural killer cells	T-lymphocytes – four main types: helper, memory, cytotoxic, regulatory (previously known as suppressor) B-lymphocytes, plasma cells (that produce antibodies) and B memory lymphocytes
Chemical mediators and humoral components	Complement Cytokines (especially interferon) Histamine Prostaglandins, kinins, pyogens	Antibodies (immunoglobulins) Cytokines (especially interleukins)

(Rote & Crippes Trask 2006, Crippes Trask *et al.* 2006, Coico *et al.* 2003)

The immune system needs to recognise pathogens. When a cell has a molecule on its surface the cell is said to express that molecule. They are known as 'markers' (this can be thought of as having an identifying flag on the outside of the cell). These 'markers' on the surface of pathogens are made up of lipopolysaccharides and other cell wall components and are more formally known as pathogen-associated molecular patterns. These trigger the release of cytokines including interferons and chemokines, which signal the cells of the immune system to respond (Murray *et al.* 2005). Some markers are unique to the pathogen. These can be recognised by specialist molecules (human leucocyte antigen, T-cell receptors) to lead to an antigen-specific response.

INNATE IMMUNITY (ALSO KNOWN AS NON-SPECIFIC)

Innate immunity is inherent in each individual and is designed to give immediate protection to the body. It includes external defences that prevent entry of microbes, chemical mediators, and cells that are involved in phagocytosis. Table 1.4 gives an overview of the components of innate immunity.

External defences

The first line of defence for invading microorganisms is the skin and mucous membranes, which act as a physical barrier. The external defences also remove microorganisms in several ways. The ciliated epithelium of the respiratory tract, for example, wafts out microbes trapped in mucus, and coughs and sneezes expel them forcefully. In the urinary tract, normal flora and changes in acidity make it difficult for invading pathogens to grow, and bacteria can be washed out with the flow of urine. Figure 1.3 identifies some of the key features of the external defence system.

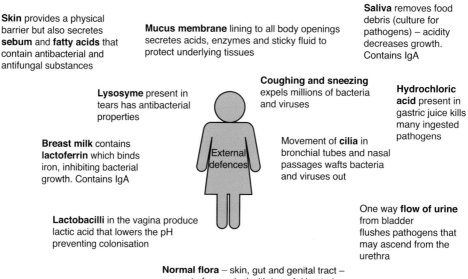

Skin provides a physical barrier but also secretes **sebum** and **fatty acids** that contain antibacterial and antifungal substances

Mucus membrane lining to all body openings secretes acids, enzymes and sticky fluid to protect underlying tissues

Saliva removes food debris (culture for pathogens) – acidity decreases growth. Contains IgA

Lysosyme present in tears has antibacterial properties

Coughing and sneezing expels millions of bacteria and viruses

Hydrochloric acid present in gastric juice kills many ingested pathogens

Breast milk contains **lactoferrin** which binds iron, inhibiting bacterial growth. Contains IgA

Movement of **cilia** in bronchial tubes and nasal passages wafts bacteria and viruses out

External defences

Lactobacilli in the vagina produce lactic acid that lowers the pH preventing colonisation

One way **flow of urine** from bladder flushes pathogens that may ascend from the urethra

Normal flora – skin, gut and genital tract – compete for survival with harmful bacteria. They also produce **bacteriocins** which act like antibiotics and suppress competing organisms

FIGURE 1.3 External defences

Cells of the innate immune system

White blood cells (WBCs) (leucocytes) are manufactured in the red bone marrow and lymphatic tissue, and are released into the blood to be transported through the body. Table 1.5 lists the cells of the innate system and their main function and Figure 1.4 illustrates the different types of cells. To be effective, white cells need to be able to move into the tissue. They are alerted to the presence of microbes by chemical mediators (*see* section 'Chemical mediators' later in this chapter) and can squeeze over the surface and between cells to reach their target and destroy them by phagocytosis (engulfment) and other mechanisms.

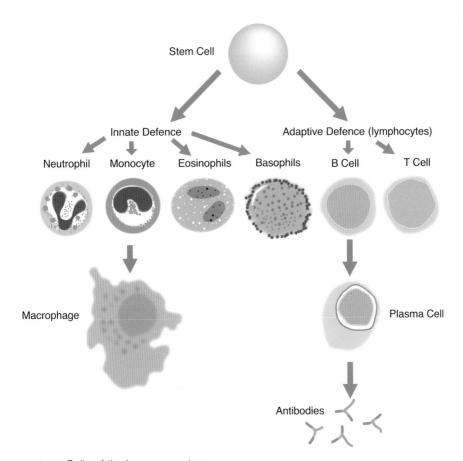

FIGURE 1.4 Cells of the immune system

Phagocytes include *neutrophils* (the most numerous of WBCs (40%–75%) and *macrophages* (derived from monocytes). They engulf foreign substances and destroy them with chemicals. Phagocytes have a molecule on their surface known as a receptor. This receptor binds on to the surface of pathogens and holds them. The phagocytes can then release proteolytic enzymes, which destroy the pathogen (Helbert 2006).

Phagocytes can then ingest particles including bacteria, fungi and viruses. Pus, a yellow discharge commonly found at a site of infection, is made up of dead and dying neutrophils and bacterial and tissue debris. Phagocytes also release *chemokines*, (including complement and histamine) which are small proteins that establish a chemical pathway, attracting more phagocytes to the site of infection.

Basophils are found in small numbers in the circulation (<0.2%). They are produced in the red bone marrow and, in a similar way to neutrophils, they can leave the blood and enter infected tissue. *Mast cells* are non-motile cells found in connective tissue, particularly in the epithelial layers of the intestinal, respiratory and urogenital tract. When activated by complement or by antibodies they produce an inflammatory response through release of histamine and other chemicals (Higgins 2007). *Eosinophils* produce enzymes that break down the chemicals released by basophils and mast cells, acting to keep the inflammatory response under control. Eosinophils also secrete enzymes that effectively kill larger pathogens such as parasites. *Natural killer cells* are large white cells found in the circulation and in most tissue. As their name implies, the main function is to deal with virus-infected cells and tumours.

TABLE 1.5 Cells of the innate immune system and their main function

Cell	Main function
Neutrophil	Small phagocyte; usually the first cell to arrive at site of infection, promotes inflammation
Macrophage (derived from monocytes)	Large and effective phagocytic cell; name means 'big eater'; important in later stages of infection and in tissue repair; involved in activation of B- and T-cells
Basophil	Motile cell that can move from blood into tissue; it releases chemicals that promote inflammation
Mast cell	Non-motile cell present in connective tissue that causes inflammation
Eosinophil	Enters tissues from the blood and releases chemicals that inhibit inflammation
Natural killer cells	Break down tumour and virus infected cells

(Seeley *et al.* 2008)

Chemical mediators of the immune system

These are molecules (rather than cells) that work alongside the cells of the immune system. They include surface chemicals such as lysozymes present in tears and saliva, cytokines (including the interferons), and other factors, including complement, that act as chemical signals to attract WBCs and promote inflammation (Seeley *et al.* 2008).

Complement is a system of approximately 20 plasma proteins that circulate in the blood in an inert form. Activation of a complement cascade involves a series of enzyme reactions activated by sugars present on the surface of pathogens. Complement works by punching holes in pathogens but also signals to bring more phagocytes to the area. Phagocytes and the complement system are effective in dealing with pathogens living outside the cells (i.e. most bacteria).

Cytokines are peptide messenger molecules used for communication between cells. All the cells of the innate and adaptive immune system can both secrete and respond to cytokines. They include interleukins, interferons and tumour necrosis factor. *Interferons* are secreted by many body cells and act by switching off the cells' mechanisms that are used in viral replication. As such they are effective at fighting viral infections. Interferons also play a role in controlling growth of some cancer cells, and genetically engineered interferons are used in cancer treatment and the treatment of some viral diseases including hepatitis C and genital warts (Seeley *et al.* 2008).

An acute inflammatory response such as that seen in wound healing involves a number of these chemical mediators and cytokines (*see* section on inflammatory response later in this chapter and also Chapter 3). Table 1.6 lists some chemical mediators and outlines their function.

TABLE 1.6 Chemical mediators and their function

Chemical	Function
Surface chemicals	Lysosome (in tears, saliva, nasal secretions and breast milk) breaks down cells and increases acidity to prevent microbial growth; creates mucus to trap microbes so they can be destroyed
Histamine	Released from mast cells, basophils and platelets; causes vasodilation, which increases blood flow; increases vascular permeability that allows movement of fluid out of the blood and into the tissue causing oedema; causes contraction of bronchiole airways; attracts eosinophils
Kinins	Cause vasodilation, increases vascular permeability, stimulates pain receptors and attracts neutrophils
Interferons	Act by switching off the cells' mechanisms that are used in viral replication
Complement	System of approximately 20 plasma proteins; they damage pathogens and promote the release of histamine and kinins and attract a range of white cells to the area
Prostaglandins	Cause smooth muscle relaxation that increases blood supply through vasodilation; they also increase vascular permeability and stimulate pain receptors
Pyogens	Chemicals released by some of the white cells that stimulate fever

(Seeley *et al.* 2008, Marieb & Hoehn 2013)

There are limitations to what the innate immune system can do. It is not completely effective against intracellular organisms (i.e. viruses and *M. tuberculosis*). Innate immunity is swift and non-specific. However, longer-lasting resistance and immunity that has a specific memory for a quicker response to the pathogen is also important.

ADAPTIVE IMMUNITY (ALSO KNOWN AS SPECIFIC OR ACQUIRED)

Adaptive immunity is a form of defence that identifies specific foreign substances (antigens) and produces long-lasting antibodies, which are present on mucosal surfaces and in the blood. Lymphocytes (so called as they were first identified in lymph) are the distinctive cells of this system, and unlike the cells of the innate immune system they carry specific surface molecules (usually referred to as receptors), which enable them to recognise foreign antigens. Lymphocytes can work in different ways. They can:

- secrete proteins called antibodies
- secrete substances that influence other cells including the release of special chemical mediators in blood (e.g. complement or interferon) that aid pathogen destruction.

See Table 1.4 for a summary of the main components of adaptive immunity.

There are three fundamental features of adaptive immunity (Coico *et al.* 2003, Marieb & Hoehn 2013).

1. *Specificity*: the adaptive immune system differentiates between different pathogens and can create specific T- and B-lymphocytes to recognise and mount an effective response to most of them.
2. *Tolerance to self*: 'avoiding friendly fire'. The immune system needs to recognise itself.
3. *Memory*: the body remembers the first contact with an infective illness so that any subsequent infection is repelled. First contact with a pathogen is slow and less aggressive but secondary response is rapid and vigorous. This is the basis for the use of vaccines.

Anatomical components of the lymphatic system

Adaptive immunity begins at the site of infection, is amplified in the lymph nodes and then spreads through the body via the lymphatic and blood system. The anatomical structures of this system include the bone marrow and the thymus (situated behind the sternum), as well as lymph nodes, spleen and mucosa-associated lymphoid tissues (*see* Figure 1.5).

This system is closely linked to the cardiovascular system. It provides a complex network of drainage, defence and storage of white cells. Lymphatic capillaries run alongside blood capillaries and remove excess interstitial fluid from tissue and that fluid becomes lymph. This lymph travels to lymph nodes through lymphatic vessels where lymphocytes respond to infection (Seeley *et al.* 2008, Vickers 2005). The lymphatic system recycles 2–4 L a day of interstitial fluid, which drains back into the venous system regulating fluid balance between the interstitial space and the vascular system (Blay *et al.* 2012). Lymphoid tissue provides support for lymphocytes and

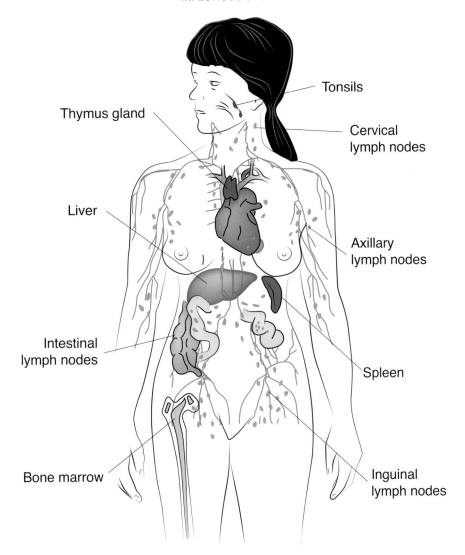

Tonsils

Thymus gland

Cervical
lymph nodes

Liver

Axillary
lymph nodes

Intestinal
lymph nodes

Spleen

Bone marrow

Inguinal
lymph nodes

FIGURE 1.5 Anatomical structures of the lymphatic system

macrophages, which can quickly squeeze through the capillary walls, enabling them to circulate in the blood and respond to invading microorganisms. Lymph nodes, full of lymphocytes that are ready to destroy pathogens, are strategically placed around the body. Antigens can be conveyed to a lymph node close to the site of infection, enabling the infection to be contained in a small area. This causes swollen, painful lymph nodes. The spleen is the largest lymphoid organ. Box 1.1 lists the main functions of the spleen. The spleen has only a thin outer capsule and is liable to rupture following blunt trauma. If damage occurs, removal is recommended to prevent life-threatening blood loss. The function of the spleen can be taken over by the liver and bone marrow, although the person is left more vulnerable to infection.

BOX 1.1 MAIN FUNCTIONS OF THE SPLEEN

- Surveillance for infection
- Circulates lymphocytes and is a site where lymphocytes respond to infection
- Filters pathogens and toxins from the blood
- Removes ageing, faulty platelets and red blood cells from the blood
- Storage of platelets
- Recycling and storage of iron for the production of red blood cells

---

Lymphocytes

Lymphocytes are the cells of the lymphatic system and spend most of their 2- to 4-year life cycle within lymphoid tissue. They originate from stem cells in the red bone marrow and account for 20%–45% of WBCs (Seeley *et al.* 2008). There are two types of lymphocytes: B-cell lymphocytes ('B' because they mature in the **b**one marrow) and T-cell lymphocytes ('T' because they mature in the **t**hymus). The B-cells make antibodies that attack bacteria and toxins, while the T-cells attack body cells that have been taken over by viruses.

T-Lymphocytes

The immunity given by T-lymphocytes is also called cell-mediated immunity. There are four main types of T-cells.

1. T helper (Th1 and Th2): these are the most common T-lymphocytes –
    a. Th1 cells help coordinate the immune response by production of cytokines, which support and promote cytotoxic T-lymphocytes and macrophages
    b. Th2 cells cooperate with B-lymphocytes to produce antibodies; mature T helper cells express the surface protein CD4.
2. T regulatory (Treg) (formerly known as T suppressor): these control the immune response to avoid friendly fire.
3. T cytotoxic (Tc): recognise and attack cells containing intracellular pathogens such as viruses. The CD8 co-receptor is predominantly expressed on the surface of these cells.
4. T memory (Tm): these cells, as the name implies, remember there was an infection, so that when there is another encounter with the same pathogen the response is rapid with the pathogen being destroyed before having a chance to cause a problem (Vickers 2005, Marieb & Hoehn 2013, DH 2013).

The importance of helper T-cells can be seen in HIV, a virus that infects cells that are CD4 positive (including helper T-cells). With progression of HIV infection the number of functional CD4-positive T-cells falls, which leads to the symptomatic stage of infection known as the acquired immune deficiency syndrome (*see* Chapter 7).

T-lymphocytes are also able to recognise and control cancerous cells (Higgins 2007).

B-lymphocytes

B-lymphocytes give rise to the type of immunity known as humoral immunity, so called because the effective components are soluble in tissue and plasma rather than being cells. B-lymphocytes are triggered into action by T helper lymphocytes, which enable them to multiply. B-lymphocytes differentiate to *plasma cells*, which produce antibodies (known as immunoglobulin). Plasma cells are found in lymphoid tissue (e.g. spleen, lymph nodes). Other B-lymphocytes are *B memory lymphocytes*.

Immunoglobulins perform several functions:

- activate the complement system
- attach themselves to the invading microorganism and 'mark' them for disposal, allowing phagocytes or other killer cells to destroy the cell
- can bind to and neutralise bacterial toxins.

Microorganisms (bacteria, viruses, and so forth) all have specific surface proteins called antigens. When antibodies bind to these surface antigens, this prevents the bacteria and viruses from invading further. In addition, bacteria that are antibody coated in this way are much more readily phagocytosed (destroyed). Antibodies can also neutralise toxins (DH 2013). Antibodies are only effective against microbes outside of the host cells, as they cannot enter cells.

Box 1.2 gives an overview of the five classes of immunoglobulin and their function.

BOX 1.2 CLASSES OF IMMUNOGLOBULIN AND THEIR FUNCTION

There are several different classes of immunoglobulin molecules and the main ones are IgM, IgG, IgA and IgE.

- **IgM** can recognise many common antigens and is particularly important during the first few days of a primary immune response. It activates components of the innate immune system stimulating complement and phagocytosis.
- **IgG** is probably the most important immunoglobulin and is the most abundant. It is present in most body compartments, including interstitial spaces and is able to activate complement and increase phagocytosis. It is the major immunoglobulin in a secondary response to infection and survives a long time. It can be measured to confirm immunity to a specific condition. IgG is a small enough molecule to cross the placental barrier, providing immunity to the newborn for up to 4 months.

- **IgA** – there are two different types of IgA: serum IgA, found in blood, and secretory IgA, found in saliva, tears, colostrum, breast milk and mucosal secretions. Consequently, IgA provides mucosal immunity and thus is protective of the respiratory passages and gastrointestinal tract. It is particularly useful in protecting the breastfed infant from intestinal pathogens.
- **IgE** binds to mast cells and basophils and stimulates the inflammatory response. Its main function is to combat intestinal worm infection in combination with mast cells. If the IgE recognises worm antigen it causes the mast cells in the host's mucosa underlying the worm to release chemicals that make the gut produce increased amounts of mucus. The gut contracts, the worm loses grip and it is expelled. In developed countries where worm infestation is rare it is mainly seen in allergic conditions.
- **IgD** is found mainly in the blood on lymphocyte surfaces. Its function is not known for certain, but is possibly related to tolerance.

(Helbert 2006,Vickers 2005, Marieb & Hoehn 2013)

B memory lymphocytes

These 'remember' antigens that have been encountered before. When subsequent infection occurs, these cells instruct plasma cells to produce the particular immunoglobulin required, bringing the infection under control quickly. Thus after a primary (first) infection that makes the person quite ill, repeat or secondary infection won't be noticed. Immunisation uses this principle and is very effective against a range of illnesses.

ACQUIRING IMMUNITY INCLUDING VACCINATION
Primary and secondary response

A first exposure to a foreign antigen produces a primary antibody response. This response is dominated by IgM antibody. The secondary response follows, and is noted by an increase in IgG. The recognition of the different type of antibody on a blood test will allow a microbiologist to determine whether a woman has immunity to a particular infection (indicated by the presence of type-specific IgG) or has had recent contact with the infection (indicated by the presence of type-specific IgM).

Adaptive immunity can be acquired by *natural* means when exposed to antigens as part of everyday living or *artificially* through immunisation. An *active* immune response that is long-lasting, involves the individual's own immune system developing immunological memory. *Passive* immunity occurs when ready made antibodies are introduced to the body instead of being made by the body's own plasma cells. The protection these 'borrowed' antibodies provide is short-lived and ends when they are naturally degraded (Marieb & Hoehn 2013). Figure 1.6 shows the different ways to acquire immunity.

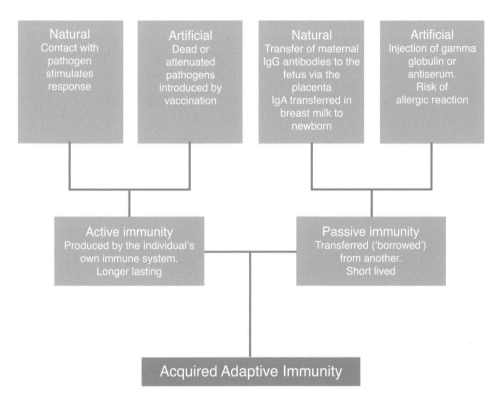

FIGURE 1.6 Acquiring adaptive immunity

Passive immunity

An important protection for newborn babies is passive immunity acquired from the mother. Transfer of immunoglobulins to the fetus or newborn means there is temporary transfer of immunological memory. Whatever organisms the mother is immune to, she transfers those IgG antibodies across the placenta. Transport of IgG begins at around 22 weeks and peaks at 32 weeks of pregnancy (Blackburn 2013). IgA antibodies present in colostrum and breast milk provide further protection. Both IgG and IgA do not last long but do offer protection for the newborn during the first 3–6 months of life (Marieb & Hoehn 2013, Vickers 2006, Blackburn 2013).

Passive immunity can be provided in the form of gamma globulin such as that used when a person is exposed to hepatitis B, or as antiserum following a spider bite. A common use of artificial passive immunity is the use of anti-D (an example of gamma globulin), which prevents a Rh-negative mother developing her own antibodies to Rh-positive cells that may enter her system from a rhesus-positive baby (Vickers 2005).

It works by destroying the fetal Rh-positive red blood cells in the mother's system before the foreign D antigen on these cells can be recognised by the mother's immune system. If that happened it would trigger formation of antibodies and, more importantly, create immunological memory that would result in a destructive antibody response to Rh-positive fetal cells in a subsequent pregnancy. Because the anti-D is passive, the body naturally degrades it and it disappears from the system (Blackburn 2013).

Vaccination

For a vaccine to be successful it needs to be safe, not cause the illness it is aiming to prevent and must be effective in protecting the person for at least several years. Vaccination uses the principle of antigen recognition and memory to augment the body's immune system and has been very successful in fighting infections. Immunological memory enables the immune system to recognise and respond to natural infection at a later date. Vaccines can be made from inactivated (killed) or live but attenuated (weakened) pathogens. Other vaccines use just a few fragments from the cell as antigens (DH 2013). Toxoids are inactivated bacterial toxins that can induce an immune response. Diptheria and tetanus are examples of toxoids. Killed vaccines have the advantage of non-infectivity but generally evoke a lowered immunogenic response and thus require several doses (Goering *et al.* 2013). DNA technology and new ways of administering vaccines via mucosal surfaces such as nasal passages are the focus of new research (Vickers 2006, Goering *et al.* 2013). Hepatitis B virus vaccine was the first vaccine for use in humans that was made using recombinant DNA technology to produce a protein antigen (Goering *et al.* 2013).

Some vaccines require two or more injections to elicit an effective antibody response. The diptheria, pertussis, tetanus vaccination is an example of this, requiring three doses for the primary course. Further reinforcement is required with booster doses to provide longer-term protection. Waning immunity was identified as a cause of the 2012 whooping cough outbreak (*see* Chapter 10).

Live attenuated vaccines such as MMR usually provide a lifelong response after one to two doses. In this form of vaccination the live organism replicates in the person and this triggers the immune system to respond in the same way as would occur following a natural infection. The virus has been developed to be weak so should not cause illness but sometimes mild symptoms like a rash may appear. Live attenuated vaccines include yellow fever, measles, mumps, rubella and bacillus Calmette–Guérin (DH 2013). MMR in particular is contraindicated in pregnancy because of potential for the attenuated virus to cause fetal damage (Blackburn 2013, Goering *et al.* 2013). Caution should also be applied regarding live vaccines and those who are immunocompromised. *The Green Book: Immunisation against Infectious Diseases* (*see* the list of useful resources at the end of the chapter for access details) provides detailed advice about specific vaccine preparations.

A small number of individuals may not mount a primary response to a vaccination and will remain vulnerable to infection. For others the primary response works but wanes over time. However, vaccination works in two ways. First, for the individual as described; second, protection is also achieved via 'herd' immunity, that aims to ensure sufficient immunity in an entire population to reduce the risk of the infection being transmitted (DH 2013).

Concerns regarding vaccines

With a reduction in many childhood illnesses, parents' concerns have moved from anxiety related to their child getting one of these illnesses to concern over the safety of the vaccines (Bloom *et al.* 2014). The Joint Committee on Vaccination and Immunisation in the UK, and similar organisations in other countries, such as the Centers for Disease Control and Prevention in the United States, review research evidence to monitor the safety record of vaccinations. Their findings are included in information leaflets for parents. Readers are directed to the useful resources for professionals provided at the end of this chapter that provide access to extensive reviews of evidence regarding vaccine safety. Midwives involved with vaccination programmes will need to be knowledgeable about the specific vaccines they are giving and be able to offer information to parents.

One of the concerns that has been expressed by parents, is regarding the number of vaccinations given, particularly the practice of combining vaccines to be given at the one time and the potential for this to 'overload' the immune system. On a daily basis from birth, babies are exposed to foreign antigens including bacteria and viruses. Eating food introduces bacteria and when the infant puts their hands in their mouth they introduce a large range of antigens from the environment. By comparison with this large amount of antigenic stimuli, vaccines provide specific stimulation to a much smaller proportion of the capacity of the immune system (DH 2013, Miller *et al.* 2003, Offit *et al.* 2002, CDC 2012a)

Parents may also ask midwives about constituents added to vaccines. Adjuvants are substances added to a vaccine to enhance the body's response to the antigen component of the vaccine. They allow a smaller amount of the inactivated virus or bacterial component to be used in the production of the vaccine. Aluminium salts or gels are used and these elements are common in the environment already, being present in air, food and water and thus are considered safe (CDC 2010, Goering *et al.* 2013). New adjuvants are being investigated including the use of cytokines (Goering *et al.* 2013).

Some vaccines used in the UK may contain traces of thiomersal, a mercury-containing preservative used in the manufacturing process to prevent bacterial growth. Links to autism, despite lack of evidence of harm, led to a reduction in its use in vaccines since 1999, although studies still have not found any evidence of a causal link (CDC 2012b, McMahon *et al.* 2008, Thompson *et al.* 2007, Price *et al.* 2010). The

Commission on Human Medicines maintains a regular review of the safety of all vaccines including those containing thiomersal. They conclude that there is a small risk of a skin rash or swelling at the injection site in thiomersal-containing vaccines but no evidence of any adverse neurodevelopmental effects (MHRA 2014).

Alterations to the immune system during pregnancy do not appear to alter the woman's response to vaccination (Blackburn 2013). (*See* individual chapters for more specific detail on relevant vaccinations for women and the newborn.)

THE INFLAMMATORY RESPONSE

The inflammatory response is the physiological response generated by the immune system in response to tissue damage and to the invasion of bacteria, viruses and other pathogens. The cardinal signs of acute inflammation are redness, heat, swelling, pain and loss of function. Inflammation isolates, inactivates and removes any pathogens and damaged tissue in order to protect the body and enable healing. Inflammatory conditions are recognised by the Latin suffix *itis*. For example, endomet*ritis* describes infection of the endometrium (lining of the uterus). (Chapter 3 provides in-depth discussion of the application of the inflammatory response in relation to wound healing.)

Chemical mediators (*see* earlier section 'Chemical mediators of the immune system'), including histamine, complement and kinins, are released from damaged cells. These dilate arterioles and local capillaries so that blood flow to the area is increased (redness). Increased blood flow brings more oxygen and nutrients for the cells and increases local temperature. The increased temperature at the site of infection has the dual benefit of inhibiting pathogen growth whilst helping the action of phagocytes. Histamine, along with prostaglandins, also cause changes to the walls of venules that allow movement of fluid out of the blood and into the tissue causing oedema.

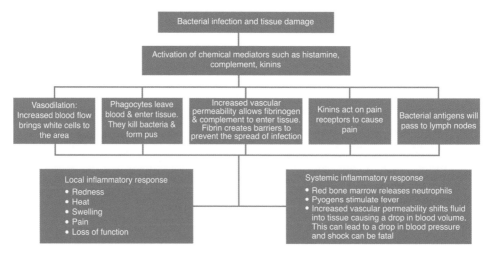

FIGURE 1.7 Stages of local and systemic inflammation

In addition, plasma proteins leave the blood, the osmotic pressure of blood falls and water moves from the blood to the tissue (Seeley *et al.* 2008). *Cytokines* (which include interferon and different classes of interleukin) are a further set of specialised proteins that prime an immune response. Their role in the signs and symptoms of the inflammatory response are elaborated in Box 1.3.

Figure 1.7 summarises some of the stages of local and systemic inflammation – these occur in a series of overlapping stages.

BOX 1.3 CYTOKINES AND SIGNS AND SYMPTOMS OF THE INFLAMMATORY RESPONSE

Receptors for cytokines in the hypothalamus trigger the autonomic nervous system, which raises body temperature and helps control replication of viruses and other pathogens. Tiredness, muscle pains, headaches and loss of appetite are common features of infection thought to be due to higher levels of cytokines. Sweating and shivering can occur with more severe infection.

The liver responds to cytokines (and thus infection) by increasing a number of acute phase proteins. C-reactive protein levels increase up to a 100 times during infection. Blood levels are used to monitor progression of infection. C-reactive protein binds to pathogens and initiates part of the complement cascade.

This increase in acute-phase proteins in the blood has the effect of increasing plasma viscosity; this is reflected in a raised erythrocyte sedimentation rate.

High levels of cytokines increase nitric oxide, which is a powerful vasodilator, causing cardiac output to fall. The resultant drop in blood pressure is characteristic of very severe infections such as septicaemia.

(Helbert 2006, Waugh & Grant 2010)

BLOOD TESTS THAT INDICATE THE INFLAMMATORY RESPONSE
White blood cell count

There are five distinct populations of white cells that are included in the WBC count. Another category known as blasts or atypical cells is also included. Total WBC count is the total number of all of these, while the differential count is a count of each one. They are reported as the absolute number of each type of cell, as well as the percentage proportion of total WBCs. Table 1.7 gives the approximate reference ranges for WBCs.

An increase in WBCs is usually a sign of infection and inflammation, although they can be raised following surgery or because of autoimmune disease or malignancy (Blann 2006). WBC volume increases slightly after 8 weeks of pregnancy.

During labour and the early postpartum period there is an increase in neutrophils, which represents a normal response to physiological stress. This returns to normal by 4–7 days postpartum (Blackburn 2013). A decreased WBC count implies a problem with immunity and thus a susceptibility to infection.

TABLE 1.7 Approximate reference ranges for white blood cell (WBC) counts in a non-pregnant adult

WBC	Percentage of total WBCs	No. of cells × 10⁹ L
Total WBC count		3.9–11.1
Neutrophils	40–75	2.5–7.5
Lymphocytes	20–45	1.5–4.0
Monocytes	2–10	0.2–0.8
Eosinophils	1–6	0.04–0.44
Basophils	<1	0.01–0.10
Blasts (atypical cells)	<1	

(Higgins 2007, Blann 2006)

C-reactive protein

C-reactive protein levels increase up to a 100 times during infection. C-reactive protein binds to pathogens and initiates part of the complement cascade.

Raised erythrocyte sedimentation rate

The increase in acute phase proteins in the blood has the effect of increasing plasma viscosity, and this is reflected in a raised erythrocyte sedimentation rate.

NEGATIVE ASPECTS OF IMMUNITY

Hypersensitivity

Inflammation is a normal response to infection. In some situations though, the immune response causes more damage than the pathogen. Hypersensitivity can also occur when the immune system responds to harmless substances. There are a number of different types of hypersensitivity provoked by immune response but this section considers only two, as they occur more commonly in the maternity population.

1. *Allergic reactions* occur immediately after exposure to an antigen (or allergen as it is usually called in this circumstance) and involves activation of mast cells. Allergic reactions are more common in individuals with an 'atopic' genetic predisposition (Helbert 2006). Examples include atopic eczema, rhinitis, asthma, anaphylaxis.
2. *Autoimmunity* The distinction between 'self' and 'foreign' is a key requirement of immunity. The thymus sifts out any T-cells that would activate against 'self' cells. Similarly, only self-tolerant B-cells leave the bone marrow. Failure of the

thymus (usually genetic) or a breakdown in peripheral tissues caused by infection can impair the mechanisms. This lack of 'tolerance' results in production of autoantibodies (antibodies that attack self). Examples of autoimmune disorders are systemic lupus erythematosus, rheumatoid arthritis and Graves' disease.

Infertility, spontaneous miscarriage, pre-eclampsia and rhesus isoimmunisation are conditions that are related to immune dysfunction and adversely impact outcomes for mother and baby (Blackburn 2013).

CHANGES TO IMMUNITY IN PREGNANCY

The fetus is essentially 'foreign' to the maternal immune system, being the result of the combined DNA contribution of mother and father and thus 50% foreign material. To avoid rejecting the fetus the maternal immune system reduces its immune response predominantly through suppression of Th1 cell activity. However, other factors are enhanced and provide protection for mother and fetus (Gibson & Lee 2008). Box 1.4 summarises some of the changes to immunity seen in pregnancy.

BOX 1.4 CHANGES TO IMMUNITY IN PREGNANCY

INNATE
- Moderate increase in neutrophils
- Decreased natural killer cell activity
- Some complement factors are increased and some (those that would reject the fetus) are decreased

ADAPTIVE
- Suppression of Th1 cell function and reduced cytokine production. This suppression of cellular immunity may be responsible for the increased susceptibility of pregnant women to infections such as chickenpox, listeria and fungal infection.
- Enhanced Th 2 cell response and increased activation of complement system enhances maternal defences against most bacterial infections.
- Humoral immunity stays the same – normal B-cell function and antibody response is maintained to pathogens and vaccines, although levels of IgG may go down in later pregnancy secondary to placental transfer to the fetus.

(Gibson & Lee 2008, Blackburn 2013)

IMMUNITY AND THE NEONATE

Babies' immune systems begin to develop during embryogenesis, within their sterile environment. Following birth, they are exposed to innumerable antigens, and within a very short time the muscosal surfaces of the gastrointestinal and respiratory tract are colonised (Favier *et al.* 2002). Colonisation in a hospital environment will differ from those babies born at home, and they will also receive antigens from caregivers' handling, as well as familiar ones from their mother.

There is some evidence that the gut flora influences the physiology of the mucosal tissue, barrier function and immunologic and inflammatory responses (Agostoni *et al.* 2004), therefore underpinning the efficiency of the immune system, and Turroni *et al.* (2012) suggest successful colonisation is directly affected by the mode of delivery and breastfeeding.

Vaginal birth is thought to promote the production of cytokines and their receptors, and therefore means that the immune system of these babies is stimulated significantly more than that of babies born by caesarean section (Malamitsi-Puchner *et al.* 2005; Aagaard *et al.* 2012). This may be an area where midwives can influence the outcome, by promoting practices that can lead to a vaginal birth.

The baby's immune system is supported by passive immunity, which is transferred from the mother during pregnancy and following delivery via breast milk (Niers *et al.* 2007). It has been suggested that breast milk is an irreplaceable immunological resource, as it not only influences passive and active immunity during infancy (Labbok *et al.* 2004) but also can have potentially life-long benefits (Niers *et al.* 2007). Promotion and support of breastfeeding is very much a key part of the midwife's role.

SUPPORT OF THE IMMUNE SYSTEM IN PREGNANCY

All childbirth includes some tissue damage needing healing, and in addition, childbirth is usually a major life stressor; therefore, the risk of a compromised immune system, and infection, for the new mother is always present. However, some women may also have additional risk factors (*see* Box 1.5) and midwives need to be aware of this when assessing and supporting women in their care.

As all women have the potential for compromise to their immune system, the midwife's practice should routinely encompass ways of supporting the immune system (*see* Box 1.6). The immune system is not a single entity, but a complex – and poorly understood – interface of varied components. Although there is little hard evidence on what actions can increase the effectiveness of an individual's immune system (Stambach 2010), there are several areas where it is likely that the midwife could potentially make a difference in the outcome, by her activities or by education and support of the woman. By her actions at this time, not only may the midwife be fulfilling her role as a health promoter but also this could be seen as preconception care for the next pregnancy, and it has the potential for long-term health benefits for the woman and her family.

BOX 1.5 CHARACTERISTICS OF THOSE AT RISK OF PREGNANCY OR POSTNATAL INFECTION

- Age >35 years
- Poorly nourished
- Underlying illness or conditions such as diabetes, anaemia, obesity
- Pre-existing infection such as chorioamnionitis
- Smoking
- Premature labour
- Prolonged rupture of membranes
- Pre-operative hospitalisation (possible compromised nutrition, lack of sleep, increased stress or increased exposure to hospital pathogens)
- Prolonged labour (increased numbers of interventions, especially vaginal examinations, as well as potential for compromised nutrition, lack of sleep and increased stress)
- Extensive perineal damage (especially with increased blood loss)
- Caesarean section delivery (in particular, emergency or urgent: usually these operations will be done either following a long, debilitating labour, or due to an emergency such as haemorrhage; for whatever reason the likelihood is that the woman will be under both physical and psychological stress – resulting in potential compromise to the immune system)
- Repeat caesarean section (frequently involving increased surgery time)
- Increased stress, either physiological or psychological

BOX 1.6 AREAS IN WHICH HEALTH PROMOTION MAY IMPROVE THE IMMUNE SYSTEM

- Nutrition and/or weight reduction
- Smoking cessation, reduction in alcohol consumption
- Maintenance of adequate sleep
- Regular exercise
- Reduction of stress
- Alternative healing and complementary therapies
- Avoidance of infection (midwifery actions and advice to women)

NUTRITION

Deficiency in nutrients in pregnancy may not necessarily impact on the fetus, but it may deplete the woman's stores so that she is prone to delayed healing and increased infection following the birth. Attention paid to the nutritional status of a woman could protect her from beginning motherhood in a compromised state.

Although it seems self-evident that a healthy diet (*see* the list of useful resources at the end of this chapter for specific guidance on what constitutes a healthy diet in pregnancy) should contribute to a healthy immune system, there are few studies that lead to specific guidelines. However, not all women may have the knowledge of what constitutes a healthy diet for pregnancy – a small study in the United States found that most women had inadequate nutritional knowledge and suboptimal diets (Fowles 2002) and this had previously also been found in the UK (Pearson *et al.* 1996). There is some evidence that women would welcome a 'healthy eating' support system during pregnancy (Olander *et al.* 2012).

Food choices can be dependent on many factors apart from knowledge as to what is a 'healthy diet'. Choice may be limited by what is affordable or available, and food eaten as children influences choices as adults. Some may avoid food that they feel was 'forced' on them, whereas other foods may be seen as a 'treat' or comfort food because of past experiences. There are many value judgements attached to foods; for instance, when eating alone people will often eat food they would not eat in company. This may influence how a woman describes her diet to a midwife, and she may only include food that she perceives will be approved of by the midwife. Overall in the UK there has been a change in how food is viewed, and with the growing trend in obesity, many foods are seen as bad and dangerous. In the postnatal period the tiredness of new motherhood may work against spending the time needed to source and prepare healthy food.

The postnatal period is a time when the immune system is highly activated in order to undertake all the necessary healing and avoid infection. However, it may also be a time when many women embark on calorie-restricted or fad diets. The majority of first-time mothers are surprised at the amount of weight retained immediately post-delivery (Stein & Fairburn 1996) and may be highly motivated to lose weight. Midwives need to ensure women are aware of what their body needs to accomplish, and that good nutrition is necessary to heal and maintain good health at a time of increased stress. Therefore, fad diets and/or decreasing valuable nutrients at this time will not be beneficial. The establishment of healthy eating and exercise is recommended to avoid long-term obesity (a risk factor for infection) although women should not try to lose weight quickly but, rather, set realistic goals for gradual weight loss based on good nutrition (NICE 2010).

Daily requirements for nutrients will vary for the individual and the circumstances. Amounts must be able to be obtained from the daily diet or from the body's stores of nutrients, and if from stores, these then need to be replaced or they will become depleted. However, it is difficult to determine what is an exact deficiency level of each nutrient, as many do not have recognised criteria of clinical deficiency, especially in pregnancy and the puerperium. Even if there were clear deficiency levels identified, it would be more useful to aim for adequate intake and stores to ensure the ability to cope with times of decreased input or increased stress. Since these would be highly individualised, it seems establishing general criteria would be of limited use. It also must be remembered that pregnancy enhances absorption of many nutrients, so any criteria would need to reflect this.

In pregnancy and the puerperium when perhaps being able to tolerate only a small intake, or when time is very limited, concentration on nutrients is vital. Pregnancy is often a time when women report altered ability to taste certain foods, or 'morning sickness' may be present in a more extreme and prolonged way, and this may also restrict their diet. If already ill, the influence of being sick may impact on intake of food – many infections include nausea as part of their symptomology, and drugs taken may also cause nausea.

There is much controversy over whether or not nutritional supplements should be advised. For those women where a specific condition is identified, such as anaemia, supplementation would be needed. A healthy woman who has regularly eaten a balanced and good-quality diet pre-pregnancy probably does not need artificial supplements except for folic acid, and perhaps vitamin D, although this is more controversial (De-Regil *et al.* 2012). However, even for this woman, some would argue that elements beyond her control (e.g. vegetables grown in nutrient-deficient soil, chemicals in the food chain) may have put her at nutritional risk. A woman who has started pregnancy with poor nutritional reserves, or finds pregnancy-related illness severely restricts what she can eat, or is living in an impoverished situation (Bhutta & Haider 2009), may need a supplement. A midwife is not a professional nutritionist and should she be concerned about any individual woman, a referral to a dietician is probably the safest and most effective option.

When talking to a woman who wishes to take nutritional supplements, it is important to ensure she understands that some supplements should be avoided in pregnancy and that by taking some unnecessary individual supplements, she may be putting herself at risk of malabsorption of other micronutrients (e.g. unnecessary iron supplementation may reduce absorption of zinc).

SMOKING

Nicotine and carbon monoxide are known to have a damaging influence on wound healing, and even limited smoking can reduce the peripheral blood flow. Smoking also reduces vitamin C, which is vital for healing. Research has demonstrated that pregnant women who were smokers had lower intakes of most micronutrients, although, after adjusting for variables, only vitamin C and carotenoid intakes were reduced (Mathews *et al.* 2000). Since there is evidence in trials of elderly patients demonstrating that vitamin C supplementation aided healing (Ellinger & Stehle 2009), perhaps others, such as smokers or teenagers (especially if the woman falls into both categories), should be advised to supplement with vitamin C, or at least to increase their dietary intake, as this vitamin is so vital to healing. Again, the midwife should seek expert advice.

LACK OF SLEEP

There is a direct link between the innate immune system and sleep (Majde & Krueger 2005, Manzar & Hussain 2012). If hospitalised prior to delivery, there is a need to encourage and enable good-quality sleep as much as possible. When antenatal ward space is limited, the midwife will have to be creative to meet the needs of those in early labour, who may need to move around and make noise, and other women, who need uninterrupted sleep. Following birth, again midwives need to be aware that as much sleep as possible will contribute to the woman's uneventful recovery.

Wound healing is predominantly an anabolic process. Sleep disturbances may inhibit wound healing as sleep encourages anabolism, the synthesis of complex molecules from simple ones. It would be very rare to find a new mother who enjoyed her full quota of sleep every night, therefore putting all midwifery clients at risk in the postnatal period, and the midwife should ensure the woman knows the importance of obtaining as much sleep as possible.

EXERCISE

There is little direct evidence that regular exercise enhances the immune system (Stambach 2010). However, it is suggested that regular moderate exercise may reduce the incidence of infection (Baltopoulos 2009) and it is known to contribute to overall good health by restricting obesity, increasing general well-being and promoting good circulation, all of which are likely to impact on the immune system.

STRESS

Psychological stress is an inevitable component of pregnancy, childbirth and the puerperium. Anxiety and concern for her own – and her baby's – health and well-being are often compounded in a first pregnancy with apprehension about her ability to care for her baby. Stress, of course, is likely to be increased even further if there is any identified complication or infectious condition present.

Studies of the effect of stress on the immune system have been numerous, but there are few related specifically to pregnant women or new mothers. A stressor can be defined as a stimulus that activates the hypothalamic-pituitary-adrenal axis and/ or the sympathetic nervous system to adapt physiologically to a threat (Black 2003). However, stress has also been described as occurring when events or environmental demands exceed an individual's perceived ability to cope (Segerstrom & Miller 2004) – and this situation can clearly be applied to childbearing in general. Models of stress include 'life stressors' such as academic examinations or marital stress, 'physical training stressors' such as primary caregiving to dementia patients or pain following surgery, and 'psychological stressors' such as feelings of loneliness and depression (Webster, Marketon & Glaser 2008). These models of stressors all contain elements relevant to childbearing and therefore observed effects on immunity may similarly affect women in pregnancy and postnatally.

Stressors can increase the risk of developing infectious disease, and they can also prolong infectious illness episodes (Glaser & Kiecolt-Glaser 2005). In laboratory tests, stressors that lasted for more than 1 month were the best predictors of developing colds (Glaser & Kiecolt-Glaser 2005).

Disorders in cytokine response (an important component of the inflammatory response) can be associated with perceived stress (Coussons-Read *et al.* 2007). There are also data that suggest that stress alters the inflammatory response to immune triggers in human pregnancy (Christian 2012). In addition, there are some animal studies that demonstrate that stress or isolation can impact on the immune system by suppressing the activity of T-cells and generating fewer antibodies (Stambach 2010). In one study, chronic stress in pregnant women was associated with an increased risk of bacterial vaginosis (Culhane *et al.* 2001). Additional stress can be caused by pain and fear, and the resulting hormone secretion (especially norepinephrine) can lead to vascular changes that result in oxygen reduction in the tissue (Bryant & Nix 2012). Increased secretion of corticosteroids can inhibit production and effectiveness of leucocytes (Workman 1995). All these actions can reduce the ability of the woman's immune system to respond rapidly and adequately.

In addition, tissue damage is inevitable in any form of childbirth and it is thought that the effect on the immune system of anxiety and stress can inhibit wound healing (Christian 2012) (*see* Chapter 3 for further discussion on wounds associated with childbirth).

Depression may occur in the puerperium, and recent literature has suggested that antenatal depression is also common (Redshaw & Henderson 2013). It has been suggested that women with depressive symptoms may be more vulnerable to negative sequelae of infectious illness during pregnancy (Christian 2012). Depression may also increase cortisol levels substantially, and these increases can cause many adverse immunological changes (Glaser & Kiecolt-Glaser 2005).

Although not undertaken specifically on childbearing women, many studies (Glaser & Kiecolt-Glaser 2005) have demonstrated that greater fear or distress before surgery is associated with poorer outcomes, including longer hospitalisation and more post-operative complications. A scenario involving emergency caesarean section for fetal distress, a very common labour ward experience, will inevitably involve anxiety and fear for the woman, and the midwife needs to be aware of the possible long-term complications of this, and use her skills to moderate the woman's distress wherever possible.

Since reduction in stress can have such wide-ranging benefits, it is considered that interventions can have substantial clinical effects (Kiecolt-Glaser *et al.* 1998). It may be that increased attention to preparation for motherhood, perhaps through parent-education classes, may help to 'prepare' new mothers, although possibly this can never be accomplished. However, good supportive midwifery care at this vulnerable time may go some way towards alleviating unnecessary stress and its consequences.

ALTERNATIVE HEALING AND COMPLEMENTARY THERAPIES

Many women will seek to use alternative and/or complementary therapies, with the belief they can boost their immune systems and/or help heal specific wounds. Most of these therapies claim a decrease in stress and anxiety and this may have positive benefits for enhancing the immune system and healing. Any therapies that can deliver increased relaxation for a new mother may have effects in supporting an efficient immune system as increased rest and sleep have a proven benefit.

USEFUL RESOURCES

- Department of Health (DH) (2013) *Immunisation against Infectious Disease (the Green Book)* [online]. Available at: www.gov.uk/government/organisations/public-health-england/series/immunisation-against-infectious-disease-the-green-book
- NHS Choices (2013) *Have a Healthy Diet in Pregnancy* [online]. Available at: www.nhs.uk/conditions/pregnancy-and-baby/pages/healthy-pregnancy-diet.aspx#close (accessed 13 May 2014).
- NHS Choices (2013) *Vaccinations* [online]. Available at: www.nhs.uk/Conditions/vaccinations/Pages/Safety-and-side-effects.aspx

REFERENCES

Aagaard K, Riehle K, Ma J, *et al.* (2012) A metagenomic approach to characterization of the vaginal microbiome signature in pregnancy. *PLoS One.* **7**(6): e36466.

Agostoni C, Axelsson I, Goulet O, *et al.* ESPGHAN Committee on Nutrition (2004) Prebiotic oligosaccharides in dietetic products for infants: a commentary by the ESPGHAN Committee on Nutrition. *J Pediatr Gastroenterol Nutr.* **39**(5): 465–73.

Baltopoulos P (2009) Exercise induced modulation of immune system functional capacity. *Biol Exerc.* **5**(1): 39–49.

Bhutta Z, Haider B (2009) Prenatal micronutrient supplementation: are we there yet? *CMAJ.* **180**(12): 1188–9.

Black P (2003) The inflammatory response is an integral part of the stress response: implications for artherosclerosis, insulin resistance, type II diabetes and metabolic syndrome. *Brain Behav Immun.* **17**(5): 350–64.

Blackburn ST (2013) *Maternal, Fetal, and Neonatal Physiology*. 4th ed. Philadelphia: Elsevier.

Blann A (2006) *Routine Blood Results Explained*. Keswick: M&K Publishing.

Blay A, Finch J, Dutton H (2012) The immune and lymphatic systems, infection and sepsis. In: Peate I, Dutton H (editors). *Acute Nursing Care: recognising and responding to medical emergencies*. Harlow: Pearson. pp. 283–327.

Bloom BR, Marcuse E, Mnookin S (2014) Addressing vaccine hesitancy [editorial]. *Science*. **334**(6182): 339.

Brankston G, Giterman L, Hirji Z, *et al.* (2007) Transmission of influenza A in human beings. *Lancet Infect Dis*. **7**(4): 257–65.

Bryant R, D Nix (2012) *Acute and Chronic Wounds: current management concepts*. 4th ed. St Louis, MO: Elsevier Mosby.

Centers for Disease Control and Preventaion (CDC) (2010) *Vaccine Safety: frequently asked questions about adjuvants* [online]. Available at: www.cdc.gov/vaccinesafety/concerns/adjuvants. html (accessed 22 May 2014).

Centers for Disease Control and Prevention (CDC) (2012a) *Vaccine Safety: frequently asked questions about multiple vaccinations and the immune system* [online]. Available at: www.cdc.gov/ vaccinesafety/vaccines/multiplevaccines.html (accessed 22 May 2014).

Centers for Disease Control and Prevention (CDC) (2012b) *Vaccine Safety: thimerosal* [online]. Available at: www.cdc.gov/vaccinesafety/Concerns/Thimerosal/Index.html (accessed 22 May 2014).

Christian L (2012) Psychoneuroimmunity in pregnancy: immune pathways linking stress with maternal health, adverse birth outcomes, and fetal development. *Neurosci Biobehav Rev*. **36**: 350–61.

Coico R, Sunshine G, Benjamini E (2003) *Immunology: a short course*. 5th ed. New Jersey: Wiley–Liss.

Coussons-Read M, Okun M, Nettles C (2007) Psychosocial stress increases inflammatory markers and alters cytokine production across pregnancy. *Brain Behav Immun*. **21**(3): 343–50.

Crippes Trask B, Rote NS, Huether SE (2006) Innate immunity: inflammation. In: McCance KL, Huether SE (editors). *Pathophysiology: the biological basis for disease in adults and children*. 5th ed. Edinburgh: Elsevier Mosby.

Culhane J, Rauh V, McCollum K, *et al.* (2001) Maternal stress is associated with bacterial vaginosis in human pregnancy. *Matern Child Health J*. **5**(2): 127–34.

Department of Health (DH) (2013) Immunity and how vaccines work. In: *Immunisation against Infectious Disease (the Green Book)* [online]. Available at: www.gov.uk/government/publica tions/immunity-and-how-vaccines-work-the-green-book-chapter-1 (accessed 17 September 2014).

De-Regil L, Palacios C, Ansary A, *et al.* (2012) Vitamin D supplementation for women during pregnancy. *Cochrane Database Syst Rev*. (2): CD008873.

Ellinger S, Stehle P (2009) Efficacy of vitamin supplementation in situations with wound healing disorders: results from clinical intervention studies. *Curr Opin Clin Nutr Metab Care*. **12**(6): 588–95.

Favier C, Vaughan E, de Vos W, *et al.* (2002) Molecular monitoring of succession of bacterial communities in human neonates. *Appl Environ Microbiol*. **68**(1): 219–26.

Fowles E (2002) Comparing pregnant women's nutritional knowledge to their actual dietary intake. *MCN Am J Matern Child Nurs*. **27**(3): 171–7.

Gibson P, Lee RV (2008) Antibiotic use, immunizations and normal physiological changes in pregnancy associated with risk of infection. In: Rosene–Montella K, Keely E, Barbour LA, *et al.* (editors). *Medical Care of the Pregnant Patient.* 2nd ed. Philadelphia: ACP Press. pp. 655–61.

Gillespie S, Bamford K (2012) *Medical Microbiology and Infection at a Glance.* 4th ed. Oxford: Wiley-Blackwell.

Glaser R, Kiecolt-Glaser J (2005) Stress-induced immune dysfunction: implications for health. *Nat Rev Immunol.* **5**(3): 243–51.

Goering RV, Dockrell HM, Walkelin D, *et al.* (2013) *Mims' Medical Microbiology.* 5th ed. Oxford: Elsevier, Saunders.

Helbert M (2006) *Flesh and Bones of Immunology.* Edinburgh: Elsevier.

Higgins C (2007) *Understanding Laboratory Investigations for Nurses and Health Professionals.* 2nd ed. Oxford: Blackwell.

Kiecolt-Glaser J, Page G, Marucha P, *et al.* (1998) Psychological influences on surgical recovery: perspectives from psychoneuroimmunology. *Am Psychol.* **53**(11): 1209–18.

Labbok M, Clark D, Goldman A (2004) Breastfeeding maintaining an irreplaceable immunological resource. *Nat Rev Immunol.* **4**(7): 565–72.

Majde J, Krueger J (2005) Links between the innate immune system and sleep. *J Allergy Clin Immunol.* **116**(6): 1188–98.

Malamitsi-Puchner A. Protonotariou E, Boutsikou T, *et al.* (2005) The influence of the mode of delivery on circulating cytokine concentrations in the perinatal period. *Early Hum Dev.* **81**(4): 387–92.

Manzar D, Hussain E (2012) Sleep-immune system interaction: advantages and challenges of human sleep loss model. *Front Neurol.* **3**: 2.

Marieb EN, Hoehn K (2013) *Human Anatomy and Physiology.* 9th ed. Boston: Pearson.

Mathews F, Yudkin P, Smith R (2000) Nutrient intakes during pregnancy: the influence of smoking status and age. *J Epidemiol Community Health.* **54**(1): 17–23.

McMahon AW, Iskander JK, Haber P, *et al.* (2008) Inactivated influenza vaccine (IIV) in children <2 years of age: examination of selected adverse events reported to the Vaccine Adverse Reporting System (VAERS) after thimerosal-free or thimerosal-containing vaccine. *Vaccine.* **26**(3): 427–9.

Medicines and Healthcare Products Regulatory Agency (MHRA) (2014) *Thiomersal (ethylmercury) Containing Vaccines* [online]. Available at: www.mhra.gov.uk/Safetyinformation/Generalsafetyinformationandadvice/Product-specificinformationandadvice/Vaccinesafety/Thiomersal(ethylmercury)containingvaccines/index.htm (accessed 22 May 2014).

Miller E, Andrews N, Waight P, *et al.* (2003) Bacterial infections, immune overload, and MMR vaccine: measles, mumps, and rubella. *Arch Dis Child.* **88**(3): 222–3.

Murray PR, Rosenthal KS, Pfaller MA (2005) *Medical Microbiology.* 5th ed. Edinburgh: Elsevier Mosby.

National Institute for Health and Care Excellence (NICE) (2010) *Weight Management Before, During and After Pregnancy.* NICE Public Health Guidance 27 [online]. Available at: http://guidance.nice.org.uk/PH27 (accessed 13 May 2014).

Niers L, Stasse-Wolthuis M, Rombouts F, *et al.* (2007) Nutritional support for the infant's immune system. *Nutr Rev.* **65**(8): 347–60.

Offit PA, Quarles J, Gerber MA, *et al.* (2002) Addressing parents' concerns: do multiple vaccines overwhelm or weaken the infant's immune system? *Pediatr.* **109**(1): 124–9.

Olander E, Atkinson L, Edmunds J, *et al.* (2012) Promoting healthy eating in pregnancy: what kind of support services do women say they want? *Prim Health Care Res Dev.* **13**(3): 237–43.

Pearson S, Dimond H, Ford C, *et al.* (1996) A survey of pre-pregnancy nutritional knowledge in family planning clinics. *Br J Fam Plann.* **22**(2): 92–4.

Playfair J, Bancroft G (2004) *Infection and Immunity.* 2nd ed. Oxford: Oxford University Press.

Playfair J, Lakhani S, Lydyard P (1998) *General Pathology, Microbiology and Immunology: for health care students.* Edinburgh: Churchill Livingstone.

Price CS, Thompson WW, Goodson B, *et al.* (2010) Prenatal and infant exposure to thimersol from vaccines and immunoglobulins and risk of autism. *Pediatrics.* **126**(4): 656–64.

Redshaw M, Henderson J (2013) From antenatal to postnatal depression: associated factors and mitigating influences. *J Womens Health (Larchmt).* **22**(6): 518–25.

Rote NS, Crippes Trask B (2006) Adaptive immunity. In: McCance KL, Huether SE (editors). *Pathophysiology: the biological basis for disease in adults and children.* 5th ed. Edinburgh: Elsevier Mosby. pp. 211–48.

Seeley R, Stephens TD, Tate P (2008) *Anatomy and Physiology.* 8th ed. Boston: McGraw Hill.

Segerstrom S, Miller G (2004) Psychological stress and the human immune system: a meta-analytic study of 30 years of inquiry. *Psychol Bull.* **130**(4): 601–30.

Stambach M (2010) *The Truth about your Immune System: a Harvard Medical School special health report.* Cambridge, MA: Harvard Health Publications.

Stanberry LR (2006) *Understanding Herpes.* Mississippi: University Press of Mississippi.

Stein A, Fairburn C (1996) Eating habits and attitudes in the postpartum period. *Psychosom Med.* **58**(4): 321–5.

Thompson WW, Price C, Goodson B, *et al.* (2007) Early thimersol exposure and neuropsychological outcomes at 7–10 years. *N Engl J Med.* **357**(13): 1281–92.

Turroni F, Peano C, Pass DA, *et al.* (2012) Diversity of bifidobacteria within the infant gut microbiota. *PLoS One.* **7**(5): e36957.

Vickers PS (2005) Acquired defences. In: Montague SE, Watson R, Herbert RA (editors). *Physiology for Nursing Practice.* 3rd ed. Edinburgh: Elsevier. pp. 685–724.

Waugh A, Grant A (2010) *Ross and Wilson: anatomy and physiology in health and illness.* 11th ed. Edinburgh: Churchill Livingstone.

Webster Marketon J, Glaser R (2008) Stress hormones and immune function. *Cell Immunol.* **252**(1–2): 16–26.

Wilson J (2006) *Infection Control in Clinical Practice.* 3rd ed. Edinburgh: Baillière Tindall.

Workman M (1995) Essential concepts of inflammation and immunity. *Crit Care Nurs Clin North Am.* **7**(4): 601–15.

CHAPTER 2

Common infections associated with childbirth

→ **Urinary tract infection**

→ **Chorioamnionitis**

→ **Post-partum endometritis**

→ **Mastitis**

URINARY TRACT INFECTION

INTRODUCTION

Urinary tract infections (UTIs) are one of the most frequent complications of pregnancy, and are also very common in the puerperium, therefore making this infection of importance to the midwife. There is a range of estimates of the number of cases of asymptomatic bacteriuria during pregnancy, from 2.5% to 15% (Meads 2011).

UTIs may be categorised as follows.

- *Lower UTI*: bacterial cystitis causing frequency, urgency and dysuria (pain on micturition). In some cases bacteria cannot be cultured by routine laboratory methods.
- *Upper UTI*: bacterial pyelonephritis. Pyelonephritis is an infection of the upper urinary tract. Symptoms, in addition to those for lower UTI, may include flu-like symptoms, pyrexia, tachycardia, nausea, backache, abdominal pain and tenderness over the costo-vertebral angle on the affected side. The right side is more commonly affected (Thorsen & Poole 2002).
- *Asymptomatic bacteriuria* (covert bacteriuria): excess bacteria are present but no symptoms are evident.

There is a distinction in the definitions of cystitis, urethritis and vaginitis but in practice, symptoms often overlap, and the infection needs eradication regardless of its primary site.

Bacteria are commonly present in the perineal area, and women are thought to be more at risk of UTIs because of the short length of the urethra and the close proximity to the rectal area. Some normal defence measures are listed in Box 2.1.

BOX 2.1 NORMAL URINARY TRACT DEFENCE MEASURES

- The flushing action of the flow of urine that removes organisms from the bladder and urethra
- Urinary pH
- Phagocytosis by polymorphs on the bladder surface
- A mucous layer containing IgA on the bladder wall prevents bacterial adherence

In health the urinary tract is usually sterile, apart from the distal region of the urethra, which may be colonised with commensal organisms, such as periurethral and faecal organisms (one reason contamination may occur in a urine specimen unless a 'midstream' specimen is used). Bacterial infection is usually acquired by the ascending route from the urethra to the bladder and, if untreated, may continue to the kidney. If the infection enters the bloodstream, septicaemia may result (Bothamley & Boyle 2009).

An increased risk of UTI including pyelonephritis occurs in pregnant women because of the anatomical and physiological changes that take place in the renal system in pregnancy. These changes include:
- increased glucose excretion with glycosuria (which is not necessarily indicative of diabetes but is a good medium in which bacteria can grow)
- elongation and dilation of the ureters and physiological hydronephrosis
- decreased bladder tone as pregnancy advances, leading to urinary stasis
- change in the angle at which the ureters enter the bladder, causing urine reflux.

The majority of UTIs are caused by bacteria, and the most usual is the common perineal inhabitant, Gram-negative rod *Escherichia coli* (or *E. coli*), probably causing about 80% of infections (Meads 2011). For childbearing women, *Candida* (a fungus – *see* Chapter 5) or group B streptococci (*see* Chapter 6) are also possible causes. Further causative agents may be other Gram-negatives such as *Klebsiella*, Gram-positives such as *Staphyloccus aureus* or *Enterococcus faecalis*, or a protozoan *Trichomonas vaginalis* (most commonly seen as a sexually transmitted condition – *see* Chapter 5). Viral infection may also occur, but this is unlikely unless another condition is present (e.g. human immunodeficiency virus, mumps).

CLINICAL FEATURES

Predisposing factors

Some women are more likely to suffer from UTIs than others – obviously those with a history of recurrent UTIs when not pregnant are highly susceptible. Other predisposing conditions include obesity (Basu *et al.* 2010) and other relevant medical conditions such as diabetes or renal disease. Labour is a time when the normal defence mechanisms of the renal system may be compromised (see Box 2.2 for potential preventive measures), and catheterisation is the major predisposing factor for UTI, both during insertion and as an in-dwelling device.

Microorganisms can enter the body in the following ways:

- if the correct aseptic technique has not been followed at insertion
- bacteria can travel along the outside of the in-dwelling catheter
- bacteria can travel along the inside of the catheter, from a catheter drainage bag that has become contaminated during sampling, disconnection of the tubing, or emptying.

For these reasons, disconnection of the tubing should never be undertaken unless there is a good reason. Midwives should take care to avoid contamination of the collecting bag, and obtain specimens via the special ports in the tubing according to the manufacturer's instructions.

BOX 2.2 POTENTIAL PREVENTION OF URINARY TRACT INFECTIONS DURING LABOUR

- Encourage good fluid intake and frequent voiding
- Ensure good hygiene is maintained (a woman with an epidural may stay in a sitting position, potentially in a damp environment if amniotic fluid is draining, for some time, and this will allow perianal contamination to increase)
- Avoid urinary catheterisation
- If catheterisation is necessary, ensure best principles are followed (*see* Chapter 14)

Diagnosis and management

Testing for asymptomatic bacteriuria is a routine part of midwifery care: 'women should be offered routine screening for asymptomatic bacteriuria by midstream urine culture early in pregnancy. Identification and treatment of asymptomatic bacteriuria reduces the risk of pyelonephritis' (NICE 2008). It has been estimated that about 25%–30% of women with untreated asymptomatic bacteriuria will develop pyelonephritis (Vazquez & Abalos 2011, Smaill & Vazquez 2007). There is a link between untreated UTIs, pyelonephritis and preterm labour.

In pyelonephritis there is usually a raised serum CRP (C-reactive protein) and high leukocytes demonstrated, and screening with blood cultures for septicaemia is also carried out. Urine cultures are positive and pyuria is found – and often seen. Women with pyelonephritis are usually hospitalised, closely monitored and treated with intravenous antibiotics. Acute respiratory distress syndrome can occur, especially in those women who have received tocolysis for threatened premature labour (Gilstrap & Ramin 2001), so monitoring of the respiratory system should take place. Other complications for the woman may include septic shock with increased risk of pulmonary oedema due to fluid shift.

As it has been identified that pyelonephritis in pregnancy is a risk factor for reoccurrence of the condition (Meads 2011), both in the current pregnancy and also in a future pregnancy, midwives should ensure that if a woman reports a history of pyelonephritis, increased surveillance should be undertaken, underpinned with appropriate record keeping.

As well as signs and symptoms noted earlier, more severe symptoms such as retention of urine, haematuria, incontinence and uterine irritability, manifesting as contractions, or premature labour can also be present.

Urine tests

Visually, urine may be cloudy due to pyuria (pus cells) and bacteria, and it may contain blood. There is also frequently an offensive smell. A dipstick examination will demonstrate varying levels of protein, and perhaps blood, as well as possibly neutrophils and leucocytes. Several rapid screening tests have been evaluated; however, none have been found to perform adequately to replace urine culture for detecting asymptomatic bacteriuria (Smaill 2007). Therefore, the gold standard test for both symptomatic and asymptomatic bacteriuria is urine culture (Meads 2011). A midstream specimen of urine needs to be obtained, and therefore the midwife must ensure the woman knows how to collect this (*see* Box 2.3). The laboratory commonly tests the urine for M, C & S.

- *Microscopy* may indicate the presence of leucocytes, erythrocytes and/or epithelial cells. Neutrophils can indicate active infection. Bacteria may be seen when present in large numbers, but that may not indicate an infection if the specimen was poorly collected or left at room temperature for a prolonged period of time.
- *Culture*: various methods can be used to quantify the number of bacteria in fresh midstream urine. However, a catheter specimen will be considered infected with minimal bacteria, and any amount can be seen as abnormal as it will not be contaminated by periurethral flora. Culture normally takes 18–24 hours to allow time for the bacteria to grow, although new rapid methods are increasingly becoming

available. If anaerobes are suspected, some of the specimen will be cultured in an oxygen-free container.

- *Susceptibility or Sensitivity*: response of the bacteria to various antibiotics.

A sample that contains two or more bacterial species and/or squamous cells from the perineum is considered to be contaminated and may not be reliable.

The success of diagnostic testing depends on the optimum collection of the specimen – for urine this will include:

- correct collection of a midstream specimen of urine (*see* Box 2.3)
- when the specimen is collected
- how the specimen is stored and handled before it reaches the laboratory.

The literature states that urine specimens need to be received by the laboratory within 2–3 hours to avoid bacterial growth and false diagnoses, and if this is not possible, specimens should be refrigerated. This may prove a challenge for midwives who may be, for example, booking women in their homes and not returning to the hospital until later that day, or those working in a clinic where pick-up of specimens is limited. However, every effort needs to be made to ensure specimens are received by the laboratories in the ideal condition (e.g. by not accepting samples women bring in from home). Specimens should ideally also be collected before antimicrobial therapy is commenced – if drugs have been taken in the previous 48 hours, this information needs to be made available to the laboratory staff.

BOX 2.3 COLLECTING A MIDSTREAM SPECIMEN OF URINE

The woman may clean her labial area to remove any potential contaminants such as vaginal discharge. This stage is debatable, as some studies have not demonstrated any benefit (Gould & Brooker 2008).

While holding the labia apart, she will then void the first part of the urine stream into the toilet, then catch the middle part in a (sterile) wide-mouthed container, finishing in the toilet.

Consideration needs to be made of the contortions necessary to undertake this when heavily pregnant. Providing a sterile jug, the contents of which can then be transferred into a universal container, may be cost-effective if it allows accurate diagnosis.

Treatment

UTIs are common in women, regardless of their pregnancy state, but whereas normally a woman may disregard mild symptoms (self-treating with increased fluid intake, and perhaps substances such as cranberry juice) in pregnancy it is important to have a rapid and effective treatment, as there is an increased risk of pyelonephritis. However, women may find self-help actions useful to supplement treatment, or perhaps to help prevent recurrent infections.

Any identified infection including asymptomatic bacteriuria will require treatment, as the evidence has demonstrated that the risk of pyelonephritis is reduced with antibiotic treatment (Meads 2011). There are no clear data available to identify which regimen or drug is superior to any other for either asymptomatic or symptomatic bacteriuria (Guinto *et al.* 2010, Vazquez & Abalos 2011), but the midwife's role is clear: she must advise that all antibiotics are taken by the woman as prescribed and the course completed. This is to ensure the antibiotics are effective and to avoid the development of antibiotic resistance. New antibiotics that are taken as a single dose may be as effective as a course of treatment (Usta *et al.* 2011) and if these are adopted as a standard UK treatment in the future, it is likely compliance would improve.

ROLE OF THE MIDWIFE

- Ensure screening is done accurately and whenever indicated
- Avoid contamination of specimens by ensuring optimal handling and teaching women how to give a specimen correctly
- Obtain and follow up all results as necessary
- Educate women about the signs and symptoms of UTIs, premature labour and signs of ill health
- Ensure women understand the importance of completing the full course of antibiotics as prescribed, even if symptoms improve

---

CHORIOAMNIONITIS

INTRODUCTION

Chorioamnionitis (also known as intra-amniotic infection, amnionitis or intrapartum infection) is the infection of the pregnant uterus, amniotic fluid, fetal membranes and/or placenta. It is the most common cause of preterm labour and therefore a source of complication for both mother and fetus (Burke 2009). The incidence is difficult to establish – American literature suggests it may occur in 0.5%–10% of all pregnancies, and 0.5%–2.0% of term pregnancies (Fahey 2008).

Chorioamnionitis is usually caused by bacteria, and is often polymicrobial. Both aerobic and anaerobic organisms can be responsible, and may derive from the blood or originate from the skin, oral cavity, gastrointestinal system or genitourinary tract. Fungi (usually *Candida*) or mycoplasma (usually *Ureaplasma urealyticum*) can cause chorioamnionitis (Redline 2012). Chorioamnionitis can also result from medical procedures such as amniocentesis; however, ascending organisms from the cervico-vaginal region are the cause in most cases (Kraus *et al.* 2004).

Infection in the uterus not only can infect the fetus but also produces endotoxins that may produce an inflammatory response, which, through a complex chemical interaction, causes a prostaglandin release from the myometrium and fetal membranes (Fahey 2008). This can lead to rupture of the membranes and/or contractions. In addition, ruptured membranes allow organisms an easier access to the uterus and fetus, and therefore signs of infection may begin, or increase, once membranes are ruptured.

Chorioamnionitis is associated with one-third of preterm labours with intact membranes, and 40%–75% of preterm pre-labour rupture of membranes (Woensdregt *et al.* 2008). It is also closely associated with prolonged rupture of membranes (PROM), as once the protective barrier is removed, infection can easily track up from the vagina. In fact, the presence of subclinical infection in the vagina may have been the cause of pre-labour rupture of membranes. However, any ascending infection can cross intact membranes to the amniotic fluid. It has been shown that in a twin pregnancy, the amniotic fluid sac closest to the os is the most usual (or only) one affected (Bergstrom 2001). It is possible that the risk of chorioamnionitis with intact membranes increases after the cervix begins to dilate (Lee *et al.* 2011a).

CLINICAL FEATURES

Predisposing factors

There are many predisposing factors associated with chorioamnionitis (*see* Box 2.4), and in clinical practice it will be noted that many of these overlap. There is also some evidence that meconium in the amniotic fluid may increase the risk for

---

BOX 2.4 PREDISPOSING FACTORS ASSOCIATED WITH CHORIOAMNIONITIS

- Preterm and/or pre-labour rupture of membranes
- Premature contractions
- Prolonged rupture of membranes
- Presence of foreign bodies (e.g. cerclage)
- Scarring from previous uterine surgery
- Multiple vaginal examinations – chorioamnionitis is associated with more than five vaginal examinations (Newton 2005)
- Fetal scalp electrodes
- Urogenital infections
- Immunologic defects (such as chronic disease, poor nutritional status or emotional stress)

chorioamnionitis, perhaps by changing the composition of amniotic fluid and therefore compromising its antimicrobial properties (Fahey 2008). However, pre-labour rupture of membranes is the highest risk for chorioamnionitis (Guinn *et al.* 2007).

MANAGEMENT ISSUES

Diagnosis

Chorioamnionitis can be diagnosed by culture of the amniotic fluid or placental tissue, but unless the membranes have ruptured and a specimen of amniotic fluid is available, it is more commonly suspected and treated according to clinical signs (*see* Box 2.5). If the membranes have ruptured, amniotic fluid can be cultured, and (for a more quickly available result) tested for white blood cell count and leucocyte esterase levels.

Some literature refers to undertaking an amniocentesis to obtain amniotic fluid to test, but this would be carried out only rarely in current UK obstetric practice. Blood test results such as a rising white blood cell count and a high or rising CRP level would contribute to the diagnosis.

BOX 2.5 POSSIBLE CLINICAL SIGNS OF CHORIOAMNIONITIS

- Pyrexia (>37.8°C–38°C)
- Maternal tachycardia
- Fetal tachycardia
- Uterine pain or tenderness
- Maternal leucocytosis
- Offensive amniotic fluid if membranes ruptured
- Changes on the CTG (cardiotocograph) may be present, and apart from fetal tachycardia, there is an association with a lack of variability (De Felice *et al.* 2004) or even fetal bradycardia (Presta *et al.* 2004).
- Placental abruption may also be associated with chorioamnionitis (Suzuki *et al.* 2011)

Chorioamnionitis can lead to a long labour, as it may adversely affect uterine function (Cheng *et al.* 2010), or it is possible that a long labour may predispose to chorioamnionitis (Lee 2011b). An American study looking at a long latent phase during induction of labour found one of the few adverse maternal outcomes to be chorioamnionitis (Rouse *et al.* 2011).

Treatment

Treatment of chorioamnionitis is by urgent administration of intravenous antibiotics and, depending on the woman's and/or fetal condition, immediate delivery of the baby. However, if induction of labour is considered, it should be noted that chorioamnionitis is associated with dysfunctional labour, even when oxytocin is used (Burke 2009).

There is no evidence that using corticosteroids in the routine dose to promote lung maturity in the premature fetus causes harm to the woman (Fishman & Gelber 2012).

OUTCOME

There is evidence that 5%–10% of women with chorioamnionitis may develop bacteraemia (Rouse *et al.* 2004) (*see* Chapter 4 for further information). Chorioamnionitis may also increase the risk of post-partum haemorrhage, wound infection, pelvic abscess and post-partum endometritis (Fahey 2008).

Chorioamnionitis is considered to be one of the leading causes of fetal and neonatal morbidity and mortality (Hagberg *et al.* 2002). As well as an increased likelihood of premature birth, chorioamnionitis is associated with intrauterine growth restriction in the fetus (Williams *et al.* 2000) and there may be a chance that some otherwise unexplained stillbirths may be due to ascending infection (Tolockiene *et al.* 2001). A study has demonstrated that the concentration of maternal CRP at admission for premature rupture of membranes is the most accurate infectious marker for prediction of early-onset neonatal infection (Popowski *et al.* 2011).

Neonatal sepsis (Buhimschi *et al.* 2008), an increased risk of cerebral palsy (Wu & Colford 2000) and bronchopulmonary dysplasia (Hartling *et al.* 2012) are also associations for the infant. When assessing outcomes for the neonate it must be noted that many of these babies will be delivered early, and prematurity carries its own range of complications. However, there is some evidence that spontaneous preterm birth (which is likely to be associated with chorioamnionitis) had a much higher rate of adverse outcomes than in those babies whose premature birth was initiated by obstetric reasons such as pre-eclampsia (Hagberg *et al.* 2002).

ROLE OF THE MIDWIFE

- Accurate diagnosis of rupture of membranes and careful assessment of symptoms
- Appropriate referral for antibiotic treatment, fetal assessment and/or induction of labour
- Vigilant monitoring of the maternal and fetal/infant well-being during labour and the immediate postnatal period.

POST-PARTUM ENDOMETRITIS

INTRODUCTION

Post-partum endometritis is also known as 'genital tract infection' or 'uterine infection', or simply 'endometritis'. Endometritis is usually a result of contamination of the endometrial cavity with vaginal organisms during labour and delivery (Bick *et al.* 2009). Post-partum endometritis may spread from the infected uterus to the cervix, vagina or perineum, or result in salpingitis, parametritis and/or generalised peritonitis, including abscess formation (Burke 2009).

The most common cause of sepsis in new mothers is endometritis associated with caesarean section: an American study identified that these women accounted for 15%–85% of cases, compared with vaginal delivery complicated by endometritis of 1%–4% of cases (Sheffield 2004). *See* Chapter 4 for an in-depth discussion of sepsis.

Mild endometritis usually only involves the decidua and superficial myometrium, and is associated with minimal pyrexia and limited symptoms, most frequently occurring between days 2 and 6 following a vaginal delivery (Cunningham 2002). Moderate to severe endometrial infection occurs most often in the first 48 hours post-partum, usually after a caesarean section (Tharpe 2008). However, severe endometritis can occur later in the postnatal period, and mild infection may become more severe. Community midwives need to be vigilant as much post-partum endometritis will become evident after discharge from hospital, and prompt identification and referral is required to avoid more severe disease.

The most common bacteria responsible for endometritis include group B beta-haemolytic streptococci, anaerobic streptococci, aerobic Gram-negative bacilli (e.g. *E. coli*), anaerobic Gram-negative bacilli, aerobic Gram-positive bacilli (e.g. clostridium) and group A streptococci, which has recently been identified as a particularly serious pathogen.

CLINICAL FEATURES

Predisposing factors

It is thought that endometritis may complicate 1%–4% of vaginal deliveries, 5%–15% of elective caesarean sections and >30% of caesarean sections undertaken after a lengthy labour and/or rupture of membranes (Ambrose & Repke 2011). Although rates vary considerably throughout the literature, the chief risk factor for endometritis appears to be caesarean section – in particular, when undertaken during active labour (Hadar *et al.* 2011). Repeat caesarean sections may carry increased risks, as operations frequently last longer, and the length of surgery is a risk factor for increased infection (Lyell 2011).

Following a vaginal birth endometritis is associated with bacterial vaginosis, PROM, prolonged labour (in particular, one that involves many interventions, including multiple vaginal examinations), significant meconium-stained amniotic fluid and low infant birthweight (French & Smaill 2004). A common cause of endometritis is retained products of conception, and these may be detected by ultrasound examination, although this may be inconclusive (Carlan *et al.* 1997).

In both caesarean section and vaginal deliveries, the general risk factors for endometritis are the same as for all infections. However, although obesity is a risk factor, it has been suggested that the risk for these women is even greater if higher parity and increased pregnancy weight gain by 28 weeks are also taken into account (Magann *et al.* 2011).

Diagnosis

Since laboratory tests are often non-specific, endometritis is usually diagnosed by clinical features and exclusion of other possible causes of post-partum pyrexia (*see* Box 2.6). The World Health Organization (WHO) (2006) and the National Institute for Health and Care Excellence (NICE) (2006) have identified lists of similar symptoms leading to diagnosis. Every maternity unit will have their own criteria for referral or escalation of care, but all of the elements in both the guidelines provided here are worthy of note and further investigation.

BOX 2.6 POSSIBLE CAUSES OF POST-PARTUM PYREXIA EXCLUDING ENDOMETRITIS

- Wound infection
- UTI
- Thrombophlebitis
- Infected haematoma or abscess
- Mastitis
- Breast engorgement (non-pathological)
- Reaction to medication ('drug fever')

WHO (2006): pyrexia >38°C plus one or more of the following:
- lower abdominal pain/general abdominal tenderness
- 'bulky' or suboptimal uterine contraction
- offensive lochia
- heavy or scant lochia
- fatigue and/or general malaise.

NICE guidelines (2006) suggest a diagnosis based on two or more of the following:
- pyrexia >38.5°C once, or >38°C on two occasions 4 hours apart
- abdominal tenderness

- uterine subinvolution
- offensive or heavy lochia
- tachycardia.

MANAGEMENT ISSUES

Prevention

Reduction in postnatal endometritis was seen following recommendations by the Royal College of Obstetricians and Gynaecologists and NICE that prophylactic antibiotics should be given routinely as a one-dose intraoperative administration during all caesarean sections following clamping of the baby's cord. However, there has been further research that has demonstrated that if the antibiotic is given 15–50 minutes before skin incision, it is more effective. There has been concern that the drug would cross to the fetus, masking any infection in the baby; however, this has not been shown to date (Sullivan *et al.* 2007). It would, however, mean the baby had been exposed to unnecessary antibiotics.

Treatment

Treatment is by intravenous antibiotics, and this may be changed to oral antibiotics as the woman's condition improves. However, about 10% of women may not be cured with the initial therapy (Woensdregt *et al.* 2008) and further investigations may reveal resistant organisms or other sites for the infection (*see* Box 2.6 for some examples). These may be suspected from careful observation by the midwife, and confirmed by laboratory or other tests.

ROLE OF THE MIDWIFE

The historical importance of observation for post-partum endometritis was underlined by the previous perceived necessity for daily postnatal visits by community midwives, undertaking routine procedures to assess for infection (temperature, pulse, assessment of involution and lochia). Current practice makes these regular visits unlikely; however, women can be at increased risk of infection now, with a growing number of women with predisposing factors, and sepsis the leading cause of maternal mortality (CMACE 2011). This will provide a challenge for midwives, who will need to ensure precise risk assessment is done for all women, identifying those who will need to receive increased professional attention, as well as ensuring all women have the information on signs and symptoms of sepsis and on how and when to self-refer.

MASTITIS

INTRODUCTION

Mastitis is an inflammatory condition of the breast tissue that may or may not be accompanied by infection (Crepinsek *et al.* 2012), and when present in postnatal women it is referred to as 'lactational' or 'puerperal' mastitis (Noonan 2010). The incidence of lactational mastitis differs in various reports but may range from <10% to 33% (WHO 2000, Jahanfar *et al.* 2009). The breadth of the range is probably contributed to by the lack of agreement in the literature of what exactly constitutes mastitis (Kvist 2010). Mastitis can be either non-infective or infective.

- *Non-infective mastitis* is described as an inflammatory response, usually to a blocked duct, engorgement or injury to the breast.
- *Infective mastitis* frequently occurs from bacteria entering through broken skin (Burke 2009) – typically, cracked nipples from breastfeeding (Crepinsek *et al.* 2012). However, bacteria are often found in breast milk and so the presence of bacteria does not necessarily indicate infection. The most common organism causing mastitis is *S. aureus*, but *Staphylococcus albus*, *E. coli* and *Streptococcus* can also be responsible.

Mastitis is a significant and common complication of lactation and contributes to a woman's decision to stop breastfeeding. It can occur at any stage of lactation (Noonan 2010), and it is considered that recurrent mastitis develops in 20%–25% of women (Scott *et al.* 2008). As such it is clearly a concern for midwives.

CLINICAL FEATURES

Predisposing factors

- Previous history of mastitis
- Birth complications
- Poor micronutrient status
- Compromised immune system
- Trauma (particularly from poor feeding techniques)
- Working outside the home
- Parity (primiparity identified in some research, but not others)

It has been suggested that any flu-like symptoms (pyrexia, headache, myalgia, nausea and vomiting, fatigue, general malaise) in a breastfeeding mother should be considered as mastitis unless proved otherwise, as symptoms specifically involving the breast often occur later than systemic symptoms (Cadwell *et al.* 2006). When symptoms in the breast do occur, usually only one breast is affected (bilateral symptoms are likely to be engorgement), and these may include:

- breast pain and tenderness
- breast feels warm and swollen
- reddened, wedge-shaped discoloration (although if untreated it may spread to the whole breast).

The upper outer quadrant of the breast is the most common site for mastitis, as the majority of the breast tissue is located there (Riordan & Wambach 2009).

Non-infective mastitis is associated with milk stasis due to blocked ducts, and milk stasis commonly occurs with poor breastfeeding techniques (*see* Box 2.7). This can usually be prevented by effective milk removal. Infective mastitis can be caused by bacteria entering the breast through damaged nipples, or through the lactiferous ducts into a lobe via haematogenous spread. Nipples can become cracked when breastfeeding through poor breastfeeding techniques, and therefore midwifery support to prevent nipple trauma can be extremely beneficial.

BOX 2.7 BREASTFEEDING PRACTICES THAT MAY CONTRIBUTE TO MASTITIS

- Poor attachment by the infant to the breast
- Restriction of the frequency or duration of breastfeeds
- Milk oversupply
- Ineffective suckling
- Blockage of milk ducts
- Obstruction of milk ducts from tight clothing or position

(WHO 2000, Riordan & Wambach 2009)

Diagnosis and treatment

It can often be difficult to distinguish between non-infective and infective mastitis, especially as cultures of the milk are usually unhelpful (Ambrose & Repke 2011). Engorgement or a blocked duct can cause local symptoms such as swelling and tenderness. Non-infective mastitis usually involves pyrexia and systemic symptoms. However, if the symptoms persist for more than a few hours after starting interventions (*see* Box 2.8), are worsening or are particularly severe, immediate referral needs to be made, as the woman probably has infective mastitis and needs antibiotic therapy. Symptoms should start to improve within 24 hours of commencing antibiotics; however, if there is not complete resolution within 5 days of antibiotic treatment, then an abscess may be the cause or a change of antibiotics may be needed. Recurrence or chronic mastitis may be caused by antibiotic-resistant infection (ABM 2008).

BOX 2.8 TREATMENT OF MILK STASIS

A blockage can be treated by changing the feeding position, ensuring that the baby's nose or chin points towards the blocked duct (Riordan & Wambach 2009), frequent feeding starting on the affected breast (more vigorous suckling is usual at the beginning of the feed) and perhaps the use of warm packs and/or gentle massage (from the blocked area towards the nipple) during the feed. The midwife may need to supervise the feeds to ensure correct attachment so the breast is properly emptied (Mohrbacher & Stock 2003). The midwife also needs to ensure that the woman understands that stopping breastfeeding may increase the problem and may lead to a risk of abscess development (Scott *et al.* 2008). Appropriate analgesia, cold packs after feeding and increased rest may also help the woman to keep breastfeeding successfully (Noonan 2010). In a study that investigated the experience of mastitis, it was reported that women found reducing their activity level was beneficial to their recovery (Wambach 2003), a finding that is not surprising, as this would contribute to supporting their immune systems, as well as providing more time to feed frequently and to concentrate on feeding technique.

The decisions of who should receive antibiotics, when they should be commenced and which antibiotic to use have little consensus (Jahanfar *et al.* 2009). However, WHO (2000) considers that effective milk removal is also an essential part of treatment.

Thrush

Thrush (candida) may cause mastitis, although there is some controversy surrounding this subject (Dixon & Khan 2011, Hale *et al.* 2009). Symptoms may include a burning sensation (Bick *et al.* 2009) or deep breast pain, particularly after the breast empties (Mass 2004). It may be clearly visible on the nipple (painful with flaky or shiny skin), and suspected if present in the baby's mouth (Francis-Morrill *et al.* 2004). Early and appropriate treatment is necessary, for both the mother and the baby. Analgesia for the mother may also be necessary until the condition resolves, and she needs to be advised concerning frequent handwashing and the need to change her breast pads often (Bick *et al.* 2009).

Breast abscess

A breast abscess is a localised collection in the breast tissue, presenting as a breast lump, and may be a result of bacterial mastitis (Cusack & Brennan 2011). The most common organism responsible is *S. aureus*, and methicillin-resistant *S. aureus* (MRSA) has been found, especially when the infection was acquired in hospital (Dixon & Khan 2011). The incidence of breast abscess is suggested to be 3%–11% (Amir *et al.* 2004).

Continuing to breastfeed through mastitis may prevent abscess formation (Ambrose & Repke 2011), but if the pain prevents this, emptying the breast via pumping may be helpful. Abscess may also be prevented by accessing appropriate treatment early during mastitis (Dixon & Khan 2011).

Breast abscess has similar symptoms to mastitis, with the addition of a tender lump that may be tense or fluctuant (Cusack & Brennan 2011), and ultrasound can diagnose the presence of pus. Treatment may be either be by surgical incision and drainage or needle aspiration. Needle aspiration under ultrasound guidance is most commonly used; however, the success may depend on the size of the abscess, and there may eventually be a need for surgical incision and drainage. There is usually a better cosmetic outcome with needle aspiration (Eryilmaz *et al.* 2005).

Surgical intervention is accompanied by antibiotic treatment. It is worth noting that recent research in the United States found 64.2% of women in a study were resistant to the most commonly used antibiotic (Lee *et al.* 2010), and methicillin-resistant *S. aureus* (MRSA) may become an increasing problem in this area (Montalto & Lui 2009, Spencer 2008). The study by Lee *et al.* (2010) also found all their subjects stopped breastfeeding; however, other literature (Martin 2009) has identified women who have been treated for recurrent breast abscess and continued to breastfeed, and this is of course to be encouraged.

ROLE OF THE MIDWIFE

The midwife has a vital role to play in teaching women correct breastfeeding techniques, identifying any breastfeeding problems as soon as possible and ensuring appropriate advice, treatment, referral and follow-up occurs. Failure to fulfil this role could lead to a woman discontinuing breastfeeding and/or suffering recurrent mastitis, permanent tissue damage, chronic inflammation and irreversible distortion of the breast (WHO 2000). It can also be a cause of maternal death, albeit rarely. CMACE (2011) reported on a woman who developed fatal septic shock from breast infection, and they emphasised the importance of frequent assessment and urgent referral to hospital if the woman is clinically unwell, has severe or unusual symptoms or does not respond to oral antibiotics within 48 hours.

USEFUL RESOURCES

- The Academy of Breastfeeding Medicine (www.bfmed.org) is an international organisation of doctors dedicated to the promotion, protection and support of breastfeeding and human lactation.

- Royal College of Midwives (2002) *Successful Breastfeeding.* 3rd ed. Edinburgh: Churchill Livingstone.
- UNICEF: details and discussion on the 'Baby Friendly' breastfeeding initiative led by UNICEF can be found online (www.unicef.org.uk/babyfriendly).

REFERENCES

Academy of Breastfeeding Medicine (ABM) (2008) *Mastitis.* ABM Clinical Protocol 4. Available at: www.bfmed.org/Resources/Protocols.aspx (accessed 27 April 2012).

Ambrose A, Repke J (2011) Puerperal problems. In: James D, Steer P, Winer C, *et al.* (editors). *High Risk Pregnancy: management options.* 4th ed. New York: Elsevier, Saunders.

Amir L, Forster D, McLachlan H, *et al.* (2004) Incidence of breast abscess in lactating women: report from an Australian cohort. *BJOG.* **111**(12): 1378–81.

Basu J, Jeketera C, Basu D (2010) Obesity and its outcomes among pregnant South African women. *Int J Gynecol Obstet.* **110**(2): 101–4.

Bergstrom S (2001) Bacterial and viral infections in pregnancy: chorioamnionitis. In: Lawson J, Harrison K, Bergstrom S (editors). *Maternity Care in Developing Countries.* London: RCOG Press. pp. 125–38.

Bick D, MacArthur C, Winter H (2009) *Postnatal Care: evidence and guidelines for management.* 2nd ed. Edinburgh: Churchill Livingstone.

Bothamley J, Boyle M (2009) *Medical Conditions Affecting Pregnancy and Childbirth.* Oxford: Radcliffe Publishing.

Buhimschi I, Zanbrano E, Pettker C, *et al.* (2008) Using proteomic analysis of the human amniotic fluid to identify histological chorioamnionitis. *Obstet Gynaecol.* **111**(2 Pt. 1): 403–12.

Burke C (2009) Perinatal sepsis. *J Perinat Neonatal Nurs.* **23**(1): 42–51.

Cadwell K, Turner-Maffei C, O'Connor B, *et al.* (2006) *Maternal and Infant Assessment for Breastfeeding and Human Lactation: a guide for the practitioner.* 2nd edition. Sudbury: Jones & Bartlett.

Carlan S, Scott W, Pollack R, *et al.* (1997) Appearance of the uterus by ultrasound immediately after placental delivery with pathologic correlation. *J Clin Ultrasound.* **25**(6): 301–8.

Centre for Maternal and Child Enquiries (CMACE) (2011) Saving mothers' lives: reviewing maternal deaths to make motherhood safer: 2006–2008. The Eighth Report on Confidential Enquiries into Maternal Deaths in the UK. *BJOG.* **118**(Suppl. 1): 1–203.

Cheng Y, Shaffer B, Bryant A, *et al.* (2010) Length of the first stage of labor and associated perinatal outcomes in nulliparous women. *Am J Obstet Gynecol.* **116**(5): 1127–35.

Crepinsek M, Crowe L, Michener K, *et al.* (2012) Interventions for preventing mastitis after childbirth. *Cochrane Database Syst Rev.* (10): CD007239.

Cunningham F (2002) Postoperative complications. In: Gilstrap L, Cunningham F, VanDorsten J (editors). *Operative Obstetrics.* 2nd ed. New York: McGraw-Hill. pp. 293–310.

Cusack L, Brennan M (2011) Lactational mastitis and breast abscess. *Aust Fam Physician.* **40**(12): 976–9.

De Felice C, Dileo L, Parrini S, *et al.* (2004) Persistent fetal heart rate hypo-variability: a presenting clinical sign of histologic chorioamnionitis at term gestation. *J Matern Fetal Neonatal Med.* **16**(6): 363–5.

Dixon J, Khan L (2011) Treatment of breast infection. *BMJ.* **342**: 484–9.

Eryilmaz R, Sahin M, Hakan M, *et al.* (2005) Management of lactational breast abscesses. *Breast.* **14**(5): 375–9.

Fahey J (2008) Clinical management of intra-amniotic infection and chorioamnionitis: a review of the literature. *J Midwifery Womens Health.* **53**(3): 227–35.

Fishman S, Gelber S (2012) Evidence for the clinical management of chorioamnionitis. *Semin Fetal Neonatal Med.* **17**(1): 46–50.

Francis-Morrill J, Heinig J, Pappagianis D, *et al.* (2004) Diagnostic value of signs and symptoms of mammary candidosis among lactating women. *J Hum Lact.* **20**(3): 288–95.

French L, Smaill F (2004) Antibiotic regimens for endometritis after delivery. *Cochrane Database Syst Rev.* (4): CD001067.

Gilstrap L 3rd, Ramin S (2001) Urinary tract infections during pregnancy. *Obstet Gynecol Clin North Am.* **28**(3): 581–91.

Gould D, Brooker C (2008) *Infection Prevention and Control.* 2nd ed. New York: Palgrave MacMillan.

Guinn D, Abel D, Tomlinson M (2007) Early goal directed therapy for sepsis during pregnancy. *Obstet Gynecol Clin North Am.* **34**(3): 459–79.

Guinto V, De Guia B, Festin M, *et al.* (2010) Different antibiotic regimens for treating asymptomatic bacteriuria in pregnancy. *Cochrane Database Syst Rev.* (9): CD007855.

Hadar E, Melamed N, Tzadikevitchy-Geffen K, *et al.* (2011) Timing and risk factors of maternal complications of caesarean section. *Arch Gynecol Obstet.* **283**(4): 735–41.

Hagberg H, Wennerholm U, Sävman K (2002) Sequelae of chorioamnionitis. *Curr Opin Infect Dis.* **15**(3): 301–6.

Hale T, Bateman T, Finkelman M, *et al.* (2009) The absence of *Candida albicans* in milk samples of women with clinical symptoms of ductal candidiasis. *Breastfeeding Med.* **4**(2): 57–61.

Hartling L, Liang Y, Lacaze-Masmonteil T (2012) Chorioamnionitis as a risk factor for bronchopulmonary dysplasia: a systematic review and meta-analysis. *Arch Dis Child Fetal Neonatal Ed.* **97**(1): F8–17.

Jahanfar S, Ng C, Teng C (2009) Antibiotics for mastitis in breastfeeding women. *Cochrane Database Syst Rev.* (1): CD005458.

Kraus F, Redline R, Gersell D, *et al.* (2004) Inflammation and infection. In: *Placental Pathology.* Washington, DC: American Registry of Pathology. pp. 75–115.

Kvist L (2010) Toward a clarification of the concept of mastitis as used in empirical studies of breast inflammation during lactation. *J Hum Lact.* **26**(1): 53–9.

Lee I, Kang L, Hsu H, *et al.* (2010) Puerperal mastitis requiring hospitalization during a nine-year period. *Am J Obstet Gynecol.* **203**(4): 332–3.

Lee S, Lee K, Kim S, *et al.* (2011a) The risk of intra-amniotic infection, inflammation and histologic chorioamnionitis in term pregnant women with intact membranes and labour. *Placenta.* **32**(7): 516–21.

Lee S, Romero R, Lee K (2011b) The frequency and risk factors of funisitis and histologic chorioamnionitis in pregnant women at term who delivered after the spontaneous onset of labor. *J Matern Fetal Neonatal Med.* **24**(1): 37–42.

Lyell D (2011) Adhesions and perioperative complications of repeat caesarean delivery. *Am J Obstet Gynecol.* **205**(6): S11–18.

Magann E, Doherty D, Chauhan S, *et al.* (2011) Pregnancy, obesity, gestational weight gain and parity as predictors of peripartum complications. *Arch Gynecol Obstet.* **284**(4): 827–36.

Martin J (2009) Breast abscess in lactation. *J Midwifery Womens Health.* **54**(2): 150–1.

Mass S (2004) Breast pain: engorgement, nipple pain and mastitis. *Clin Obstet Gynecol.* **47**(3): 676–82.

Meads C (2011) *Screening for Asymptomatic Bacteriuria in Pregnancy: external review against programme appraisal criteria for the UK National Screening Committee (UK NSC). Version 2* [online]. Available at: www.screening.nhs.uk/policydb_download.php?doc=169 (accessed 18 September 2014).

Mohrbacher N, Stock J (2003) *The Breastfeeding Answer Book.* Illinois: La Leche League International.

Montalto M, Lui B (2009) MRSA as a cause of postpartum breast abscess in infant and mother. *J Hum Lact.* **25**(4): 448–50.

National Institute for Health and Care Excellence (NICE) (2006) *Postnatal Care: routine postnatal care of women and their babies.* NICE Clinical Guideline 37. London: NICE.

National Institute for Health and Care Excellence (NICE) (2008) *Antenatal Care.* NICE Clinical Guideline 62. London: NICE.

Newton E (2005) Preterm labor, preterm premature rupture of membranes and chorioamnionitis. *Clin Perinatol.* **32**(3): 571–600.

Noonan M (2010) Lactational mastitis: recognition and breastfeeding support. *Br J Midwifery.* **18**(8): 503–9.

Popowski T, Goffinet F, Maillard F, *et al.* (2011) Maternal markers for detecting early-onset neonatal infection and chorioamnionitis in cases of premature rupture of membranes at or after 34 weeks of gestation: a two-center prospective study. *BMC Pregnancy Childbirth.* **11**: 26.

Presta G, Rosati E, Giannuzzi R, *et al.* (2004) Prolonged fetal bradycardia as the presenting sign in *Streptococcus agalactiae* chorioamnionitis. *J Perinat Med.* **32**(6): 535–7.

Redline R (2012) Inflammatory response in acute chorioamnionitis. *Semin Fetal Neonatal Med.* **17**(1): 20–5.

Riordan J, Wambach K (2009) Breast-related problems. In: Riordan J, Wambach K (editors). *Breastfeeding and Human Lactation.* 4th ed. Sudbury: Jones & Bartlett. pp. 291–324.

Rouse D, Landon M, Leveno K, *et al.* (2004) The maternal-fetal medicine units caesarean registry: chorioamnionitis at term and its duration – relationship to outcomes. *Am J Obstet Gynecol.* **191**(1): 211–16.

Rouse D, Weiner S, Bloom, *et al.* (2011) Failed labor induction: toward an objective diagnosis. *Obstet Gynecol.* **117**(2): 267–72.

Scott J, Robertson M, Fitzpatrick J, *et al.* (2008) Occurrence of lactational mastitis and medical management: a prospective cohort study in Glasgow. *Int Breastfeed J.* **3**: 21.

Sheffield J (2004) Sepsis and septic shock in pregnancy. *Crit Care Clin.* **20**(4): 651–60.

Smaill F (2007) Asymptomatic bacteriuria in pregnancy. *Best Pract Res Clin Obstet Gynaecol.* **21**(3): 439–50.

Smaill F, Vazquez J (2007) Antibiotics for asymptomatic bacteriuria in pregnancy. *Cochrane Database Syst Rev.* (2): CD000490.

Spencer J (2008) Management of mastitis in breastfeeding women. *Am Fam Physician.* **78**(6): 727–31.

Sullivan S, Smith T, Chang E, *et al.* (2007) Administration of cefazolin prior to skin incision is superior to cefazolin at cord clamping in preventing postcesarean infectious morbidity: a randomized, controlled trial. *Am J Obstet Gynecol.* **196**(5): 455.e.1–5.

Suzuki S, Satomi M, Hiraizumi Y, *et al.* (2011) Clinical significance of singleton pregnancies complicated by placental abruption occurred at preterm compared with those occurred at term. *Arch Gynecol Obstet.* **283**(4): 761–4.

Tharpe N (2008) Postpregnancy genital tract and wound infections. *J Midwifery Womens Health.* **53**(3): 236–46.

Thorsen M, Poole J (2002) Renal disease in pregnancy. *J Perinat Neonatal Nurs.* **15**(4): 13–26.

Tolockiene E, Morsing E, Holst E, *et al.* (2001) Intrauterine infection may be a major cause of stillbirth in Sweden. *Acta Obstet Gynecol Scand.* **80**(6): 511–18.

Usta T, Dogan O, Ates U, *et al.* (2011) Comparison of single-dose and multiple-dose antibiotics for lower urinary tract infection in pregnancy. *Int J Gynecol Obstet.* **114**(3): 229–33.

Vazquez J, Abalos E (2011) Treatments for symptomatic urinary tract infections during pregnancy. *Cochrane Database Syst Rev.* (1): CD002256.

Wambach K (2003) Lactation mastitis: a descriptive study of the experience. *J Hum Lact.* **19**(1): 24–34.

Williams M, O'Brien W, Nelson R, *et al.* (2000) Histologic chorioamnionitis is associated with fetal growth restriction in term and preterm infants. *Am J Obstet Gynecol.* **183**(5): 1094–9.

Woensdregt K, Lee H, Norwitz E (2008) Infectious diseases in pregnancy. In: Funai E, Evans M, Lockwood C (editors). *High Risk Obstetrics: the requisites in obstetrics and gynecology.* New York: Mosby, Elsevier. pp. 287–316.

World Health Organization (WHO) (2000) *Mastitis: causes and management.* WHO/FCH/CAH/00.13. Geneva: WHO.

World Health Organization (WHO) (2006) *Pregnancy, Childbirth, Postpartum and Newborn Care: a guide for essential practice.* Geneva: WHO.

Wu YW, Colford JM Jr (2000) Chorioamnionitis as a risk factor for cerebral palsy: a meta-analysis. *JAMA.* **284**(11): 1417–24.

CHAPTER 3

Wound infection

INTRODUCTION

Wound healing is the process of replacement and restoration of function to damaged tissues. Underpinning all effective wound assessment is a knowledge of the theory of wound healing, and it is therefore important for a midwife to have an understanding of this subject on which to base her care.

For the new mother, many of the normal physical components of the postnatal period involve healing to some degree and return to the non-pregnant state. Much of the process is concerned with involution of the uterus and healing of the placental site (a large 'wound'). The successful resolution of this is vital for the woman's health, but apart from nutritional guidance – and this should ideally have been done in the antenatal period – and basic advice regarding hygiene and lifestyle, there is little the midwife can do to influence this process.

However, other wounds are also very common following childbirth, and the midwife has a key role in giving advice and care concerning them, as well as being knowledgeable about the factors that could lead to infection, plus the signs and symptoms of developing infection. Perineal wounds affect about three-quarters of women following a vaginal birth, and of course they are more likely after an instrumental delivery. Caesarean section wounds have become a common part of a midwife's responsibility (Boyle 2001) and despite much effort to reduce the rate of caesarean sections, it seems unlikely these numbers will decline significantly. Therefore, wound assessment falls clearly within the midwife's remit, with her accountability for caring for women in the postnatal period (NMC 2012).

STAGES OF WOUND HEALING

All actions in wound healing are regulated by a complex series of chemical reactions that initiate, control or inhibit various factors, and all actions are inter-related. The immune system is vital to all stages of this cascade, and a compromised immune system (see Chapter 1) can significantly delay the process of wound healing, causing many adverse consequences. Although many actions overlap, for the purpose of explanation, the stages of wound healing can be divided as follows.

Immediate (*vasoconstriction, activation of clotting, platelets and endothelial cells, haemostasis, clot formation*)

Immediately following an injury, the blood vessels constrict around the site, and this vasoconstriction provides a rapid reduction in bleeding. The cellular disruption exposes blood to air and this helps activation of the coagulation process (Flanagan 2000). Platelets attach themselves to the exposed sub-endothelium of the injury and clump together (aggregation) and with fibrin, form a clot, filling the space of the injury and bringing the sides together (Dealey 2012). The fibrin (blood protein) clot contains mostly red blood cells but can also incorporate dead tissue or even foreign matter.

Vasoconstriction and blood coagulation are followed by platelet activation and the release of platelet-derived growth factors, in addition to the release of chemo-attractant factors such as cytokines and chemokines, which promote the migration of phagocytes and other cells to the wound site, starting the proliferative phase.

Inflammation

An acute inflammatory response happens within hours of the injury and its effect can last 5–7 days. Tissue damage and the resultant activation of clotting factors cause the release of various chemical mediators such as prostaglandins and histamine, which lead to increased vasodilation and increased permeability of the blood vessels as well as stimulation of pain fibres (Dealey 2012).

The fibrin clot acts to attract leucocytes and within the first 24 hours specifically neutrophils (to attack and remove bacteria and damaged cells) and monocytes (scavenger cells – once in the tissue these are called macrophages) appear. Neutrophils ingest and kill foreign matter and in the process many die. These dead cells, in infection, are part of the constituents of pus.

Macrophages play an important part in most phases of wound healing, not only in clearing the wound site but also in the production of growth factors and other substances that control the processes. New capillaries begin to grow into the wound (angiogenesis), thus resulting, most importantly, in the formation of a new connective tissue matrix – *see* fibroblast activity under 'collagen' in the next section (Bale & Jones 2006).

Vasodilation not only enables neutrophils and monocytes to be easily delivered to the site but also produces exudate that may lead to oedema. There is leakage of serous fluid into the wound bed and normal wound healing requires the growth factors, nutrients and bacterial activity factors present in this inflammatory exudate (Dealey 2012). However, depending on where the wound is, such as the perineum, the pressure of even a slight amount of excess fluid may cause some pain.

Depending on the wound's position, this increase in blood flow may cause the area to appear red. The vasodilation and additional metabolic activity can also produce heat, making the area feel warm to the touch. The increased temperature at the site has the dual benefit of inhibiting pathogen growth, while helping the action of the phagocytes.

Therefore, *normal inflammation* consists of:

- redness (erythema)
- maybe some swelling
- a slight local increase in temperature (or with a large wound, a systemic pyrexia)
- perhaps some pain.

However, an exaggeration of these signs may indicate infection (*see* 'infection', later in this chapter). *See* Chapter 4 for details of extreme inflammatory response.

During the move from the inflammatory phase to the proliferative phase, the number of inflammatory cells declines and fibroblasts increase.

Proliferation (*reconstruction, granulation, angiogenesis, collagen production, epithelialisation, contraction*)

In the proliferation phase, new blood vessels continue to form throughout the wound (angiogenesis or neovascularisation). This process is vital, as no new tissue can be built without new blood vessels supplying oxygen and nutrients. Angiogenic growth factors, secreted by macrophages (probably in response to the tissue hypoxia), stimulate the endothelium to divide and organise the growth of the new blood vessels. Intact vessels around the wound 'bud' new vessels and they spread throughout the wound and multiply.

Macrophages seem to need less oxygen than other cells, and can therefore move further into the wound (Bale & Jones 2006). As they divide within the wound site to kill microbes and clear dead tissue, the rise in macrophages also attracts fibroblasts – cells that produce collagen.

Collagen: a primary protein of connective tissue providing strength

Fibroblasts proliferate from about day 2 to day 4, and produce a matrix (a scaffold-like structure) of collagen around the new vessels. They are stimulated to produce collagen by lactate and ascorbate (a form of ascorbic acid), which are present in the hypoxic wound bed (Dealey 2012). The fibroblasts crawl over the matrix, granulation tissue (including fibroblasts, collagen, new blood vessels and macrophages) proliferates and epithelialisation occurs, commencing restoration of the epithelial barrier functions of the skin.

Epithelialisation: epidermal cells migrating over the surface

The epidermis is a multilayer epithelium consisting of epidermal cells. Epithelial cells migrate as a complete moving sheet or by 'leap-frogging' over viable tissue. Epithelial cells cannot move across a dry surface or necrotic tissue, so an open wound needs to be full of granulation tissue before epithelialisation can take place. The presence of 'crusting' or scabs also forms a barrier to epithelial cells, and they are forced to burrow underneath (Flanagan 2000). In ideal circumstances, wound epithelialisation may occur within 24–72 hours. Also contributing to the wound closure is the bringing together of the wound edges, which decreases the size of the wound (Bale & Jones 2006). Suturing following a surgical incision brings tissue together, which minimises the need for collagen synthesis and cell migration.

Maturation (*remodelling*)

The initial fibrin clot is replaced by granulation tissue, which – after expanding until it fills the defect and being covered by a viable epidermal surface – undergoes remodelling. This is usually about 20 days after injury, although this can vary according to size, site and/or individual circumstances. During remodelling the density of macrophages and fibroblasts reduces, the growth of capillaries stops and the blood flow and metabolic activity decreases. Also, during remodelling the excess collagen is removed and the original collagen is gradually replaced with stronger and better-organised collagen, laid down in a more orderly fashion along the lines of mechanical stress, although it may never be as well organised as the original. The remodelling phase begins at different times within different areas of the wound, and this can continue for up to a year or even longer. So, although the wound may look healed, the rebuilding process below continues (Dougherty & Lister 2008), and remodelled tissue may never become as strong as before the injury.

Scars

The remodelling of granulation tissue may be the most important contributor to problems developing from scarring. During remodelling the density of the fibroblasts diminishes and matures into a scar. The epidermis of a scar is different from normal skin; after healing it is thick compared with undamaged skin, although not as thick as that of freshly closed wounds. Hair follicles and sebaceous or sweat glands do not regenerate in the scar.

The dermis of a healed wound is also different – the arrangement of the organised collagen fibre bundles may be altered. The degree of the disruption is dependent on factors such as the location of the wound and inherited influences. The healed quality of the scar can vary in terms of appearance, amount and whether there is full function. A caesarean section scar needs to be strong to deal with stresses such as support, weight gain and exercise, whereas a perineal scar needs to be flat and pliable to maximise comfort.

Dehiscence is the opening of surgically closed wounds and may involve only part of the skin layer or the entire wound – for example, major dehiscence in a caesarean section wound would include exposure of abdominal organs (Baxter 2004). It usually occurs when, for whatever reason, the wound is not strong enough to withstand the forces placed on it – *see* Box 3.1 for some of the reasons a wound may be at risk of dehiscence.

BOX 3.1 WHAT MAY CAUSE SURGICAL WOUNDS TO OPEN?

- Infection
- Increasing fluid levels or pressure (e.g. haematoma)
- The presence of a foreign body
- Underlying disease process
- Uterine scar: due to the force of contractions during labour

---

Dehiscence or breakdown of a sutured perineum is always a cause for distress. The most usual reason is infection, and the most common treatment has involved antibiotic therapy and leaving the wound to heal by secondary intention. However, there is evidence that early re-suturing of the wound can give a good outcome (Uygur *et al.* 2004), although this may need further research, especially in evaluation of the management of these wounds prior to re-suturing.

HOW WOUNDS HEAL

Wounds can heal by *primary intention*, which occurs when wound edges are brought together (approximated) by suturing. When a wound is sutured, there is a close approximation of the tissues and no 'dead space', and therefore there is less granulation tissue necessary. The epithelium will migrate over the suture line, and healing is primarily by connective tissue deposition. If there is a high bacterial count present, however, this infection will prevent healthy granulation tissue forming and therefore if sutured, it is likely to break down (Vuolo 2006). Healing by *secondary intention* (where there is a tissue deficit) needs the formation of granulation tissue and wound contraction. This can result in increased dense, fibrous scar tissue and also takes longer to heal.

When these issues are considered, it is clear that accurate assessment of perineal tears is vital when deciding whether or not to suture. If the perineal wound is not approximated and/or if there is a tissue deficit that will result in a 'dead space', there will be healing by secondary intent with increased granulation and the possibility of increased scar formation, as well as a longer healing time predisposing to infection.

Although all childbearing women will need healing to some degree, many women will be vulnerable to less efficient healing. *See* Box 3.2 for some women, in addition to those who have general risk factors for infection, who may be considered to be at high risk of poor healing and infection.

BOX 3.2 FACTORS IN WOMEN AT INCREASED RISK OF WOUND INFECTION

- Obesity
- Other conditions such as diabetes, anaemia, etc
- Preoperative hospitalisation
- Lengthy labour
- Emergency caesarean section
- Instrumental delivery
- Preterm birth
- Repeat caesarean section (or increased surgery time for other reasons)
- Increased blood loss at delivery
- Prolonged healing time

Optimum environment for healing

The most effective environment for successful wound healing is:

MOIST AND WARM

Since the 1960s it has been accepted that the optimum environment for wound healing is moist and warm (Winter 1962, Bryan 2004). Exposed wounds usually form a thick, dry crust and crusted wounds epithelialise more slowly than covered wounds, and therefore often require more time and metabolic activity to heal. This is perhaps why perineal wounds tend to heal rapidly, although uncovered, as the woman's anatomy ensures the temperature remains constant and the perineal area is rarely completely dry. Efficient wound healing during the regenerative phase depends on a stable, moist environment; this environment also results in less infection, and there is some evidence that it reduces wound pain (Vuolo 2006).

Warmth, the other necessary component for optimum healing, encourages the necessary leucocyte activity (Russell 2000). The ideal wound temperature is 37°C, and a lower temperature may inhibit activity of cells involved in the healing process. Although baths or showers certainly may benefit a new mother in many ways, the exposure of the wound to temperature fluctuations may compromise healing (Parker 2000). Pathogens in hospital, especially in baths or bidets, may also put a woman with an exposed wound prior to complete epithelialisation at risk of infection (Wilson 2006).

A wound produces exudate until epithelialisation is complete. This can be seen as a pale yellowish stain on a dressing and is a normal part of the healing process. The exudate contains many substances to enhance healing, and it is vital for the formation of granulation tissue and for activating growth factors. It has also been shown that the white blood cells in exudate kill bacteria and therefore reduce infection (Williams & Young 1998).

INFLUENCES ON WOUND HEALING

General health will have a profound effect on wound healing, and aspects underpinning this are discussed in Chapter 1. However, in addition to these, some influences specific to wounds are listed in Box 3.3.

BOX 3.3 INFLUENCES ON WOUND HEALING

- Nutritional status
- Obesity
- Smoking
- Amount of sleep
- Medical conditions and therapies
- Tissue perfusion and oxygen
- Mechanical stress on wound
- Presence of infection
- Presence of haematoma, necrosis or foreign body
- Suboptimal wound care
- Stress, including pain

Nutrition

Good nutrition underpins a strong immune system (*see* Chapter 1). Malnutrition in general can lead to reduced strength of the wound, increased wound dehiscence and increased susceptibility to infection and poor quality scarring. Specific nutrient deficiencies can have an effect on healing – for example, zinc deficiency reduces rates of epithelialisation, reduces collagen synthesis and therefore reduces wound strength. Essential unsaturated fatty acids are involved in the inflammatory phase, and fat is a component of cell membranes. Vitamin A is important in cell differentiation, and epithelial keratinisation and a deficiency of vitamin A equals a deficiency of collagen and delayed epithelialisation. Vitamin A deficiency is known to increase susceptibility to infection, and vitamin C is also important, as collagen formed without adequate vitamin C is weaker. Several B vitamins, iron, copper and manganese also have significant contributions to make.

Advice on optimising nutrition should be given routinely in the antenatal period, but if a woman's condition necessitates hospitalisation prior to delivery, midwives may need to support and advise her concerning her nutrition intake, especially if the woman is ill or worried. There is evidence from some dated research that even a short period of preoperative fasting can significantly reduce nutrient levels (Goodson *et al.* 1987), and since frequently women have emergency caesarean sections after many hours in labour when food has been severely restricted, this emphasises that women should be aware that beginning labour with the best possible nutrient level would be advantageous.

There has been a general movement recently towards early feeding after caesarean section. Evidence from a survey of UK maternity units shows that in most cases midwives decide when women eat and drink post-operatively, and the time period ranged from <1 hour to >24 hours (Worthington *et al.* 1999). A Cochrane review (Mangesi & Hofmeyr 2002) reported there appears to be no reason to limit oral intake routinely following caesarean section under regional anaesthesia, although many of the trials they reviewed defined 'early' feeding as 6–8 hours post surgery. Avoiding hunger and thirst may improve women's well-being generally, and may influence earlier mobility and initiation of breastfeeding (Al-Takroni *et al.* 1999)

One of the main worries for the midwife of initiating early, or indeed immediate, feeding of post-caesarean section women is the issue of paralytic ileus. The evidence does not appear to support this concern (Kramer *et al.* 1996) although one study showed an increase in mild ileus symptoms in women whose caesarean section lasted longer than 40 minutes (Patolia *et al.* 2001). Since it is suggested that handling of the bowel may predispose to a paralytic ileus, it may be useful for the midwife caring for the woman immediately post-operatively to know the extent to which this occurred, and to adapt her care concerning offering oral intake accordingly. It would also be sensible for the midwife to introduce food gradually, starting with low fibre, fat and acidity, increasing intake as the woman demonstrates tolerance.

Obesity

The increase in obesity among midwives' clients has had a severe impact on midwifery care. Since instrumental and operative deliveries are more common in obese women (Sheiner *et al.* 2004), it is obvious they have more healing to do, but issues prior to the delivery, such as poor nutrition and co-morbidities, often compound this. In areas where a specialist midwife is in post, she should be involved in care from an early stage, to potentially optimise outcome.

The risk factors associated with obesity have been clearly highlighted in recent literature. Obesity, which can mask an impaired nutritional state, as well as provide individual risk factors such as decreased tissue perfusion, potentially reduced mobility and increase in the length of labour or surgery, is known to be a risk factor for success in wound healing (Wloch *et al.* 2012). While those who are obese may lack nutrients vital for healing, it also appears that there is a relationship between infection/wound breakdown and obesity. It is suggested this may be due to a technically more difficult operative procedure, and the fact that blood vessels within fat are more easily torn (Martens *et al.* 1995).

It has been demonstrated that although drains are not usually recommended, they may reduce infection in obese women (Allaire *et al.* 2000).

It has been suggested that the higher risk for women with a raised body mass index can be more refined if parity and increased pregnancy weight gain by 28 weeks are also taken into account (Magann *et al.* 2011).

Smoking

Nicotine and carbon monoxide are known to have a damaging influence on wound healing (Bale *et al.* 2000), and even limited smoking can reduce the peripheral blood flow. Smoking also reduces vitamin C, which is vital for healing (*see* Chapter 1 for more information).

Lack of sleep

Sleep disturbances may inhibit wound healing as sleep encourages anabolism (the synthesis of complex molecules from simple ones) and wound healing includes anabolic processes. It would be very rare to find a new mother who enjoyed her full quota of sleep every night, therefore putting all midwifery clients at risk.

Pain may also interfere with sleep (East *et al.* 2010), which also influences healing, and slower healing not only prolongs the pain but also predisposes to infection. Pain relief taken immediately before sleep may be more effective than at a pre-specified 'drug round' time.

Stress

Stress and anxiety levels can compromise the immune system (*see* Chapter 1) and inhibit wound healing (Bale *et al.* 2000), so midwives need to ensure they do everything possible to make the woman feel relaxed and confident – for example, by talking her through the information she needs or allowing her partner flexibility in visiting.

Medical conditions and therapies

Various medical conditions can influence a woman's ability to heal wounds. Recent sepsis or malnutrition, specific diseases such as AIDS, cardiac, renal or hepatic disease or drugs such as corticosteroids can lead to a woman having compromised ability to regulate growth factors, inflammatory and proliferative cells for wound repair.

In diabetic women angiopathic changes, which result in impaired perfusion, may cause a delay in wound healing. Also, the inflammatory response, fibroblast proliferation and collagen deposition can be impaired in a high-glucose environment. Since statistically diabetic women are more likely to have caesarean sections, and may have trouble regulating their drug regimen following surgery, the importance of avoiding hyperglycaemia to enable effective healing must be emphasised.

Anaemia can also impair wound healing, as red blood cells are necessary to carry oxygen to the tissues. It is not known exactly how much blood loss will be detrimental to an individual woman's condition but it would be sensible to ensure she is not anaemic either before or after the birth, especially if this involves caesarean section with the usual increased blood loss, as this may impair wound healing.

Surgical procedures and operative and post-operative care

Contribution of staff procedures to wound infection is clear. One piece of research done in the United States compared caesarean section wound infection rates before and after an education programme, refresher course and retraining in aseptic and scrub techniques was carried out. Infectious morbidity decreased from 6.4% to 2.5% (Salim *et al.* 2011).

It is known that if the operative site is shaved more than 12 hours preoperatively there is an increased risk of infection (Parker 2000). If shaving is necessary it should be done immediately before the surgery, or ideally clippers should be used (Tanner *et al.* 2006).

It is thought that the majority of bacterial contamination is from the patient's own microbial flora (Wilson 2006). It has been demonstrated in general surgery settings that a bath or shower preoperatively can reduce the number of bacteria on the skin, and therefore reduce the risk of these entering the wound during surgery. As most women undergoing an emergency caesarean section are unlikely to be able to take a preoperative shower, and, if the operation is for failure to progress (dystocia), she may have been relatively immobile in labour for many hours (with many different staff undertaking many aspects of hands-on care). A wash with soap and water preoperatively will serve to remove most of the transient bacteria she has acquired (Babb 2000).

As already noted, more lengthy surgery will put the woman at increased risk, as the length of time tissue is exposed provides an increasing risk of airborne bacteria contaminating tissue or the operators' hands or instruments (Wilson 2006). During the operation, theatre doors should remain closed and the movement of people in the operating room kept to a minimum in order to reduce the number of airborne particles.

In the UK it is recommended that all women undergoing caesarean section receive intravenous antibiotic prophylaxis during surgery (Smaill & Gyte 2010). This is based on clear evidence that it decreases the rate of post-operative endometritis and wound infection. This has historically been given following cord clamping to ensure it does not cross to the baby, but there is current controversy regarding this, as it seems to be more efficient if given prior to commencement of the operation, although the debate concerning the potential effect on the baby is also under discussion (Lamont *et al.* 2011). There is, however, an argument that queries why these mostly young healthy women undergoing 'clean' surgery are prone to infection. Perhaps greater attention to support of the immune system would change the necessity for prophylaxis.

It has been suggested that there is an increased surgical wound infection rate associated with blood transfusion. This is thought to be due to an adverse effect on cell-mediated immunity, and the risk increases with each unit administered. It is significantly lower when autologous blood is used (Wilson 2006). However, since anaemia can also predispose to poor healing and infection, blood transfusion may be necessary.

Tissue hypoxia

Tissue hypoxia from peripheral vascular disease is unlikely in childbearing women, but it may result from ill health, emergency procedures or other circumstances. *Hypovolaemia, hypothermia* (*see* Box 3.4) and *vasoconstriction* can all limit oxygen to tissues and may occur in a woman who has had traumatic labour experiences such as a post-partum haemorrhage. Tissue hypoxia – whether from long-term medical causes, an acute situation or from stress – is hard to quantify, as it can occur before measurable parameters (blood pressure, pulse, temperature or urinary output) change and when arterial oxygen levels are adequate (Bryant 1992). Tissue oxygenation can be

---

BOX 3.4 HYPOTHERMIA

Pre- and post-operative hypothermia has been suggested to increase the risk of infection through a suppression of the immune system (McNally *et al.* 2001). Hypothermia affects platelet function and suppresses neutrophils – preoperative hypothermia is probably not relevant to childbearing women going to caesarean section, especially in the normal warm environment of the labour ward, but intra-operatively (Tipton *et al.* 2012) and post-operatively it is an important consideration (Melling *et al.* 2001, Edwards *et al.* 2003). In particular, if there has been a significant blood loss treated with large amounts of unwarmed fluids, hypothermia may become relevant and is an area where the midwife can have direct influence. Midwives need to ensure this possibility is recognised and prevented, with the use of blankets or 'bear huggers' as necessary, as well as recommending the use of warmed intravenous fluids when appropriate.

supported through supplemental oxygen administration, the use of warming devices, good pain control and attention paid to moderation of stress (Ueno *et al.* 2006).

The first indication of tissue hypoxia may be a poorly healing wound and/or infection. A skilled midwife, however, could have anticipated the potential problem, and by ensuring the woman is well hydrated, warm, pain-free and nutritionally maintained, as well as psychologically supported, these complications may be prevented.

Wound care

Various activities undertaken by carers can influence efficient wound healing.

Regarding *dressings*, caesarean section wounds will normally be covered with a non-stick adhesive dressing while in theatre. Normal wound healing physiology suggests that in ideal circumstances the sutured wound will become impervious to bacteria entry within a few hours, although the dressing is usually left intact for 24–48 hours. When the dressing is removed the wound may be seen to continue to exude serous fluids, and this will be evidence that it is not normally sealed and will be vulnerable to contamination (Wilson 2006). This may be particularly so in obese women, as poor perfusion of the wound site can slow the healing process (Wilson & Clark 2003). Maintaining a sealed sterile covering will protect this wound, and if an appropriate clear film dressing is used, the site can continue to be observed, and the woman may shower, without disturbing the wound healing environment (Boyle 2001).

Wound cleaning should only be undertaken when there is an excessive amount of discharge that may cause excoriation of the surrounding tissue. Swabbing or cleaning wounds can result in organisms being redistributed around the area, cotton wool or gauze shedding fibres into granulating tissue and disruption of newly formed tissues. Foreign bodies in a wound, even as small as a hair, can cause a sinus-type wound (Miller & Collier n.d.). Cleaning of the wound, if necessary, should ideally be done by irrigation, using a prepacked single-use irrigation device. All wound assessment or cleaning should of course by carried out under aseptic technique (*see* Chapter 14).

SPECIFIC MIDWIFERY CARE INFLUENCING WOUND HEALING AND INFECTION REDUCTION

Support of the woman in labour

Duration of labour preoperatively can predispose a woman to poor healing and infection. When assessing the infection rate relating to caesarean section it is relevant to differentiate between elective and 'emergency' caesarean sections and to note how long labour was pre-surgery. Women undergoing caesarean section for 'failure to progress' (dystocia), may have been labouring for many hours, without nutrition, perhaps without adequate hydration, without sleep, without mobility (in the presence of an epidural) and with multiple interventions, many invasive (indwelling catheters, intravenous lines, multiple vaginal examinations) and many different caregivers. All these elements will add to the risk for infection post caesarean section, and these same elements may be present for some women's labours that end in a vaginal delivery. The midwife may not be able to change these circumstances but her awareness may allow her to influence activities to potentially enable a better outcome.

Specific care around the time of caesarean section, such as attention paid to pre-, intra- and post-operative warming, maintaining normoglycaemia, correcting volume deficits, providing adequate pain control and ensuring rigorous adherence to aseptic technique when necessary may also benefit the woman.

Perineal trauma

At present it is estimated that about 75% of women with vaginal births will receive perineal sutures; therefore, care of these wounds is a common part of all midwives' postnatal care. Post-partum perineal infection is most often associated with midline episiotomy, third- or fourth-degree tear or episiotomy extension and vaginal haematoma (Tharpe 2008).

There is some evidence that not all third- and fourth-degree tears are correctly diagnosed at delivery (Andrews *et al.* 2004), although it is not clear whether this is from a lack of knowledge by the carer or because of the difficulty of the diagnosis. Accurate identification to enable the woman to access appropriate ongoing care is vital to achieve the best outcome. There is a good argument that third- and fourth-degree tears, especially if complicated, should only be repaired by experienced professionals such as colorectal surgeons and the woman should be followed up until 12 months after the birth. Some maternity units have access to specialist colorectal nurses who may have a valuable part to play. Women with perineal infection may need a vaginal and rectal examination to rule out occult rectal injury. This has potential to lead to rectovaginal fistula formation and therefore must be diagnosed without delay.

The method of suturing used by the midwife may have an influence on the degree of pain and rate of healing. Over-tightness of sutures can lead to necrosis and weaker wounds (Morrison 1992). If suturing is necessary it should be done as soon as possible. When looking at the experiences of women who needed stitches, Garcia *et al.* (1998) found that while 47% were sutured straight away, 14% waited from 20 to 60 minutes and 8% waited more than 60 minutes. Of course it is difficult from a purely statistical analysis to draw exact conclusions (maybe some of the women who had to wait had more urgent needs being dealt with, such as a relaxed uterus or the baby needing resuscitation) but the potential of even a small increase in blood loss, which may compromise the woman's ability to efficiently heal, should lead to every midwife aiming to have suturing completed as a matter of urgency. There may be a psychological benefit to not delaying suturing also, as the wait may produce increased stress in the woman.

Even later in the puerperium, when a midwife considers the wound 'well healed' a woman may continue to feel pain – Glazener *et al.* (1993) along with many other researchers found a substantial number of women reporting perineal pain for extended periods. Long-term perineal pain and dyspareunia are not uncommon and can affect up to 20% of those who have suffered trauma. When it is considered that epithelialisation happens long before the underlying structures have successfully remodelled, this is not surprising.

Caesarean section wounds

The rate of wound infection following caesarean section is very hard to evaluate. Research done in 1992 has shown that only 47% of infection had occurred by the seventh day, with 78% occurring by day 14 and 90% occurring by day 21 (Weigelt *et al.* 1992), and there is no reason to suspect this pattern has changed. More recent research done in the East Midlands suggested 84% of caesarean section wound infection developed after discharge from hospital (Ward *et al.* 2008). After caesarean section women are frequently discharged home from hospital as early as day 2 or 3, and therefore it is unlikely an infection will be diagnosed at this stage. Research on general surgical wound infections demonstrate they can develop at any time after surgery, but the most common time is 4–10 days, and these are probably a result of infection introduced during surgery (Wilson 2006).

Many infections will be suspected by the community midwife but diagnosed and treated by the general practitioner, and the general practitioner alone will see many more infections, as the community midwife may no longer be visiting. Therefore, unless specific research is undertaken, the infection rate for caesarean section by individual units (or, indeed, individual surgeons) is impossible to evaluate. One large audit that assessed women post caesarean section for 30 days found a 1.3% rate of infection while in hospital but about 15% following discharge (Health Protection Scotland 2010).

A midwife's role in routine caesarean section wound care can be vital and multifold. All midwives know that new mothers have a tendency to neglect their own physiological needs in favour of those of their newborn, and therefore to begin with there is a role for education: women need to know that the best way to care effectively for their new baby is by ensuring their own health is optimal, and this involves attention to their own sleep and nutritional needs. Support of the immune system is discussed in Chapter 1 and may provide a basis for the midwife when educating the woman. Awareness of the influences on successful wound healing (*see* Box 3.3) may also allow the midwife to make timely interventions when appropriate.

Some caesarean section wounds may become complicated. Wound care has changed and is continuing to develop rapidly and the care of a difficult wound is outside a midwife's remit. Most hospitals will have expert nurse practitioners – tissue viability nurses or infection control nurses – who will have an up-to-date expertise that the midwife can access when dealing with a difficult wound. When the woman is at home, community midwives often call on district nurses, who also have relevant experience and expertise.

Analgesia

In the immediate postnatal period, most women following vaginal delivery – including those with intact perinea – report some degree of perineal pain (Albers *et al.* 1999, East *et al.* 2012), and women post caesarean section will definitely require analgesia. Pain can increase wound healing time (causing prolonged pain, a vicious circle) by impeding the immune system, and lengthy wound healing predisposes to infection. Pain can also cause emotional stress that may likewise compromise an effective immune system response (Solowiej *et al.* 2009, Woo 2012). Good pain control is necessary, especially following discharge, to enable sleep and to increase mobility – difficult mobility can lead to a woman neglecting her own needs, especially nutrition. Increased ability to mobilise comfortably can also lead to more positive feelings, increased confidence in childcare and enhanced self-esteem, all of which contribute to a healthy immune system.

If women self-administer their drugs, there is some evidence they are more satisfied with the pain management (Moffat *et al.* 2001). It would also give the midwife time to ensure women were taking their medication effectively and to make suggestions for analgesia use after discharge. Midwifery time spent with the woman may in itself have an analgesic effect. As Jennifer Sleep (1995) wrote, 'The quality of personal individualised post-partum care is likely to be a major influence in reduced perineal pain and speeding recovery.'

For perineal pain there are various comfort measures that are in common use, and recommended either by midwives or non-professionals, and some of these may not be ideal when considered from a strict 'wound healing' perspective. There is no doubt that the perineum is an ideal healing environment – warm and moist with a good blood supply – so any interventions should not interrupt this. Warm water and bathing, herbal remedies, local pharmacological therapies and ice packs or other cold therapy may be used by women and suggested by midwives; although these may disrupt the maintenance of constant temperature, they need to be balanced against the advantage of the woman feeling comfortable and the physical advantages of better sleep, mobility and the psychological benefits.

It has been suggested that pelvic floor exercises not only can prevent, or treat, urinary incontinence (Glazener *et al.* 2001) but also may help perineal healing, perhaps due to the increased blood supply. These exercises have also been reported to reduce pain (Sleep & Grant 1987), perhaps by keeping the area flexible.

INFECTION

Wound infections may come via the woman's own flora from skin or genital tract (endogenous), from direct contact with contaminated equipment and the hands of healthcare workers, or from many microbes, in particular skin squames, which can be carried on air currents and land on open wounds.

Wound infection involves a prolonged and modified inflammatory action. With mild symptoms there can easily be confusion between the normal inflammatory response and a response to invasive organisms. It is often difficult to tell whether a wound is *contaminated* (organisms present in exudates but not multiplying or entering tissues), *colonised* (organisms multiplying but without systemic reaction) or *infected* (systemic symptoms as well as spreading cellulitis) (Hampton & Collins 2003). Most signs and symptoms of a wound infection (*see* Box 3.5) are an exaggeration of normal wound healing physiology.

BOX 3.5 SIGNS AND SYMPTOMS OF INFECTION

- Increasing erythema – in particular, spreading cellulitis
- Increasing swelling
- Change in exudate – volume, colour, malodour
- Increasing tenderness and pain
- Increasing white blood cell count
- Pyrexia and tachycardia
- Generalised malaise

- *Erythema* (redness) may be the normal inflammatory process, but may progress to cellulitis.
- *Oedema* may be part of the normal healing process, or even a local reaction to suture material, or a sign of infection.
- *Discharge* – a small amount of serous fluid may be normal, but large amounts or the presence of pus is not.
- *Pain* or tenderness of the wound may be normal (and especially in a woman who is trying to care for her baby, with little sleep or nutrition, in the early postnatal period); however, increasing pain (especially when resting) would be a worrying sign.
- *Pyrexia* may indicate a wound infection, or an infection elsewhere in the woman – or, indeed, may be connected with breastfeeding and engorgement. Ongoing assessment is necessary to establish the cause.
- *Malaise* is a common postnatal and post-operative symptom; however, it may also

indicate a woman who is unwell. Assessment of progression (women should be expected to feel better day by day) and degree is important.

- *Microbiology culture* can be positive, not only when infection is present but also due to contamination or colonisation. *See* Box 3.6 for discussion regarding wound swabs.

BOX 3.6 WOUND SWABS

Wound swabs need to be taken without contamination by skin flora. Swabbing a doubtful wound may not always give a clear answer. All open wounds are contaminated but only excessive amounts of bacteria indicate there is a significant likelihood of infection (Baxter 2004). However, it should be noted that beta-haemolytic streptococcus can compromise healing at lower levels than other bacteria (*see* Chapters 4 and 6).

It has been suggested that without evidence of systemic infection, a report showing bacteria present in the wound bed should not result in antibiotic treatment (Williams & Young 1998). Even when there is extensive contamination, it has been noted that wounds usually heal without infection in women with normal immune system function; however, this would of course need close monitoring, with the knowledge that serious group A beta-haemolytic streptococcus infection may develop and spread very rapidly (*see* Chapter 4).

A wound swab can be taken to establish the microorganisms present, in order to enable appropriate antibiotics to be prescribed – if the only sign is serous discharge (a normal part of wound healing), a swab may grow various microorganisms, but these will only determine colonisation, not infection. Persistent pyrexia and continued signs of infection despite adequate antibiotics prescribed will need referral for evaluation of the antibiotics (and a possible change), surgical assessment of the wound and/or evacuation of abscess or haematoma (ultrasound or magnetic resonance imaging may be necessary to confirm diagnosis).

A wound infection may involve:

- spontaneous discharge of pus before or after suture removal
- the opening of a wound
- non-purulent discharge containing pathogens such as coliform or *S. aureus*
- spreading cellulitis.

Wound infection may present at various times, although groups A and B beta-haemolytic streptococcus may appear within 1–2 days. However, the majority will first become evident after discharge and within the first 3 weeks of the postnatal period. This confirms the importance of the midwife giving advice and information to the woman about wound healing and signs of infection, as early discharge from hospital and reduced postnatal visits limit the amount of professional observation available.

Antibiotics are the first-line treatment for any infection; however, unfortunately and probably due to many years of misuse, many antibiotics are not effective as strains of antibiotic-resistant bacteria increase. Midwives can influence the effectiveness of treatment by ensuring the timing of antibiotic administration is optimum to maintain a constant level in the blood, and providing women with the knowledge of the importance of taking full courses of antibiotics, and adhering to the times of administration.

ROLE OF THE MIDWIFE

- Care for the woman should reflect effective support of the immune system, in particular in high-risk situations such as post-operatively.
- Ensure practice conforms to good wound care principles, including strict asepsis as appropriate and attention to surgical procedures.
- Teach women about the use of antibiotics as appropriate.

USEFUL RESOURCES

- Boyle M (2006) *Wound Healing in Midwifery*. Oxford: Radcliffe Publishing.
- Dealey C (2012) *The Care of Wounds: A Guide for Nurses*. 4th edition. London: Wiley-Blackwell.
- Franz M, Robson M, Steed D, *et al.* Wound Healing Society (2008) Guidelines to aid healing of acute wounds by decreasing impediments of healing. *Wound Repair Regen.* **16**(6): 723–48.
- National Institute for Health and Care Excellence (NICE) (2008) *Surgical Site Infection: prevention and treatment of surgical site infection*. NICE Clinical Guideline 74. London: NICE. Available at: www.nice.org.uk/guidance/cg74

REFERENCES

Albers L, Garcia J, Renfrew M, *et al.* (1999) Distribution of genital tract trauma in childbirth and related postnatal pain. *Birth.* **26**(1): 11–15.

Allaire A, Fisch J, McMahon M (2000) Subcutaneous drain vs suture in obese women undergoing caesarean delivery: a prospective randomized trial. *J Reprod Med.* **45**(4): 327–31.

Al-Takroni A, Parvathi C, Mendis K, *et al.* (1999) Early oral intake after caesarean section performed under general anaesthesia. *J Obstet Gynaecol.* **19**(1): 34–7.

Andrews V, Thakar R, Sultan A (2004) Are midwives adequately trained to identify anal sphincter injury? *International Continence Society UK Proceedings.* 11th Annual Scientific Meeting: 34.

Babb J (2000) Decontamination of the environment, equipment and the skin. In: Ayliffe G, Fraise A, Geddes A, *et al.* (editors). *Control of Hospital Infection.* 4th ed. London: Arnold. pp. 92–128.

Bale S, Harding K, Leaper D (2000) *An Introduction to Wounds*. London: Emap Healthcare.

Bale S, Jones V (2006) *Wound Care Nursing: a patient-centred approach*. 2nd ed. Edinburgh: Mosby, Elsevier.

Baxter H (2004) Surgical wounds and their care. In: Maxwell D (editor). *Surgical Techniques in Obstetrics and Gynaecology.* Edinburgh: Churchill Livingstone. pp. 27–40.

Boyle M (2001) Caesarean section wound management: a challenge for midwives. *Pract Midwife.* **4**(2): 20–2.

Bryan J (2004) Moist wound healing: a concept that changed our practice. *J Wound Care.* **13**(6): 227–8.

Bryant R (1992) *Acute and Chronic Wounds: nursing management.* London: Mosby Year Book.

Dealey C (2012) *The Care of Wounds: a guide for nurses.* 4th ed. London: Wiley-Blackwell.

Dougherty L, Lister S (2008) *The Royal Marsden Hospital Manual of Clinical Nursing Procedures.* Oxford: Blackwell.

East C, Sherburn M, Nagle C, *et al.* (2012) Perineal pain following childbirth: prevalence, effects on postnatal recovery and analgesia use. *Midwifery.* **28**(1): 93–7.

Edwards R, Madani K, Duff P (2003) Is perioperative hypothermia a risk factor for post-cesarean infection? *Infect Dis Obstet Gynecol.* **11**(2): 75–80.

Flanagan M (2000) The physiology of wound healing. *J Wound Care.* **9**(6): 299–300.

Garcia J, Redshaw M, Fitzsimons B, *et al.* (1998) *First Class Delivery: a national survey of women's views of maternity care.* London: Audit Commission.

Glazener C, Abdulla M, Russell I, *et al.* (1993) Postnatal care: a survey of patients' experiences. *BMJ.* **1**(2): 67–74.

Glazener C, Herbison G, Wilson P, *et al.* (2001) Conservative management of persistent postnatal urinary and faecal incontinence: a randomised controlled trial. *BMJ.* **323**(7313): 593–6.

Goodson WH 3rd, Lopez-Sarmiento A, Jensen J, *et al.* (1987) The influence of a brief preoperative illness on postoperative healing. *Ann Surg.* **205**(3): 250–5.

Hampton S, Collins F (2003) *Tissue Viability.* London: Whurr Publications.

Health Protection Scotland (2010) *Pan Celtic Collaboration Surgical Site Infection Surveillance Report: surveillance of surgical site infection for caesarean section procedures performed in Northern Ireland, Scotland and Wales in 2008.* Glasgow: Health Protection Scotland.

Kramer R, van Someren J, Qualls C, *et al.* (1996) Postoperative management of caesarean patients: the effect of immediate feeding on the incidence of ileus. *Obstet Gynecol.* **88**(1): 29–32.

Lamont R, Sobel J, Kusanovic J, *et al.* (2011) Current debate on the use of antibiotic prophylaxis for caesarean section. *BJOG.* **118**(2): 193–201.

Magann E, Doherty D, Chauhan S, *et al.* (2011) Pregnancy, obesity, gestational weight gain and parity as predictors of peripartum complications. *Arch Gynecol Obstet.* **284**(4): 827–36.

Mangesi L, Hofmeyr G (2002) Early compared with delayed oral fluid and food after caesarean section. *Cochrane Database Syst Rev.* (3): CD003516.

Martens M, Kolrud B, Faro S, *et al.* (1995) Development of wound infection or separation after cesarean delivery: prospective evaluation of 2,431 cases. *J Reprod Med.* **40**(3): 171–5.

McNally H, Cutter G, Ruttenber A, *et al.* (2001) Hypothermia as a risk factor for pediatric cardiothoracic surgical site infection. *Pediatr Infect Dis J.* **20**(4): 459–62.

Melling A, Ali B, Scott E, *et al.* (2001) Effects of preoperative warming on the incidence of wound infection after clean surgery: a randomised controlled trial. *Lancet.* **358**(9285): 876–80.

Miller M, Collier M (n.d.) *Understanding Wounds.* London: Professional Nurse, Emap Healthcare.

Moffat H, Lavender T, Walkinshaw S (2001) Comparing administration of paracetamol for perineal pain. *Br J Midwifery.* **9**(11): 690–4.

Morrison M (1992) *A Colour Guide to the Nursing Management of Wounds.* London: Walfe Publishing.

Nursing and Midwifery Council (NMC) (2012) *Midwives Rules and Standards.* London: NMC.

Parker L (2000) Applying the principle of infection control to wound care. *Br J Nurs*. **9**(7): 394–404.

Patolia D, Hilliard R, Toy E, *et al.* (2001) Early feeding after cesarean: randomized trial. *Obstet Gynecol*. **98**(1): 113–16.

Russell L (2000) Understanding physiology of wound healing and how dressings help. *Br J Nurs*. **9**(1): 10–21.

Salim R, Braverman M, Berkovic I, *et al.* (2011) Effect of interventions in reducing the rate of infection after caesarean delivery. *Am J Infect Control*. **39**(10): e73–8.

Sheiner E, Levy A, Menes T, *et al.* (2004) Maternal obesity as an independent risk factor for caesarean section delivery. *Paediatr Perinat Epidemiol*. **18**(3): 196–201.

Sleep J (1995) Postnatal care revisited. In: Alexander J, Levy V, Roch S (editors). *Aspects of Midwifery Practice: a research based approach*. Basingstoke, UK: McMillan Press. pp. 180–95.

Sleep J, Grant A (1987). West Berkshire perineal management trial: three year follow up. *Br Med J (Clin Res Ed)*. **295**(6601): 749–51.

Smaill F, Gyte G (2010) Antibiotic prophylaxis versus no prophylaxis for preventing infection after caesarean section. *Cochrane Database Syst Rev*. (1): CD007482.

Solowiej K, Mason V, Upton D (2009) Review of the relationship between stress and wound healing: part 1. *J Wound Care*. **18**(9): 357–66.

Tanner J, Woodings D, Moncaster K (2006) Preoperative hair removal to reduce surgical site infection. *Cochrane Database Syst Rev*. (3): CD004122.

Tharpe N (2008) Postpregnancy genital tract and wound infections. *J Midwifery Womens Health*. **53**(3): 236–46.

Tipton AM, Cohen SA, Chelmow D (2012) Wound infection in the obese pregnant woman. *Semin Perinatol*. **35**(6): 345–9.

Ueno C, Hunt T, Hopf H (2006) Using physiology to improve surgical wound outcomes. *Plast Reconstr Surg*. **117**(7 Suppl.): S59–71.

Uygur D, Yesildaglar N, Kis S, *et al.* (2004) Early repair of episiotomy dehiscence. *Aust N Z J Obstet Gynaecol*. **44**(3): 244–6.

Vuolo J (2006) Assessment and management of surgical wound in clinical practice. *Nurs Stand*. **20**(52): 46–56.

Ward V, Charlett A, Fagan J, *et al.* (2008) Enhanced surgical site infection surveillance following caesarean section: experience of a multicentre collaborative post-discharge system. *J Hosp Infect*. **70**(2): 166–73.

Weigelt J, Dryer D, Haley R (1992) The necessity and efficiency of wound surveillance after discharge. *Arch Surg*. **127**(1): 77–82.

Williams C, Young T (1998) *Myth and Reality in Wound Care*. Salisbury: Quay Books.

Wilson J (2006) *Infection Control in Clinical Practice*. 3rd ed. Edinburgh: Baillière Tindall, Elsevier.

Wilson J, Clark J (2003) Obesity: impediment to wound healing. *Crit Care Nurs Q*. **26**(2): 119–32.

Winter G (1962) Formation of the scab and the rate of epithelialisation of superficial wounds in the skin of the young domestic pig. *Nature*. **193**: 293–4.

Wloch C, Wilson J, Lamagni T, *et al.* (2012) Risk factors for surgical site infection following caesarean section in England: results from multicentre cohort study. *BJOG*. **119**(1): 1324–33.

Woo K (2012) Exploring the effects of pain and stress on wound healing. *Adv Skin Wound Care*. **25**(1): 38–44.

Worthington L, Mulcahy A, White S, *et al.* (1999) Attitudes to oral feeding following caesarean section. *Anaesthesia*. **54**(3): 292–6.

CHAPTER 4

Sepsis

INTRODUCTION

Puerperal sepsis, formerly known as 'childbed fever', was responsible for around two-thirds of deaths of women in the eighteenth and nineteenth centuries. Handwashing, aseptic techniques, improved general health and antibiotic treatment all contributed to a dramatic improvement in safety for mothers during childbirth (Lucas *et al.* 2012), although in resource-poor settings, poverty and health inequality continue to contribute to maternal deaths from infection (Acosta & Knight 2013). However, in the UK, the rate of maternal mortality from sepsis has doubled in the last 20 years (Acosta *et al.* 2012), and the report of the Confidential Enquiries into Maternal Deaths (CEMD) in the United Kingdom for 2006–08 stated that sepsis had become the leading direct cause of maternal deaths (CMACE 2011). Deaths occurred during pregnancy as well as in the postnatal period. A virulent organism, Lancefield group A beta-haemolytic streptococcus (GAS) was responsible for nearly half of the deaths (13 out of 29) (CMACE 2011). Figures for maternal death reflect a much larger incidence of morbidity.

The CEMD report emphasised the need for awareness of symptoms of sepsis among health professionals and called for a 'back to basics' approach (CMACE 2011). Symptoms of sepsis may be less distinctive, and may progress more rapidly in pregnant and postpartum women (RCOG 2012a, b). The responsibility for midwives is the effective assessment of women to identify any signs and symptoms of sepsis. This will enable prompt referral for urgent medical treatment (Bick *et al.* 2011). It is important to prevent infection and to ensure treatment of any infection before it progresses to sepsis.

DEFINITIONS AND COURSE OF THE DISEASE

Sepsis, severe sepsis and septic shock are terms used to describe the progress of disease following infection. Sepsis involves a systemic inflammatory reaction that triggers pathophysiological changes that can lead to septic shock. Box 4.1 lists definitions in relation to the development of septic shock.

BOX 4.1 STAGES OF CLINICAL RESPONSE TO SEVERE INFECTION

Infection: invasion by pathogenic organisms that reproduce and multiply, which then generates an immune response

⇩

Bacteraemia: the presence of bacteria in the blood; this presence may be sustained or transient.

⇩

Systemic inflammatory response syndrome (SIRS)*: the presence of any two of the following features –

- temperature: >38°C or <36°C
- tachycardia: heart rate >90 beats per minute
- tachypnoea: respiratory rate >20 breaths per minute or $PaCO_2$ <32 mmHg
- white blood cell count: raised (>12 × 10^9 cells/L) or low (<4 × 10^9 cells/L)
- sugar: blood glucose >7.7 mmoL in the absence of diabetes.

⇩

Sepsis: this arises from the systemic response to infection and is defined as the presence of a number of the clinical signs of SIRS (listed earlier) alongside an identifiable infection. It is challenging to treat and it is life-threatening.

⇩

Severe sepsis – multiple organ dysfunction syndrome: sepsis is considered severe when associated with organ dysfunction, hypoperfusion or hypotension. The generalised inflammatory response and procoagulant changes lead to organ dysfunction. Neurological impairment, lactic acidosis and acute renal, liver, heart or respiratory failure may occur.

⇩

Septic shock: this includes the characteristics of multiple organ dysfunction syndrome listed earlier and the persistence of hypoperfusion and hypotension despite adequate fluid replacement.

* As a memory aid, SIRS is referred to as '3 Ts with white sugar' (Tripathi *et al.* 2011) (*see* Figure 4.1).

(Anthony 2011, Ferns 2007, Parsed & Sunnah 2007)

Systemic Inflammatory Response Syndrome (SIRS) assessment

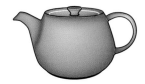

3 Ts with white sugar
- **Temperature (>38 or <36C)**
- **Tachycardia (>90/min)**
- **Tachypnoea (>20/min)**

- **White cell count (<4 or >12)**
- **Blood glucose (>7.7 mmol in absence of diabetes)**

FIGURE 4.1 3 Ts with white sugar

PATHOPHYSIOLOGY OF THE DEVELOPMENT OF SEPTIC SHOCK

Inappropriate fluid shift and vasodilation are the key pathophysiological features of systemic infection (Ferns 2007, Lucas *et al.* 2012). Vasodilation and reduced systemic resistance are normal physiological features of pregnancy. The combined effect of the pathological processes of sepsis superimposed on the physiological demands of pregnancy make pregnant women particularly vulnerable to sepsis (Lucas *et al.* 2012). The result of this is hypoxia of tissues, acidosis, hypotension and hypovolaemia. Compensatory mechanisms such as an increased heart rate and an increased respiratory rate aim to increase cardiac output and correct acidosis, but as these fail to work, underperfusion to the organs occurs. As organs start to fail, renal damage occurs and coagulation disorders further compromise function (Ferns 2007).

In response to invading pathogenic bacteria the immune system activates macrophages and neutrophils as well as other factors such as cytokines, tumour necrosis factor and interleukins (*see* Chapter 1). This is usually effective at controlling the spread of infection. However, if the infection does spread, the inflammatory response increases and this can have a serious impact on the cardiovascular system. The inflammatory mediators act on the endothelial lining of blood vessels, causing an increased production of the powerful vasodilator, nitric oxide. Eventually, the response will involve the release of platelets and stimulation of the coagulation, complement and kinin systems. The blood vessels dilate and cause a significant drop in blood pressure.

The heart rate will increase in an effort to compensate for the drop in blood pressure. In addition, activation of the coagulation system can result in disseminated intravascular coagulation. The tendency to clot formation on top of already-existing pro-coagulation of pregnancy predisposes pregnant and postpartum women with sepsis to microvascular clot formation. The combination of ischaemia from low blood pressure and clot formation can result in organ dysfunction. Fluid shifts can be dangerous. Pregnant women are at greater risk of developing pulmonary oedema due to the pregnancy-induced changes in colloid osmotic pressure, which governs the fluid shift in the lungs. As sepsis progresses there will be reduced blood flow to the uterus, with consequent reduced oxygenation to the fetus (Hayes 2007).

There are two phases recognised in the progress of septic shock: warm shock followed by cold shock. Box 4.2 lists the features of the progressive stages of septic shock.

BOX 4.2 FEATURES OF SEPTIC SHOCK

INITIAL: WARM SHOCK

- Warm peripheries (peripheral vasodilation)
- Low blood pressure
- Raised and bounding heart rate
- Temperature instability
- Increased respiratory rate
- Altered mental state

LATE STAGES: COLD SHOCK

- Cold peripheries (peripheral vasoconstriction)
- Sweating
- Weak, thready pulse

ORGAN DYSFUNCTION

- Impaired renal function: oliguria, anuria, electrolyte imbalance, raised creatinine
- Neurological compromise: confusion, agitation and possibly coma
- Cardiopulmonary impairment: cyanosis and adult respiratory distress syndrome
- Haematological changes: reduced platelet count, disseminated intravascular coagulation
- Metabolic acidosis with raised serum lactate
- Liver impairment: increased serum bilirubin and increased alkaline phosphatase
- Gastrointestinal: diarrhoea, paralytic ileus

(Hayes 2007, Raynor 2012)

SITES OF INFECTION

Sepsis can arise from many sources and is not limited to infections beginning in the genital tract. Figure 4.2 indicates the obstetric and non-obstetric sites of infection that may lead to sepsis. The commonest causes of severe sepsis are septic abortion, chorio-amnionitis, endometritis, wound infection, pyelonephritis and respiratory infections (Ferns 2007, Anthony 2011). Postpartum, the uterus and birth canal remain suscep-tible to invasion by organisms for several days following birth. Sepsis occurs when these organisms invade the lining of the uterus, adjacent structures, the lymphatics and the bloodstream. Caesarean section (CS) is a significant risk factor for serious puerperal infection and yet sepsis can occur following uncomplicated vaginal delivery (Acosta & Knight 2013, Bick *et al.* 2011). CMACE (2011) highlighted the potential risk of sepsis following contact with young children who had a sore throat or upper respiratory tract infection. Poor hand hygiene resulting in contamination of the peri-neal area has been implicated as a possible route for infection.

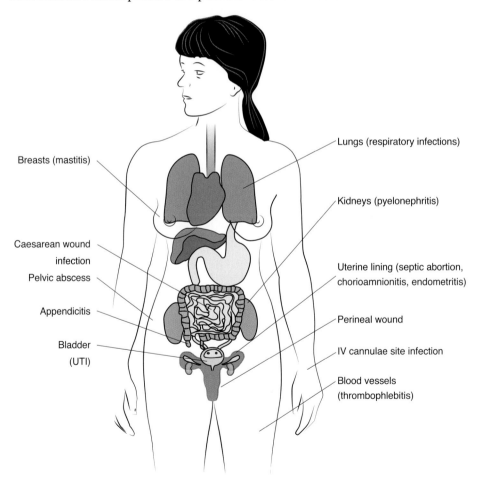

FIGURE 4.2 Sites of infection

A woman died as a result of complications of mastitis in the 2006–08 CEMD report (CMACE 2011) and consequently mastitis has been highlighted as a source of infection that may be overlooked. Mastitis can lead to breast abscess, necrotising fasciitis and toxic shock syndrome (RCOG 2012b).

Women who are unwell and are suspected of having sepsis should be examined for skin and soft tissue infection. Areas where the skin or mucosa has been broken, such as intravenous cannulae sites, CS or perineal wounds, drains or arterial line sites, should be examined and swabs taken of any discharge. When practical, lines should be removed and their tips sent for culture.

Seeding of streptococci from uterine infection can produce limb pain similar to that of deep vein thrombosis (RCOG 2012b). Associated complications of invasive infection include pelvic cellulitis, septic ovarian vein thrombosis, pelvic abscess or invasion of the infection into the joints, causing septic arthritis (Gourlay *et al.* 2001).

CLINICAL FEATURES AND DIAGNOSIS OF SEPSIS

Signs and symptoms of initial infection will depend on the source of the infection, and identification of that source is an important part of diagnosis and management. Genital tract sepsis can present as constant severe abdominal or perineal pain and tenderness that is disproportionate to that which would normally be expected, and which is not relieved by usual analgesic medication. Diarrhoea in addition to this pain is characteristic of sepsis (Lucas *et al.* 2012, RCOG 2012a). In pregnancy, maternal infection will quickly affect the fetus and an abnormal heart rate pattern or intrauterine fetal death may indicate maternal disease (Lucas *et al.* 2012).

Pyrexia is common when infection is present, but in sepsis a normal temperature or hypothermia can be found. The white cell count normally rises in response to infection. In pregnancy and in particularly in labour, the white cell count normally increases and then falls to pre-pregnancy levels within 1 week. In severe sepsis, the white cell count following delivery fails to decrease or conversely decreases rapidly (Lucas *et al.* 2012).

One of the earliest signs of sepsis is an increased respiratory rate. The respiratory rate will go up in response to pyrexia and lactic acidosis, and is a result of cytokine-mediated (immune response) effects on the respiratory centre (Lucas *et al.* 2012).

Toxic shock syndrome caused by staphylococcal or streptococcal exotoxins can produce an array of confusing symptoms including nausea, vomiting, diarrhoea, severe pain due to necrotising fasciitis, watery vaginal discharge and a generalised maculopapular rash (RCOG 2012a).

CAUSATIVE ORGANISMS ASSOCIATED WITH SEPSIS

The genitourinary tract is colonised with a wide variety of organisms but most will not cause infection and women who develop sepsis are likely to be infected with more than one organism. Box 4.3 lists some of the most frequently occurring microorganisms responsible for maternal sepsis.

BOX 4.3 COMMON MICROORGANISMS RESPONSIBLE FOR MATERNAL SEPSIS

- GAS, also known as *Streptococcus pyogenes*
- Group B *Streptococcus*
- *Escherichia coli*
- *Staphylococcus aureus*
- *Streptococcus pneumoniae*
- Methicillin-resistant *S. aureus*
- *Clostridium septicum*
- *Mycobacterium tuberculosis*

(RCOG 2012b, Lucas *et al.* 2012, Acosta & Knight 2013)

GAS is a community-acquired infection that has significantly contributed to the recent rise in rates of maternal mortality (CMACE 2011). It is a particularly serious organism, as it produces a virulent exotoxin A, which causes a rapid skin and soft tissue necrosis known as necrotising fasciitis (*see* Box 4.4 for an explanation of necrotising fasciitis).

The natural reservoir for GAS is the nasopharynx and it is a cause of pharyngitis ('strep throat') and scarlet fever as well as genital tract sepsis. Approximately 5%–30% of the population are asymptomatic carriers of the infection. Transmission is via aerosolised droplets and occurs more frequently in the winter months. Women may acquire the infection from family members, particularly children. Colonisation of the genital tract may occur via improper handwashing with subsequent contamination of the perineum (Acosta & Knight 2013).

The damage caused by GAS progresses rapidly to septic shock and multi-organ failure and it has a mortality rate of up to 25% (Gourlay *et al.* 2001). A concerning feature of GAS infections is that initially the infection has few symptoms but can progress rapidly to fulminant infection and multi-organ involvement. The CEMD report gives examples of the rapid progression of the infection. Even where health professionals recognised the illness and acted promptly, sadly some women still died, despite excellent care (CMACE 2011).

Prompt treatment with broad-spectrum antibiotics, surgical removal of damaged tissue (possibly hysterectomy) and admission to an intensive care unit offers the best chance of recovery (Gourlay *et al.* 2001).

> ### BOX 4.4 NECROTISING FASCIITIS
>
> Necrotising fasciitis is characterised by widespread necrosis of subcutaneous tissue associated with CS and perineal damage. It is usually caused by infection with GAS. Distinctive features of this serious condition include the presence of copious smelly discharge, dusky skin colouration and agonising pain (Lucas *et al.* 2012).

RISK FACTORS FOR THE DEVELOPMENT OF INFECTION AND SEPSIS

Box 4.5 lists risk factors for the development of infection and sepsis. These include characteristics of the woman that make her vulnerable to infection. Some of these features are known to reduce the immune response, such as human immunodeficiency virus, while others make the woman vulnerable to developing infection such as diabetes. There is a significantly higher incidence of sepsis in women with sickle-cell disease, probably due to poor function of the spleen (Villers *et al.* 2008). Explanations related to the increased risk of sepsis among obese women include impaired glucose tolerance, increased incidence of CS, poor wound healing, and an increase in genital tract infections (Acosta *et al.* 2012). However, obesity was found to be an independent risk factor, even after controlling for mode of delivery (Acosta *et al.* 2012). Black women, women from poor socio-economic groups and women from ethnic minority groups are over-represented in those who died from sepsis, indicating that lack of equality of access to care is an area of concern (CMACE 2011, Bick *et al.* 2011). Deaths from sepsis increase during December to April and were often preceded by a sore throat or upper respiratory tract infection. A third of deaths occurred in the first half of pregnancy, although most deaths were in the puerperium following CS (CMACE 2011). However, sepsis can occur in previously healthy women following uncomplicated pregnancy and vaginal birth (Bick *et al.* 2011).

The inclusion of women with anaemia in those at risk, alongside factors such as obesity and vulnerability, may indicate problems of nutrition, although causal links are likely to be multifactorial. The midwife's role in education and health promotion, particularly to vulnerable women, is nevertheless evident (*see* section 'Support of the immune system' in Chapter 1).

The next group of risk factors relate to events occurring during pregnancy, labour and the puerperium. Organisms require a portal of entry and many events during childbirth provide the opportunity for this. The delivery of the placenta leaves the lining of the uterus vulnerable to endometritis. The opportunity for ascending infection, and access to a good uterine blood supply, create the conditions for the development of sepsis. CS is a risk factor with an even more enhanced risk from emergency CS. CS wounds are just one site for potential infections. The development of infection

BOX 4.5 RISK FACTORS FOR DEVELOPMENT OF INFECTION AND SEPSIS

FEATURES OF THE WOMAN
- Obesity
- Impaired glucose tolerance or diabetes
- Impaired immunity; e.g. human immunodeficiency virus, immunosuppressive medication
- Anaemia or sickle-cell disease
- Women from poor socio-economic groups
- Black or minority ethnic group origin
- History of pelvic infection or vaginal discharge
- History of group B *Streptococcus* infection
- Intravenous drug misuse

FACTORS RELATED TO PREGNANCY AND CHILDBIRTH
Pregnancy:
- septic miscarriage or termination of pregnancy
- cervical sutures
- prolonged spontaneous rupture of membranes
- amniocentesis and other invasive procedures

Labour and puerperium:
- induction of labour
- preterm birth
- CS
- operative vaginal delivery
- prolonged rupture of membranes or chorioamnionitis
- retained products of conception
- prolonged labour with multiple (more than five) vaginal examinations
- urinary tract infection or catheterisation
- mastitis
- GAS infection among family members

OTHERS
- Winter months
- Failure to recognise severity

(Bick *et al.* 2011, Kramer *et al.* 2009, Anthony 2011, Lucas *et al.* 2012, CMACE 2011,
Acosta *et al.* 2012, Acosta & Knight 2013)

can take place anywhere the immune system defences are breached, including catheterisation and intravenous cannulation. Septic abortion may occur following either a spontaneous miscarriage or induced termination of pregnancy (Hayes 2007).

MIDWIFERY ASSESSMENT

Be aware of sepsis
Beware of sepsis

FIGURE 4.3 'Be aware of sepsis – beware of sepsis'

The phrase 'Be aware of sepsis – beware of sepsis' (*see* Figure 4.3) (CMACE 2011) reminds us of the potential for rapid deterioration for the woman with sepsis and that all staff, including community-based staff, require education on the early recognition of sepsis. The early warning signs of sepsis should trigger a rapid response with immediate transfer to hospital and/or appropriate referral to a senior obstetrician and anaesthetist (Hayes 2007, CMACE 2011, Raynor 2012).

Identifying a woman who is unwell involves:
- assessment of physical signs
- assessment of her current condition and history
- intuition that the woman is 'not quite right'.

Intuition arises from experience, where patterns are observed from previous experiences, and should be followed up with more objective assessment.

Midwifery assessment will include the four classic vital observations: (1) temperature, (2) pulse, (3) respiratory rate and (4) blood pressure. Midwives should observe the woman generally, enquire how she is feeling and carry out these observations. Assessment of oxygen saturation, pain, neurological function, skin perfusion and

urine output are further important aspects of assessment (Ferns 2007). The identification and treatment of the source of infection is paramount (RCOG 2012b). A
general history and examination should be carried out to try to identify the source
of the infection (RCOG 2012b). Abdominal pain, offensive lochia and diarrhoea are
particular features to be identified (Bick *et al.* 2011). A quick assessment of Airway,
Breathing and Circulation (ABC) is fundamental to midwifery assessment, but in
most cases there will be no obvious compromise in these areas and the midwife will
need to elicit more subtle features of deteriorating condition. Box 4.6 provides more
detail on how the midwife conducts the initial assessment.

**BOX 4.6 DETAILS OF THE INITIAL MIDWIFERY ASSESSMENT THAT
AIMS TO UNCOVER SUBTLE FEATURES OF DETERIORATING HEALTH**

The midwife will ask the woman how she feels. The evaluation of the woman's response to
this question covers a number of aspects of initial assessment, both in the content of her
response and the physical aspects of the way she communicates. Her airway is assessed.
Does she have to pause to breathe or find it difficult to talk? This will indicate increased
respiratory effort and give an indication of her level of pain. Does her response indicate any
level of confusion or neurological impairment? What are the features of her condition and
sense of well-being that are important to her?

The midwife should carry out observations of her vital signs. In many hospital situations,
the taking of observations is delegated to maternity care assistants. Where the midwife is
concerned about the woman, it is helpful that the midwife does this assessment. Subtle
changes such as bounding or thready pulse will be felt. When the pulse is taken, what does
her skin feel like – cold, hot, clammy, sweaty? Does she look pale or flushed? Is there any
rash evident? Can the midwife detect any unusual odours – offensive lochia, the smell of
diarrhoea?

MEOWS (modified early obstetric warning system) charts provide a standard to
record maternal observations with the aim of identifying serious illness early and
activating appropriate referral and management. They provide a template to record
basic observations of heart and respiratory rate, temperature, blood pressure, level
of consciousness and other observations. However, these charts should not replace,
but rather supplement, effective clinical assessment of the mother by the midwife.
To enable prompt care, midwifery assessment will aim to detect early signs that the
woman is developing illness and make prompt referral (Bick *et al.* 2011).

Box 4.7 lists signs and symptoms midwives should readily identify, if present,
during their assessment of a woman. They include general signs and symptoms and
those that relate to determining the focus of the infection. Box 4.8 highlights 'red flag'

BOX 4.7 SIGNS AND SYMPTOMS OF SEPSIS THAT MIDWIVES SHOULD IDENTIFY DURING ASSESSMENT

SIGNS

- Pyrexia (although may not be present)
- Hypothermia
- Tachycardia
- Tachypnoea
- Hypoxia
- Hypotension
- Oliguria
- Impaired neurological state

SYMPTOMS

- Fever or rigors
- Diarrhoea
- Vomiting
- Abdominal or pelvic pain
- Generalised rash

SYMPTOMS RELATED TO FOCUS OF INFECTION

- CS or perineal wound infection
- Symptoms of urinary tract infection
- Delay in involution, heavy lochia, offensive vaginal discharge
- Productive cough
- Mastitis

(RCOG 2012b)

features that warrant urgent referral. If the woman is at home and appears seriously unwell, then this would be by emergency ambulance.

Following on from basic observations, a range of secondary assessments includes the testing of the urine for infection and evidence of ketosis as well as measuring urine output and fluid balance. Urine output is a useful non-invasive indication of circulatory volume. A urine output of less than 30 mL per hour may indicate reduced circulatory volume. Constant abdominal pain and tenderness that are not relieved by usual analgesia should prompt the midwife to seek urgent medical review (RCOG 2012b).

BOX 4.8 'RED FLAG' FEATURES THAT WOULD PROMPT URGENT REFERRAL FOR MEDICAL ASSESSMENT

- Pyrexia of more than 38°C
- Sustained tachycardia more that 90 beats per minute
- Breathlessness (respiratory rate more than 20 breaths per minute)
- Abdominal or chest pain
- Diarrhoea and/or vomiting, dehydration
- Uterine or renal angle pain and tenderness
- Woman is generally unwell or seems unduly anxious or distressed

(RCOG 2012b)

Depending on the stage of pregnancy or puerperium, the usual fetal assessment, antenatal examination or postnatal checks should be done.

PREVENTION OF SEPSIS

Hand hygiene, aseptic techniques, prevention and prompt treatment of underlying causes, and prophylactic antibiotics are just a few of the ways to prevent sepsis developing. In 1846 a physician named Ignaz Semmelweis, practising in Vienna, identified that infective agents could be passed by staff. He ordered that medical attendants wash their hands in chlorinated water before attending births. This action led to a dramatic decrease in deaths from sepsis, and handwashing and aseptic techniques remain an important strategy in infection control (Hayes 2007) (*see* Chapter 14).

Acosta *et al.* (2012), drawing on findings from their case-control study, advocate measures to prevent sepsis including enhanced assessment of women who are obese or at high risk using MEOWS charts, improved aseptic technique during operative vaginal deliveries and limiting induction of labour to clearly indicated cases. These recommendations were in addition to usual practices of strict aseptic technique, infection control measures and antibiotic prophylaxis for CS. The National Institute for Health and Care Excellence guideline for CS (NICE 2011) recommends antibiotics for all women undergoing a CS. This guidance is based on findings from a systematic review that reported that prophylactic antibiotics in women undergoing CS substantially reduced the incidence of wound infection, endometritis and serious maternal infectious complications (Smaill & Gyte 2010).

Transmission of GAS is usually through direct contact with saliva or nasal secretions. Contamination of the perineum can occur when the organism is transferred from the upper respiratory tract via the woman's hands. Postpartum women are advised to wash their hands both before and after going to the toilet and when changing sanitary towels (CMACE 2011).

MANAGEMENT

The 'Surviving Sepsis Campaign' is an international effort to improve recognition and management of sepsis (Dellinger *et al.* 2013). Clinicians should refer to the full guidance. In addition, the Royal College of Obstetricians and Gynaecologists has developed guidelines on management of sepsis specifically for pregnancy and the puerperium. These documents and details of how to access them are listed in the 'useful resources' section at the end of the chapter. Box 4.9 outlines the key elements of the recommended management of sepsis and Box 4.10 lists the key investigations that may be undertaken.

BOX 4.9 KEY ELEMENTS OF MANAGEMENT OF SEPSIS FROM THE 'SURVIVING SEPSIS CAMPAIGN' AND GUIDELINES ON MANAGEMENT OF SEPSIS ISSUED BY THE ROYAL COLLEGE OF OBSTETRICIANS AND GYNAECOLOGISTS

- Early recognition and prompt management
- Obtain two blood cultures and other appropriate swabs and specimens prior to commencement of antibiotics
- Measure serum lactate
- Prompt treatment with adequate dose of appropriate intravenous antibiotics – the aim is that antibiotics should start within 1 hour of suspecting sepsis and after samples have been obtained for culture
- Restoration of haemodynamic status to restore adequate oxygen delivery to tissues; this may include fluid replacement and use of medication to maintain blood pressure – careful management of fluid balance is required to prevent fluid overload
- Oxygen saturation monitoring, facial mask oxygenation or ventilation
- Clear and detailed documentation of signs and treatment; use MEOWS charts and a pain scoring system and/or a specific chart designed for use in high dependency care
- Multidisciplinary management with senior clinical leadership to direct care; the team in addition to senior maternity unit staff will include an intensive care specialist, general surgeon and microbiologist
- Use of critical care outreach team
- Admission to intensive care unit as indicated by condition
- Delivery of the baby, or surgery to remove the focus of infection; hysterectomy may be required as a life-saving measure

(Dellinger *et al.* 2013, RCOG 2012a, b)

BOX 4.10 INVESTIGATIONS FOR SEPSIS

- Blood culture
- Serum lactate
- Full blood count, urea and electrolytes, and C-reactive protein
- Samples and swabs taken as indicated by clinical suspicion of the focus of infection (*see* Box 4.11)
- Imaging: chest X-ray, pelvic ultrasound scan, computed tomography

(RCOG 2012b)

A delay in commencing antibiotics has been consistently cited as an area of substandard care that has contributed to increased mortality in sepsis. Reasons for the delay of antibiotics include prescription errors, waiting for senior review, and delay when transferring between hospital departments (Appelboam *et al.* 2010). In addition to blood cultures, other swabs and specimens should be taken as indicated (*see* Box 4.11) (RCOG 2012a). The collection of swabs should not delay the commencement of antibiotics. Box 4.12 provides further detail on medical treatment with antibiotics and

---

BOX 4.11 SWABS AND SPECIMENS THAT MAY BE USEFUL IN INVESTIGATING THE SOURCE OF INFECTION

SWABS
- Throat
- High vaginal swab
- CS or perineal wound site
- From the neonate

SPECIMENS
- Midstream urine, catheter specimen urine
- Placenta
- Sputum
- Cerebrospinal fluid
- Expressed breast milk
- Stool sample

(RCOG 2012b)

intravenous immunoglobulin. Close attention to fluid balance in critically ill pregnant and postpartum women is essential, as the physiological changes of pregnancy make them susceptible to pulmonary oedema.

BOX 4.12 ANTIBIOTICS AND IMMUNOGLOBULIN

ANTIBIOTICS

The Royal College of Obstetricians and Gynaecologists (RCOG 2012a, b) provides information for the prescribing doctor on the range of effectiveness for various antibiotics. This knowledge and local policy will dictate initial treatment that will aim to cover a broad spectrum and which can be adjusted once the causative organism is identified. Blood cultures need to be taken before (but should not delay) the commencement of antibiotics. Liaison with a microbiologist will be helpful.

INTRAVENOUS IMMUNOGLOBULIN

Advice from the Royal College of Obstetricians and Gynaecologists (RCOG 2012a) advocates that intravenous immunoglobulin can be used in cases of severe invasive streptococcal or staphylococcal infections where other therapies have failed. It has the potential to neutralise the superantigen effect of exotoxins, thereby moderating tissue damage. It is made available through the blood transfusion department, who will provide protocols and advice on its use. The use of intravenous immunoglobulin is still in the experimental stages, and consultation with infectious disease consultants and microbiologists is advised when considering using this (Palaniappan *et al.* 2012).

Monitoring the fetus and considerations regarding the timing of delivery

CTG monitoring of the fetus is advised when the woman is unwell although this will depend on the gestation. Changes to the CTG, including decelerations and loss of baseline variability, may prove sensitive indicators of deteriorating maternal condition and therefore should prompt reassessment of both mother and baby (RCOG 2012a).

When a pregnant woman is critically ill, a senior obstetrician will need to consider the appropriate time to deliver the baby. Delivery may be beneficial to the woman or to the baby or to both. The decision will be made in consultation with other members of the multidisciplinary team involved, and with the woman, although this may be difficult where she is critically unwell. Attempting delivery when the mother is haemodynamically unstable is unsafe for both mother and baby, but delivery of the baby will aid recovery of the mother where the fetus, placenta and membranes are the source of infection and will be an essential part of management in the context of a mother's deteriorating condition (RCOG 2012a).

When preterm delivery is anticipated, the neonatal team should be alerted and detailed information including microbiology findings passed on. Caution is advised when considering use of corticosteroids to aid fetal lung maturity in the context of maternal sepsis (RCOG 2012a).

It is more likely that delivery by CS will be under general anaesthetic, as it is recommended that epidural or spinal anaesthesia be avoided in women with sepsis (RCOG 2012a). There is a concern for the increased risk of epidural abscess or meningitis.

These conditions might arise from the direct introduction of microorganisms on the needle or via local infection at the puncture site. The control of a drop in blood pressure of an already septic hypotensive woman and the presence of coagulation problems will further complicate use of spinal or epidural anaesthesia (Lucas *et al.* 2012). Careful individual assessment by an experienced, senior anaesthetist will determine the choice of anaesthetic weighing up the risks and benefits (Lucas *et al.* 2012). Midwives caring for women whose babies have been delivered under general anaesthetic when they are unwell have observed the need for particular psychological support. The use of diaries to document events has been suggested, enabling the woman to 'fill in the gaps' when she has recovered (Aitkin *et al.* 2013).

Psychological support

Postnatal care will involve continued assessment of the woman and management directed by the multidisciplinary team until physical recovery is evident. The midwife will, however, need to be mindful of the tremendous strain this level of ill health will place on the woman and her family in both social and psychological terms. The array of specialist input, invasive interventions and possible admission to the intensive care unit will be an experience they will find difficult to comprehend. It will be far removed from the expectations of normal childbirth and the welcoming of the new baby into the family that was anticipated.

Sepsis may occur in pregnancy or it may strike in the early days after birth. Either way, the impact on emotional health and adaptation to parenthood will be great. Partners may be at greater risk as they watch events unfold and may fear for their partner's life making them vulnerable to the development of post-traumatic stress disorder (Hallewell 2011). There are likely to be both short- and long-term anxieties regarding the health of the baby, particularly when the sepsis occurs in pregnancy. Concerns regarding preterm delivery, admission to neonatal intensive care and separation of mother and baby will compound both the physical and emotional recovery of the mother.

Midwives will need to tailor care that is supportive, empathic, respectful and kind. They should communicate effectively and listen to concerns, aiming to keep the woman and her family fully informed. Midwives are well placed to promote the 'normal' aspects of parenthood within the context of ill health. Skin-to-skin contact between mother and baby will be beneficial, if possible, but the father may benefit from this as an alternative. An interruption to the establishment of breastfeeding may occur, which will require additional support by the midwife. Follow-up, after discharge from hospital, will be important for both the physical and the psychological aspects of recovery following sepsis.

INFECTION CONTROL MEASURES AND THE IDENTIFICATION OF CLOSE CONTACTS IN CASES OF GAS INFECTION

Where invasive GAS is identified as the infecting organism, additional infection control measures and identification of close contacts is advised. The woman should be isolated and strict infection control procedures followed to minimise contact with other mothers and babies (RCOG 2012a, b). The midwife needs to request the specialist advice and support of the local infection prevention and control team. Transmission is through direct contact with saliva and nasal secretions or from the infected lesions of those with GAS sepsis (Palaniappan *et al.* 2012).

The neonatologist should be informed and close monitoring of the fetal or newborn condition and prophylactic antibiotics are advised (RCOG 2012a, b).

BOX 4.13 SUMMARY OF RECOMMENDATIONS FROM GAS GUIDELINE DEVELOPMENT WORKING GROUP ON THE CONTROL AND PREVENTION OF SPREAD OF GAS INFECTION IN ACUTE HEALTHCARE SETTINGS

- Cases of GAS should be referred to the infection prevention and control team, and the local health protection specialist informed.
- The woman should be isolated and healthcare workers should wear disposable protective equipment, including gloves and aprons, when in contact with the woman and in the vicinity of where she is located.
- Strict hand hygiene is essential.
- Visitors will need instruction and supervision so they follow the required procedures, including vigilant handwashing.
- Prophylaxis should be considered for healthcare workers who sustain needlestick injury with potentially infectious material.
- Healthcare workers in contact with a case of GAS should be alert to symptoms including a sore throat, skin infection or lesion or vaginitis. If these symptoms appear around this time, they should present to occupational health for screening with a view to antibiotic treatment.

(Steer *et al.* 2012)

Midwives need to take measures to protect themselves, ensure they don't pass the organism to others and provide information and instruction to other staff, such as maternity care assistants and domestic staff and to the woman's friends and family. Healthcare workers have been identified as a source of hospital-acquired GAS infection. The particular strain of GAS can be identified and if more than one case of GAS puerperal sepsis occurs in the same unit within 6 months, and has the same strain, there is a possibility that a birth attendant has been the source of infection (Palaniappan *et al.* 2012).

Specific guidelines for the control and prevention of the spread of GAS infection in healthcare settings, including maternity units, are available (Steer *et al.* 2012). The key recommendations are summarised in Box 4.13 and access details to the full guidance are provided in the useful resources section at the end of this chapter. The infection prevention and control team will need to provide specialist advice for the woman's close community contacts such as her family.

ROLE OF THE MIDWIFE

- Regular assessment of all women that includes basic observations when indicated
- Early recognition of the features of infection and/or sepsis and any indication of deteriorating illness
- Ensure prompt and effective referral of women with signs of sepsis and/or deteriorating illness
- Work alongside the multidisciplinary team to instigate the elements of the 'Surviving Sepsis Campaign' in a timely manner
- Keep accurate documentation of the ongoing assessment of the woman
- Attend to elements of infection control
- Provide psychological support for the woman and her family

USEFUL RESOURCES

- Hallewell E (2011) Psychological considerations for 'emergencies around childbirth'. In Boyle M (editor) *Emergencies Around Childbirth* (2nd ed). London: Radcliffe Publishing.
- Dellinger RP, Levy MM, Rhodes A, Annane D, Gerlach H, *et al.* (2013) Surviving Sepsis Campaign: international guidelines for management of severe sepsis and septic shock: 2012 *Crit Care Med.* **41**(2): 580–637.
- Royal College of Obstetricians and Gynaecologists (RCOG) (2012a) *Bacterial Sepsis in Pregnancy. Green-top Guideline 64a*. London: RCOG.
- Royal College of Obstetricians and Gynaecologists (RCOG) (2012b) *Bacterial Sepsis following Pregnancy. Green-top Guideline 64b*. London: RCOG.

- Steer JA, Lamagni T, Healy B, *et al.* (2012) Guidelines for prevention and control of group A streptococcal infection in acute healthcare and maternity settings in the UK. *J Infection.* **64**(1): 1–18.
- Surviving Sepsis Campaign guidelines provide up-to-date guidance on management and educational resources for diagnosis, management and treatment of sepsis. Available at: www.survivingsepsis.org/Guidelines/Pages/default.aspx

REFERENCES

Acosta CD, Bhattacharya S, Tuffnell D, *et al.* (2012) Maternal sepsis: a Scottish population-based case-control study. *Br J Obstet Gynaecol.* **119**(4): 474–83.

Acosta CD, Knight M (2013) Sepsis and maternal mortality. *Curr Opin Obstet Gynecol.* **25**(2): 109–16.

Aitken LM, Rattray J, Hull A, *et al.* (2013) The use of diaries in psychological recovery from intensive care. *Crit Care.* **17**: 253.

Anthony J (2011) Critical care of the obstetric patient. In: James D, Steer PJ, Weiner CP, *et al.* (editors). *High Risk Pregnancy: management options.* 4th ed.New York: Elsevier.

Appelboam R, Tilley R, Blackburn J (2010) Time to antibiotics in sepsis. *Crit Care.* **14**(Suppl. 1): 50.

Bick D, Beake S, Pellowe C (2011) Vigilance must be a priority: maternal genital tract sepsis. *Pract Midwife.* **14**(4): 16–18.

Centre for Maternal and Child Enquiries (CMACE) (2011) Saving mothers' lives: reviewing maternal deaths to make motherhood safer: 2006–2008. The Eighth Report of the Confidential Enquiries into Maternal Deaths in the United Kingdom. *Br J Obstet Gynaecol.* **118**(Suppl. 1): 1–203.

Dellinger RP, Levy MM, Rhodes A, *et al.* (2013) Surviving Sepsis Campaign: international guidelines for management of severe sepsis and septic shock: 2012. *Crit Care Med.* **41**(2): 580–637.

Ferns T (2007) Shock and the critically ill woman. In: Billington M, Stevenson M (editors). *Critical Care in Childbearing for Midwives.* Blackwell: Oxford. pp. 140–66.

Gourlay M, Gutierrez C, Chong A, *et al.* (2001) Group A streptococcal sepsis and ovarian vein thrombosis after an uncomplicated vaginal delivery. *J Am Board Fam Pract.* **14**(5): 375–80.

Hallewell E (2011) Psychological considerations for 'emergencies around childbirth'. In: Boyle M (editor). *Emergencies Around Childbirth* (2nd ed). London: Radcliffe Publishing. pp. 193–214.

Hayes M (2007) Sepsis. In: Dob D, Cooper G, Holdcroft A (editors). *Crisis in Childbirth: why mothers survive; lessons from the confidential enquiries into maternal deaths.* Oxford: Radcliffe Publishing. pp. 168–86.

Kramer HMC, Schutte JM, Zwart JJ, *et al.* (2009) Maternal mortality and severe morbidity from sepsis in the Netherlands. *Acta Obstet Gynecol Scand.* **88**(6): 647–53.

Lucas DN, Robinson PN, Nel MR (2012) Sepsis in obstetrics and the role of the anaesthetist. *Int J Obstet Anesth.* **21**(1): 56–67.

National Institute for Health and Care Excellence (NICE) (2011) *Caesarean Section.* Clinical Guideline 132. London: NICE. Available at: www.nice.org.uk/guidance/CG132 (accessed 2 October 2014).

Palaniappan N, Menezes M, Wilson P (2012) Group A streptococcal puerperal sepsis: management and prevention. *Obstetrician Gynaecologist.* **14**(1): 9–16.

Parsed BGR, Sunnah GV (2007) Sepsis. In: Grady K, Howell C, Cox C (editors). *Managing Obstetric Emergencies and Trauma*. 2nd ed, London: RCOG Press. pp. 205–12.

Raynor M (2012) *Sepsis*. In: Raynor M, Marshall J, Jackson K (editors). *Midwifery Practice: critical illness, complications and emergencies case book*. Maidenhead: McGraw Hill. pp. 175–92.

Royal College of Obstetricians and Gynaecologists (RCOG) (2012a) *Bacterial Sepsis in Pregnancy. Green-top Guideline 64a*. London: RCOG.

Royal College of Obstetricians and Gynaecologists (RCOG) (2012b) *Bacterial Sepsis following Pregnancy. Green-top Guideline 64b*. London: RCOG.

Smaill FM, Gyte GM (2010) Antibiotic prophylaxis versus no prophylaxis for preventing infection after cesarean section. *Cochrane Database Syst Rev*. (1): CD007482.

Steer JA, Lamagni T, Healy B, *et al.* (2012) Guidelines for prevention and control of group A streptococcal infection in acute healthcare and maternity settings in the UK. *J Infection*. **64**(1): 1–18.

Tripathi L, Tingi E, Parry N, *et al.* (2011) *Development of a Mnemonic for the Training of Sepsis in Pregnancy* [poster presentation]. Ninth International Scientific Meeting of Royal College of Obstetricians and Gynaecologists – Joint Meeting with the Hellenic Obstetric and Gynaecological Society, 28–30 September 2011, Megaron Athens International Conference Centre, Athens, Greece. Available at: www.epostersonline.com/rcog2011/?q=node/2770 (accessed 1 April 2014).

Villers MS, Jamison MG, De Castro LM, *et al.* (2008) Morbidity associated with sickle cell disease in pregnancy. *Am J Obstet Gynecol*. **199**(2): 125.e1–5.

CHAPTER 5

Genital and sexually transmitted infections

→ Overview
→ Gonorrhoea
→ Chlamydia
→ Herpes simplex virus
→ Syphilis
→ *Trichomonas vaginalis*
→ Genital warts and human papilloma virus
→ Bacterial vaginosis
→ Vulvovaginal candidiasis (thrush)

OVERVIEW

Sexually transmitted infections (STIs) are increasingly common in the UK and cause a considerable burden of disease worldwide. Some can have serious consequences for mothers and babies although many are asymptomatic. Preterm birth is the most prevalent and most costly complication of genital tract infection in pregnancy both in economic and human terms (Stamm *et al.* 2008) (*see* Box 5.1).

Genital tract mucosa are part of the larger mucosal immune system that provides the first line of defence against invading genital infections. The vagina and endocervix are lined with commensal flora, including lactobacilli, which, along with cervical mucus, act as an effective barrier that protects the upper reproductive tract. However, hormonal fluctuations strongly influence the immune response and there is thought to be an increased susceptibility to ascending infection in pregnancy. Some genital tract infections such as bacterial vaginosis (BV) and candidiasis are caused by changes to the normal flora and are not sexually transmitted, although they may be associated with sexual activity and have irritating symptoms.

Pregnancy is a time when normal precautions regarding contraception are relaxed and condom use would seem irrelevant to most couples. Women may not know their partner's sexual profile, making them unaware of potential risk. This makes pregnancy a potentially vulnerable time for women to be exposed to STIs, including the human immunodeficiency virus (HIV). Therefore midwives have a role in screening for STIs, recognising symptoms, and providing appropriate referral for effective treatment. However, reticence to discuss sexual practice and genital-related symptoms may mean symptoms and risk remain undisclosed. Midwives should take opportunities to provide sexual health education for women and their partners and encourage open dialogue. This will be particularly important for midwives working with vulnerable groups of women including teenagers. Genitourinary medicine (GUM) clinics provide key specialist resources for the treatment of STIs and effective liaison between GUM specialists, HIV specialists and obstetric and midwifery caregivers is recommended.

Women with a genital or STI may suffer low self-esteem and the management of their condition in pregnancy may involve a complex array of psychological, relationship and confidentiality issues (Peate 2005). Continuity of care by a known midwife may be an effective strategy to provide support. This chapter aims to give midwives a background in the tenets of sexual health promotion and knowledge of genital and STIs and their impact on pregnancy. The British Association for Sexual Health and HIV (BASHH) provides full guidance on the management of STIs, and midwives requiring detailed up-to-date information should refer to the latest online guidelines published by this group (*see* the list of useful resources at the end of this chapter).

BOX 5.1 RISK TO MOTHER AND FETUS OR NEWBORN FROM GENITAL TRACT INFECTION

Mother	Fetus or newborn
Infertility	Stillbirth
Miscarriage	Low birthweight, prematurity
Preterm delivery	Congenital abnormalities
Preterm rupture of membranes	Conjunctivitis
Post-partum infection	Pneumonia
Puerperal sepsis	Breathing difficulties
Enhanced transmission of HIV	
Reduced self-esteem	

(Khare & Khare 2007, Goldenberg *et al.* 2010, Stamm *et al.* 2008)

RANGE OF SEXUALLY TRANSMITTED INFECTIONS

Box 5.2 classifies common genital and STIs according to source organism. Table 5.1 gives an overview of the common STIs discussed in this chapter, identifying the impact of these conditions in pregnancy.

One STI can co-exist with others – for example, gonorrhoea and chlamydia – and therefore diagnosis of one will prompt screening for others including HIV. There is an up to tenfold increase in the risk of acquiring HIV if an STI is present (Hay & Kieran 2009) (*see* Chapter 7).

BOX 5.2 CLASSIFICATION OF GENITAL INFECTION BY SOURCE ORGANISM

VIRAL INFECTIONS
- HIV
- Herpes simplex virus (HSV) type 1 and type 2
- Human papilloma virus (HPV)

BACTERIAL INFECTIONS
- Syphilis
- Gonorrhoea
- Chlamydia
- *Trichomonas vaginalis*
- BV

YEAST INFECTIONS
- Candida

TABLE 5.1 Summary of the common sexually transmitted infections (STIs) discussed in this chapter and their impact on pregnancy

Infection	Impact on pregnancy: mother and fetus or newborn	Comments
Gonorrhoea	*Mother*: infertility, ectopic pregnancy, preterm labour, chorioamnionitis, sepsis *Newborn*: ophthalmia neonatorum, which can lead to permanent loss of vision and septic arthritis (rare)	Effective treatment under threat because of increasing antibiotic resistance
Chlamydia	*Mother*: may be asymptomatic and if left untreated may lead to preterm birth, endometritis, pelvic inflammatory disease and infertility *Newborn*: ophthalmia neonatorum, otitis media and *Chlamydia pneumoniae*	Most common STI in the UK; women under 24 years of age and others practising 'unsafe' sex should be referred to the NCSP programme for screening

(*continued*)

Infection	Impact on pregnancy: mother and fetus or newborn	Comments
HSV-1 and HSV-2	*Mother:* miscarriage, preterm labour, spread of HSV into bloodstream (rare) *Newborn:* damage to brain, skin and eyes; high morbidity and mortality	First-time infection of mother during later stages of pregnancy confers greatest risk of transfer to neonate
Syphilis	*Mother:* may not be aware of primary infection but may develop serious morbidity long term *Fetus and newborn:* congenital syphilis – intrauterine death, skeletal deformity and damage to brain, liver, kidney, eyes and hearing	Syphilis is easily treated and thus the serious morbidity and mortality of this distressing illness can be avoided
T. vaginalis	*Mother:* premature rupture of membranes *Fetus and newborn:* problems of low birthweight and prematurity	Co-existing infections including HIV should be considered
Genital warts and HPV	*Mother:* lesions may appear for the first time and/or grow more rapidly in pregnancy *Newborn:* complications are rare but may develop warts on the larynx or genital area	Lesions likely to regress after delivery so a non interventionist approach is usually adopted
Bacterial vaginosis	*Mother:* preterm labour, preterm rupture of membranes, endometritis, post-caesarean section infection *Newborn:* complications of prematurity	May be prevented by avoidance of vaginal douching which interrupts the protective normal vaginal flora
Candidiasis	*Mother:* distressing symptoms but not associated with any particular problems *Newborn:* infection of umbilicus, mouth and nappy area may occur; cause of serious sepsis in low birthweight babies due to immunosuppression	More common in pregnancy due to alterations in vaginal mucosa

NCSP = National Chlamydia Screening Programme

RATES OF SEXUALLY TRANSMITTED INFECTION AND THOSE AT RISK

The incidence of STI in the UK has followed peaks and troughs. Following the Second World War rates increased as service men returned home. A further peak occurred with the introduction of the oral contraceptive pill in the 1960s, which heralded a new era of sexual freedom. Rates of STIs dropped significantly in the late 1980s when HIV awareness and fear was at its peak. However, since then there has been a steady and steep increase alongside a return to high-risk sexual behaviour (Hay & Kieran 2009). Figure 5.1 shows the rates of diagnosis of STI among women in England, 2003–12.

There are no reliable figures for rates of STI among pregnant women in the UK. Box 5.3 sets out those groups considered to be most at risk for STI in the general population. Chlamydia is the most common STI and, as with all STIs, is more common in the under-25-year-old age group. There has been a steady increase in the diagnosis of first-episode genital herpes in women since 2005. In addition, there was a 21% increase in new diagnoses of gonorrhoea in 2012. Antibiotic resistance to gonorrhoea

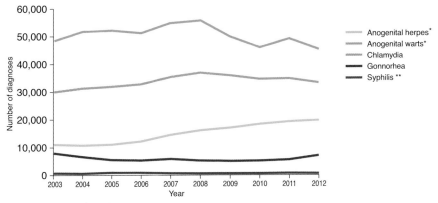

- Data from routine GUM clinic returns
- *First episode: ** Includes diagnosis of primary, secondary and early latent syphilis
- Chlamydia data from 2012 are not comparable to data from previous years
- Data type: service data

FIGURE 5.1 Rates of diagnosis of sexually transmitted infection among women in England, 2003–12 (reproduced with permission of Public Health England) (PHE 2012))

makes this an area of particular concern. A fall in cases of genital warts among young women may be attributed to vaccination for HPV (PHE 2014a). Worldwide the highest rates of STI, with the greatest economic burden, occur in South Asia and South East Asia, sub-Saharan Africa, Latin America, the Caribbean and in areas of political conflict (Fenton & Rogstad 2011). Higher rates of STI are seen in deprived urban areas of London and among black ethnic communities, demonstrating the inequality of sexual health in the population (PHE 2014a).

BOX 5.3 THOSE CONSIDERED MOST AT RISK OF GETTING A SEXUALLY TRANSMITTED INFECTION

- Age range: 15–24 years
- Those attending clinics aimed at sexual health advice including GUM clinics, family planning and termination of pregnancy (TOP) clinics
- Multiple partners, especially over a short period of time
- Little or no use of barrier contraception
- History of previous STI
- Paying or receiving money for sex
- Intravenous drug abuse
- Those living in deprived urban areas
- Travel (or partner's travel) to a country with high incidence of STI

(Hay & Kieran 2009, Adams *et al.* 2004, Fenton *et al.* 2001, PHE 2014a)

SEXUAL HEALTH PROMOTION

The control and prevention of STIs requires a number of strategies ranging from supporting behavioural change of individuals to broader government policy and legislation. *A Framework for Sexual Health Improvement in England* (DH 2013) sets out the agenda of public policy to improve the sexual health of the general population. Specific strategies of sexual health promotion aim to reduce the rate of STIs, the spread of HIV and a reduction in unintended pregnancies, alongside support for rights of sexual equality, freedom and respectful sexual relationships (WHO 2010). Sexual health promotion includes raising awareness of sexual health issues, providing information and education and access to services such as HIV and STI testing and treatment. The promotion of the correct use of condoms and contraception, as well as access to emergency contraception, is included (Peate 2005). The emphasis is on empowering individuals and communities with the knowledge, skills and opportunities to make positive health choices (DH 2003, 2013).

Key policies such as the implementation of the UK National Chlamydia Screening Programme (NCSP) in 2003 (HPA 2012), the Infectious Diseases in Pregnancy Screening Programme (UK NSC 2010), and the worldwide WHO strategy against congenital syphilis (WHO 2007) set a framework for service provision in maternity settings. Box 5.4 lists various strategies to prevent and control the spread of STIs.

BOX 5.4 GENERAL STRATEGIES TO PREVENT AND CONTROL THE SPREAD OF SEXUALLY TRANSMITTED INFECTIONS

- Health education that informs people of the benefits of discriminate and safer sex
- Health education that aims to improve low self-esteem, address power and sex inequalities, and identify the influence of drugs and alcohol on sexual choice and behaviour
- Health education on recognition of symptoms of STI and long-term consequences
- Easy access to services that provide rapid diagnosis, quick effective treatment and sensitively handled contact tracing if required
- Social and structural interventions to improve the lives of women, making them less vulnerable to sexual exploitation
- Encourage use of condoms

(Cowan & Bell 2011, Peate 2005, Hay & Kieran 2009, DH 2013)

THE ROLE OF THE MIDWIFE IN PROMOTING SEXUAL HEALTH

Midwives should take opportunities to promote sexual health and screen for STIs during pregnancy. Routine antenatal screening in the UK includes serology for syphilis, hepatitis B, and HIV antibody testing with pre-test discussion. At antenatal booking the midwife will enquire about any history or present symptoms of STI, although the effectiveness of that questioning will be variable. Booking clinics are busy with many aspects of care to be discussed. This coupled with general reticence to discuss sexual matters may mean the priority of discussion regarding sexual health may be low. Pregnancy implies a period of stable relationship and responsibility and the midwife will not want to risk causing offence to women by insensitive questioning. A check-list approach that includes questions about genital infections is a useful approach but may not allow the women the time and safety to divulge intimate details. Disclosure by women that the pregnancy was unplanned may set a foundation for sexual health education regarding reliable contraception and safe sex.

The terminology related to sexual-related illness is problematic, with use of such expressions as 'sore down below'. Further detailed questioning will be needed to elicit what the woman means. There may be a mismatch between the terms the mid-wife may use and colloquial terms the woman understands. Implied meanings may be misinterpreted. This is made more difficult when using interpreters. Professional translators will, like all people, have more difficulty conveying intimate questions and answers and the translation of colloquial sexual terms may be problematic. In addi-tion, many ethnic communities are relatively close-knit and issues of confidentiality and freedom to discuss concerns may be compromised. Use of family members as interpreters would obviously be even more difficult and inappropriate. The woman may not be as forthcoming with information if the partner is present and yet joint consultations allow safe sex to be considered as a joint responsibility.

A woman experiencing symptoms consistent with an STI may be reluctant to seek out help. Equally, her symptoms may not be pronounced – slight vaginal discharge, post-coital bleeding. The midwife, prompting for information regarding these symp-toms, may enable the woman to discuss her concerns (Fletcher & Ball 2006). Concern over health of the baby may encourage women to seek help.

BOX 5.5 USEFUL QUESTIONS IN SCREENING FOR SEXUALLY TRANSMITTED INFECTIONS IN PREGNANCY

- Have you ever experienced a burning sensation when passing urine?
- Have you had any discharge from your vagina?
- Have you had any rash or lumps around your genital area?
- Have you ever had a STI?
- Do you think you are at risk of getting a STI?

(Adapted from Peate 2005)

Box 5.5 provides some example questions that may be used by midwives to ascertain an effective sexual health history. These questions will provide a platform for dialogue regarding STIs but will also uncover symptoms of urinary tract infection, thrush and the normal vaginal discharge associated with pregnancy.

Antenatal clinics have always been proposed as testing venues for the NCSP for those under the age of 25, but this doesn't seem to have translated into the regular role of the midwife and antenatal care, except perhaps for specialist midwives working with teenagers (Fletcher & Ball 2006). This may represent a missed opportunity to improve surveillance.

Midwives are not professional counsellors but should use effective communication and counselling skills to offer help and advice to women who have been affected by STIs. Appropriate referral, confidentiality and information are fundamental (BASHH 2013a). The midwife needs to be genuine, accepting and empathetic. Peate (2005) maintains the premise for promoting sexual health is the positive endorsement of sexual activity as life-enhancing and normal. This sets the scene for discussions that take a matter-of-fact approach. Privacy should be assured and discussion should be relaxed but professional, friendly and non-judgemental. Peate (2005) also argues that all nurses should be able to discuss sex in a routine way, similar to asking the patient if she has had her bowels open. This could similarly be extrapolated to midwives in discussion with pregnant and postnatal women. Women may be psychologically vulnerable when disclosing information about STIs and it is important that the midwife offers time, respect and attention (Peate 2005). Midwives may benefit from further training in relevant skills for health promotion (Hay & Oakeshott 2005, BASHH 2013a).

The management of a STI in pregnancy will include screening for other pathogens and will include the offer of a further HIV test. Other aspects of management are the inclusion of counselling regarding safe sex, possible long-term complications and contact tracing. This is a specialist area, generally outside the remit of the midwife. Referral to medical colleagues and particular referral to specialist GUM clinic is recommended (Hay & Oakeshott 2005, Kieran & Hay 2006). Close collaboration between midwives and GUM clinics will improve care for women (Hay & Oakeshott 2005).

Some midwives – for example, those working with vulnerable groups such as teenagers – will take on a more specialised role with regard to sexual health promotion. Binge drinking and use of recreational drugs in adolescent women has been linked to risky sexual behaviour, unintended pregnancies and a higher rate of chlamydia infection in this group (Hay & Oakeshott 2005, McMunn & Caan 2007). For many young women, antenatal care provides their first opportunity to address sexual health issues (Fletcher & Ball 2006). Targeted midwifery care supported by the Royal College of Midwives for this vulnerable group includes a proactive role in health promotion (DH 2008). Midwives working with teenagers aim to empower young women to make positive choices regarding future pregnancies. Midwives may also participate in health education initiatives in schools and community groups (Hay & Oakeshott 2005).

Poor sexual health correlates to inequality of health related to poor social circumstances including unemployment and poverty, and risk of domestic violence (Bauer *et al.* 2002, PHE 2014a). Models of midwifery care that promote continuity aim to support vulnerable women to improve a range of physical and psychological outcomes, which will include sexual health. Rates of STIs are also higher in women with intravenous drug addiction and specialist midwives work with this group. Many units now also have specialist midwives to work with women diagnosed with hepatitis and HIV.

PSYCHOLOGICAL IMPACT OF A SEXUALLY TRANSMITTED INFECTION

Those infected with a STI, particularly those that are difficult to treat such as genital herpes, may experience a range of psychological and psychosexual reactions to the diagnosis including loss of self-worth, difficulties in relationships and fear of transmitting infection to others (Stanberry 2006). They need time and support from others, including health professionals, to re-establish an appropriate balance of attitude to sexual relationships. Knowledge and education with regard to managing the condition will aid psychological recovery. Strategies with regard to telling partners are needed (Stanberry 2006, McMillan & Ogilvie 2002a). Specialist counselling through a GUM clinic is advised. Midwives will need to ensure a non-judgemental, empathetic and professional response to women that will help build the woman's confidence and avoid feelings of guilt with regard to any risk to neonatal transmission.

GONORRHOEA

EPIDEMIOLOGY

There has been an increase in the number of people diagnosed with gonorrhoea in recent years. The highest rates are in men aged 20–24 but a substantial number have been in women aged 16–19. It is the second most common bacterial STI in the UK (chlamydia is highest). These increasing rates are of particular concern, as the effective treatment for gonorrhoea is under threat because of increasing antibiotic resistance (PHE 2014a).

CAUSATIVE ORGANISM

Gonorrhoea is the condition caused by *Neisseria gonorrhoeae*, which is a Gram-negative diplococcus bacteria. The primary site of infection is the mucous membrane of the cervix (85%–95%) and the urethra (65%–75%). Other sites include the rectum, oropharynx and conjunctiva (McCathie 2006).

CLINICAL FEATURES IN WOMEN

- Many are asymptomatic (up to 50%)
- Increased or altered vaginal discharge
- Mucopurulent cervicitis
- Lower abdominal pain (25%)
- Dysuria usually without frequency (12%)
- 30%–40% of women with gonorrhoea will also be infected with chlamydia; trichomoniasis and candidiasis may also be present
- Disseminated gonococcal infection (rare) can cause fever, rash, arthralgia, arthritis.

(Bannister *et al.* 2006, McCathie 2006, Peate 2005, Young & McMillan 2002, Bignell *et al.* 2011)

TRANSMISSION

- Spread through direct contact of secretions from one mucous membrane to another. It is transmitted easily through vaginal, anal and oral sex. Women are more likely to catch it from infected men (60%–90%) rather than vice versa (Young & McMillan 2002).
- Vertical transmission occurs during vaginal delivery from the mother's cervical secretions to the eyes of the fetus.
- Infection can be spread from the genital area, via fingers, to the eyes.

Soap and water, and other cleansing or antiseptic agents, easily kill *N. gonorrhoeae* (Young & McMillan 2002).

INCUBATION

The incubation period is 1–14 days, but many cases are asymptomatic.

COMPLICATIONS RELATED TO PREGNANCY

Mother

- Preterm delivery
- Preterm rupture of membranes
- Chorioamnionitis
- Post-partum sepsis
- Infertility and increased risk of ectopic pregnancy.

(Wilson 2011, McCathie 2006, Stamm *et al.* 2008)

Fetus and newborn

Complications for the infant will include those associated with an increased incidence of preterm delivery. Intrapartum infection occurs in about 30%–50% of babies born to mothers who have not been treated and can cause a serious conjunctivitis ('sticky eye') – ophthalmia neonatorum. This condition is not exclusively caused by *N. gonorrhoeae* and is now more commonly caused by other organisms, including *Chlamydia trachomatis.* It usually presents within 48 hours of birth. The eyelid swells and pus collects in the conjunctival sac. Permanent loss of vision can occur if not treated (Wilson 2011, Young & McMillan 2002) (*see* Box 5.6).

DIAGNOSIS AND MANAGEMENT

Commercial kits for diagnosis that utilise nucleic acid amplification tests and test for both *C. trachomatis* and *N. gonorrhoeae* are recommended. Cultures should be taken in all cases of gonorrhoea prior to commencing antibiotics so that antibiotic sensitivity testing can be performed (BASHH 2012a). This is important because of the evolving antibiotic resistance to *N. gonorrhoeae* (Bignell *et al.* 2011). Samples for testing are taken from the cervix or vagina, and liaison with the GUM clinic with regard to sample collection is advised (Lazaro 2013).

If the woman or her partner has a history of gonorrhoea or other STI, the midwife should ensure appropriate referral is made, which would include involvement of GUM clinicians. The woman should be tested at booking and the test should be repeated in the third trimester. The paediatrician should be informed if gonococcal infection has occurred in late pregnancy (Khare & Khare 2007).

Treatment with antibiotics should be directed by a medical practitioner, ideally a GUM physician, and in accordance with current BASHH guidelines (Bignell *et al.* 2011) (*see* the list of useful resources at the end of this chapter). Recent surveillance data have shown that antimicrobial resistance is occurring, which threatens the effectiveness of treatment regimens. A test of cure is now recommended in all cases to assess problems of emerging resistance (Bignell *et al.* 2011) and treatment failures must be reported to Public Health England (HPA 2013).

Screening for other STIs and treatment of the woman's partner is essential to prevent reinfection, and both should refrain from sexual intercourse until they have completed treatment and follow-up. A full explanation of the condition is needed, with particular reference to long-term complications for the woman (pelvic inflammatory disease) and her male partner/s (epididymitis, difficult urination) if left untreated. Clear, accurate written information should supplement verbal discussion (Bignell *et al.* 2011).

CHLAMYDIA

EPIDEMIOLOGY

Chlamydia is the most common sexually transmitted infection in the UK (Manavi 2006), with the highest rates occurring in London. The prevalence is highest among young sexually active adults – specifically, women aged 16–24 years and men aged 25–34 years (Fenton *et al.* 2001, Adams *et al.* 2004, Manavi 2006, PHE 2014a). In addition to young age, risk factors for chlamydia infection include recent partner change, multiple partners and lack of consistent use of condoms (BASHH 2006, Fenton *et al.* 2001, McMillan & Ballard 2002).

The prevalence in pregnancy varies from 2% to 14% (Oakeshott *et al.* 2002a, Pimenta *et al.* 2003, McMillan & Ballard 2002, Adams *et al.* 2004).

CAUSATIVE ORGANISM

C. trachomatis is a small Gram-negative bacteria that needs living cells to replicate in a similar way that a virus does.

CLINICAL FEATURES AND COMPLICATIONS IN WOMEN

Clinical features in women

- Asymptomatic in approximately 70% of women and the cervix frequently appears normal
- Sites of infection include urethra, cervix, rectum, pharynx, conjunctiva
- Mucopurulent cervicitis, cervix bleeds easily during intercourse
- Bleeding between periods or heavier periods
- Lower abdominal pain
- Purulent vaginal discharge
- Dysuria

(Hay & Kieran 2009, Stamm *et al.* 2008, McMillan & Ballard 2002, BASHH 2006)

Complications

- 20%–40% of infected women are at risk of developing pelvic inflammatory disease (PID) (Khare & Khare 2007, Manavi 2006)
- Chronic pelvic pain
- Adult conjunctivitis
- Arthritis
- Inflammation of the liver capsule
- Chlamydia infection may help the transmission of HIV and those with HIV are more vulnerable to chlamydia
- Chlamydia co-exists with other infections such as BV and gonorrhoea (Oakeshott *et al.* 2002b).

TRANSMISSION

The key route of transmission is through vaginal intercourse but chlamydia can be transmitted via anal or oral–genital route or occasional accidental transfer to the eye. As *C. trachomatis* is frequently asymptomatic, and thus unrecognised, ongoing transmission is sustained in the community (BASHH 2006).

Vertical transmission occurs from mother to baby during vaginal delivery.

INCUBATION PERIOD

The incubation period is around 1–3 weeks after exposure, but many cases are asymptomatic, making early diagnosis and treatment difficult.

COMPLICATIONS RELATED TO PREGNANCY
Mother

- Infertility as a result of PID
- Ectopic pregnancy (Bakken *et al.* 2007)
- Miscarriage
- Amnionitis
- Post-partum endometritis
- Post-partum PID
- Premature rupture of membranes
- Preterm delivery (Andrews *et al.* 2000)

Fetus and newborn

About 75% of infants born vaginally and 20% born by caesarean section (with intact membranes) to mothers infected with chlamydia become infected (McMillan & Ballard 2002). These rates will be reduced where the mother was treated during pregnancy. The most frequent presenting symptom of neonatal chlamydia infections is infectious conjunctivitis (ophthalmia neonatorum) (Wilson 2011). The features of ophthalmia neonatorum are described in Box 5.6.

Up to 80% of infants infected with chlamydia will also have nasopharyngeal infection, which is often asymptomatic, and a third of those will develop pneumonitis (Lazaro 2013). Infection of the middle ear, the gut and vagina can also occur (Wilson 2011, McMillan & Ballard 2002). Infants with *C. pneumoniae* usually present between 3 and 12 weeks of age with rapid respirations, distinctive staccato cough and/or failure to thrive but are usually afebrile (Rours *et al.* 2009). Low birthweight is more common because of premature delivery.

BOX 5.6 OPHTHALMIA NEONATORUM

- Conjunctivitis that develops within 21 days of birth
- Mucopurulent discharge, inflammation and possibly oedema of the eyelids
- Chlamydia is the more common cause (usually presents 5–12 days post delivery) but it may be gonorrhoea (usually presents 2–5 days post delivery)
- As it is not possible to distinguish clinically, tests must be taken to exclude gonococcus infection, as untreated gonococcal infection can lead to corneal ulceration, perforation and blindness.
- Diagnosis is by culture of swab taken from the conjunctiva

(Wilson 2011, McMillan & Ballard 2002, Bannister *et al.* 2006)

SCREENING FOR CHLAMYDIA

The NCSP was set up in 2003 to improve the uptake of screening tests and treatment for this infection. Screening venues have been extended beyond GUM clinics to family planning clinics, general practice surgeries and high street pharmacies but not usually antenatal clinics. Opportunistic screening is recommended for those considered most at risk (*see* Box 5.7).

BOX 5.7 WOMEN AT RISK OF CHLAMYDIA INFECTION AND RECOMMENDED FOR OPPORTUNISTIC SCREENING

- Sexually active women under 25 years of age
- Older women with two or more partners or a partner change within the preceding year
- Following TOP
- Sexual partners of chlamydia-positive individuals
- Those previously diagnosed with chlamydia
- GUM clinic attendees.

(SIGN 2009)

In 2011, the UK National Screening Committee reviewed the evidence with regard to adopting a screening programme for chlamydia in pregnancy (UK NSC 2011). This review concluded that there was insufficient evidence that screening and treating women would significantly reduce adverse pregnancy outcome and that routine screening for chlamydia in pregnancy should not be offered. The National Institute for

Health and Care Excellence, in its guideline for antenatal care (NICE 2010), makes a similar recommendation with the suggestion that health professionals should provide women under 25 years of age with information about chlamydia testing, and how to access a test from venues offered under the NCSP.

Fletcher and Ball (2006) have published a recommended integrated pathway midwives could use to effectively screen and treat those affected by chlamydia. The pathway includes information, testing, treatment, follow-up of results and partner screening (*see* the list of useful resources at the end of this chapter). They argue that lack of midwife involvement in screening represents a 'missed opportunity' to prevent long-term complications for women that includes PID, ectopic pregnancy and future infertility. The argument for not having a national policy for routine screening of chlamydia, for all pregnant women, centres on a lack of proven benefit, organisational constraints and the prioritising of resources on those considered higher risk (SIGN 2009). However, there may be a premise for local policies among high-risk populations as advocated by Fletcher and Ball (2006). In the absence of a screening programme it becomes even more important for midwives to identify those at risk and those with symptoms and to ensure appropriate testing, referral and follow-up. Screening in pregnancy for gonorrhoea, chlamydia, and trichomonas should be considered in women at high risk for STIs (Wilson 2011).

DIAGNOSIS AND MANAGEMENT

Collecting specimens

Testing will be carried out for those who present with symptoms and for opportunistic screening in those considered at risk (*see* Box 5.7) but have no evident symptoms. DNA amplification technology has improved the sensitivity and specificity for tests for chlamydia (Sheffield *et al.* 2005). These new tests, known as nucleic acid amplification tests, allow less-invasive samples to be used, and tests for gonorrhoea and chlamydia can be performed on the same sample (McCathie 2006, BASHH 2010).

In women, chlamydia can be tested on specimens taken from the cervix, the vagina or from first-catch urine (FCU) (BASHH 2010). Cervical specimens need to be taken during a speculum examination. A swab, from the manufacturer's pack, is inserted gently into the opening of the cervix and rotated for a few seconds. Alternatively, the woman can obtain a vaginal specimen herself. The swab needs to be inserted about 2 inches into the vagina and gently rotated for 10–30 seconds (BASHH 2010). Vulval specimens are not recommended. Vaginal specimens have been shown to be as sensitive as samples taken from the cervix (Schachter *et al.* 2003) and are more acceptable than swabs taken during speculum examination (Hay & Oakeshott 2005).

A FCU sample involves the women collecting the first 15–50 mL of urine passed at any time of the day. She needs to have not passed urine in the previous 1–2 hours. FCU is thought to be a less-sensitive test than cervical or vaginal specimens (BASHH 2010).

When obtaining an eye swab from a newborn with 'sticky eye', the lower lid should be everted, and the swab taken by drawing it gently along the mucosal surface. Swabs should be taken from upper lids also if possible (McMillan & Ballard 2002).

Treatment of the woman and her partner

In common with other STIs, GUM clinic specialists, in liaison with obstetric and midwifery teams, should direct the management. Treatment of *C. trachomatis* infection involves a course of prescribed antibiotics. BASHH provides guidance on regimens most suitable for pregnancy (BASHH 2006) (*see* the list of useful resources for access details).

Partner notification is essential to prevent reinfection. The most recent sexual partners and those who have been at risk in the preceding 6 months should be encouraged to attend screening (McMillan & Ballard 2002). The incidence of reinfection is estimated to be 15%–30% at 1 year for women in the UK (Lamontagne *et al.* 2007). Couples should refrain from sexual intercourse for at least 7 days after single-dose treatment or until completion of a multiple-dose course (BASHH 2006). However, involvement of partners may prove a problem for women who perceive that their partners are difficult and unlikely to attend a clinic (Melvin *et al.* 2009). Patient-delivered partner medication, which involves the woman delivering antibiotic therapy directly to her sexual partner, has been suggested. This may improve the control of spread of chlamydia, although it presents a problem with regard to regulations covering the administration of prescribed medication (Melvin *et al.* 2009).

A full explanation of the condition is needed with particular reference to the long-term complications for the woman and her partner/s. Clear, accurate written information should supplement verbal discussion (BASHH 2006) and those under the age of 25 years treated for chlamydia should be offered a repeat test for chlamydia 3 months after the completion of treatment (BASHH 2013b). However, in pregnancy, this 'test of cure' is advised to occur 5 weeks after completion of antibiotic treatment and repeat screening in the third trimester is recommended (BASHH 2010, Allstaff & Wilson 2012). A follow-up visit for this retest offers the opportunity to ascertain if the antibiotic course has been completed and to reinforce sexual health advice (McMillan & Ballard 2002).

In many individuals who are infected with chlamydia, it is thought that spontaneous resolution of the infection eventually occurs. However, those with persistent infection are those most likely to develop long-term complications (McMillan & Ballard 2002).

There is significant correlation between chlamydial infection and viral shedding of HIV and therefore identification and treatment of chlamydia may reduce the transmission of HIV (Manavi 2006). In common with other STIs, those diagnosed with chlamydia infection should be offered an HIV test and screened for other STIs (BASHH 2006).

Treatment of infant

Paediatricians should be informed of chlamydia infection in the mother, as some infants may develop infection despite apparently successful treatment (SIGN 2009). There will also be cases where chlamydia infection in the newborn will be the presenting indicator of infection in the mother and her partner, so appropriate follow-up as described earlier will be indicated. Sensitivity will be required, as mothers will find this a distressing situation, particularly where the baby is unwell.

Antibiotic eye ointments are not effective on chlamydia conjunctivitis, nor do they treat other sites such as the nasopharynx that may be colonised. General antibiotic therapy is indicated, which will also treat any concurrent chlamydial pneumonia or genital pneumonia infection (Mårdh 2002, Lazaro 2013). It is recommended that a further eye swab be taken 3 weeks after treatment, as antibiotic therapy is not always effective. A paediatrician should direct care, as complications can arise.

HERPES SIMPLEX VIRUS

EPIDEMIOLOGY

In 2013 there were nearly 20 000 women diagnosed with first-episode anogenital herpes in England. This represents a steady increase in diagnoses since 2005, with rates highest among those aged 20–24 years (PHE 2014a). Eighty per cent of people who are positive for herpes simplex virus (HSV) type specific antibodies are unaware they have been infected with the virus (Lazaro 2013). There are no reliable recent figures for numbers of pregnant women who are seropositive for HSV. However, the estimated prevalence of neonatal HSV is low (4 in 100 000) (Tookey & Peckham 2006). This provides a source of reassurance to parents and clinicians regarding the impact of this condition for the newborn.

CAUSATIVE ORGANISM

Herpes simplex virus type 1 and type 2.

- Type 1 (HSV-1): This is the usual cause of infections seen on the face and lips commonly known as 'fever blisters' or 'cold sores'. It is usually transmitted during childhood via non-sexual contact with family members. Most of these first infections are asymptomatic, although they may be associated with an outbreak of an ulcer in the throat or on the lips accompanied by fever and generally feeling unwell. Flare-ups are thought to occur during times of stress, sunburn or febrile illness. During these flare-ups viral shedding lasts up to a week (Roos & Baker 2011).
- Type 2 (HSV-2): Infections associated with the genitalia, although there are an increasing number of genital herpes infections that are caused by HSV-1. HSV-2 can cause oral herpes.

CLINICAL FEATURES IN WOMEN

- Asymptomatic (50%)
- Tingling, itching and burning sensation
- Blistering, painful ulceration of the external genitalia although lesions may be on the cervix or rectum (*see* Box 5.8)
- Flu-like illness with fever, headache and muscle pain
- Dysuria
- Swollen lymph nodes in the groin.

(Conlon and Snydman 2004, Peate 2005, Goering *et al.* 2013)

HSV may feature typical fluid-filled blisters on an erythematous base described collo-quially as 'dew drops on a rose petal', although it more commonly presents as painful papules and ulcers (Stamm *et al.* 2008). Average duration of lesions is about 20 days for women. There is considerable variation in the presentation and number of lesions a person will develop. They may also appear as abrasions, innocuous fissures or just a mild reddened area (Lazaro 2013, Stanberry 2006, Stamm *et al.* 2008).

BOX 5.8 CHARACTERISTIC STAGES OF HERPES LESIONS

Tingling, burning, itching

⇩

Small blister-like fluid-filled vesicle; skin surrounding may be slightly reddened

⇩

Loses thin skin covering, leaving ulcer (shallow erosion)

⇩

Develops crust with thin scab covering

⇩

Healed when crust disappears

(Lazaro 2013, Stamm *et al.* 2008)

TRANSMISSION

Transmission of HSV-2 is mostly through sexual intercourse with a person who has the virus, genital-to-genital and oral-to-genital. As HSV can be asymptomatic it is possible to acquire the infection from someone who doesn't know he or she has it. This may cause tension and conflict during the course of contact tracing, as the origin of infection may be unknown (Roos & Baker 2011). Women are more likely than men to get genital herpes. Female genitalia have a greater surface of mucosa cells than the male, where the mucosa surface is confined to the urethra. Mucosal cells are more easily infected than skin cells. It is also thought that changes during the menstrual cycle may alter the local mucosal immune barrier (Stanberry 2006).

Vertical (mother-to-child) HSV transmission is rare. As stated earlier, estimated prevalence of neonatal HSV is about 4 in 100 000 (Tookey & Peckham 2006). Risk of vertical transmission is greatest when the mother acquires a primary genital HSV infection in the third trimester, with neonatal infection occurring as a result of direct contact with secretions around the time of birth. Transplacental intrauterine infection is rare (BASHH 2014a). There is a risk of postnatal transmission to the infant from parents or close relatives with an active cold sore, from kissing and close contact (Tookey & Peckham 2006).

PATHOPHYSIOLOGY OF HERPES SIMPLEX VIRUS INFECTION

Primary infection with HSV results in lifelong latent infection with periods of reactivation. A person will acquire the infection when the virus is transmitted across a mucosal surface such as the genitalia or through interruptions in the skin (Gupta *et al.* 2007). The replication of the virus, along with the host immune response, results in the characteristic small blisters of herpes (*see* Box 5.8), although for many people the infection will be unnoticed or asymptomatic.

With the initial infection the virus enters the tiny peripheral sensory nerves that are present in the skin. These sensory nerve cells extend to the spinal cord and transmit sensations of touch, temperature and pain. The virus DNA moves to the nucleus of the neurons (nerve cells) located in the dorsal root ganglia and essentially 'hides' from the immune system in an inactive form termed latent infection (Gupta *et al.* 2007). During reactivation the virus sheds and is transported back down nerve endings. It is not clear what triggers reactivation of the latent virus, although many people cite stress as a factor. The process of reactivation may cause tingling or odd sensations in the skin known as prodromal symptoms, indicating that an outbreak is imminent. However, these symptoms, in common with the blisters, are variable and may be non-existent. Once thought of as a way to indicate when infectious, it is now known this is unreliable, as the virus can be shed when no symptoms are present and virus replication may occur more frequently than previously thought (Stanberry 2006, Schiffer *et al.* 2011). Replication allows the virus be passed to a new host (Hay & Kieran 2009).

With reactivation, symptoms can occur in any area covered by the network of nerve fibres of the sacral dermatome and this includes locations distant to the place of first contact such as thighs, buttocks and the anal area (Gupta *et al.* 2007). It is generally thought that over time those with HSV will have fewer outbreaks, especially after the first year. Recurrent episodes tend to be less severe than the first (Hay & Kieran

2009). Prior infection with HSV-1 may offer some protection against HSV-2 infection (Gupta *et al.* 2007).

INCUBATION PERIOD

The period from infection to symptoms is 7–14 days (average 5 days), although approximately half of primary infections are asymptomatic (Conlon & Snydman 2004, Bannister *et al.* 2006, Hay & Kieran 2009).

COMPLICATIONS RELATED TO PREGNANCY

Mother

Maternal primary HSV infection during pregnancy is associated with the following factors.

- Preterm labour
- Miscarriage
- Although rare, HSV can spread through the bloodstream (disseminated herpes) and cause more serious complications including encephalitis and liver infection. This is more likely in pregnancy, which may be due to the altered immunity of pregnancy. It is also more likely in women who are HIV positive (Stanberry 2006).
- Women with HIV may have more severe and frequent episodes of HSV during pregnancy and are more likely to shed HSV at term. Co-infection of these two viruses increases the replication of both and thus increases the risk of perinatal transmission of both HSV and HIV (Roos & Baker 2011, BASHH 2014a).

Fetus and newborn

Herpes simplex infection is a rare but serious infection in the neonate. The site of infection will determine the extent of complications and rate of mortality. Infection may lead to damage to the brain (encephalitis), skin and eyes (Stamm *et al.* 2008, Bannister *et al.* 2006). Disseminated herpes with multiple organ involvement has a poor prognosis and is more common in preterm infants (Tookey & Peckham 2006).

The risk for transmission to the neonate from a primary HSV infection during pregnancy is less than 3%. The greatest risk to the neonate is when the mother acquires the primary HSV infection within 6 weeks of delivery (BASHH 2014a). The risk to the neonate from past infection is much less, about 1 in 2000–20 000 (Stamm *et al.* 2008). In most cases of vertical transmission of HSV to the neonate, mothers are not aware of the infection (Stamm *et al.* 2008, Tookey & Peckham 2006). Congenital herpes can occur as a result of the virus crossing the placenta, although this is very rare.

Factors influencing vertical transmission include:

- the type of maternal infection – primary HSV infection is more likely to result in transmission of the virus than a recurrent infection, as transplacental maternal antibodies provide some protection to the neonate

- duration of rupture of the membranes
- use of fetal scalp electrode
- mode of delivery.

DIAGNOSIS AND MANAGEMENT

Referral to the GUM clinic is recommended for accurate diagnosis. Diagnosis can be made on clinical appearance of typical vesicles and confirmed by viral polymerase chain reaction. Women will require specialist counselling, preferably at the GUM clinic regarding the implications of the diagnosis. BASHH provides guidance on the management of HSV infection in women (*see* the list of useful resources at the end of this chapter for access details for up-to-date BASHH guidelines). Box 5.9 lists some of the issues to be discussed at that time.

Routine screening in pregnancy for herpes is not advocated, as this will not predict viral shedding at delivery. Gardella and Brown (2011) suggest that new rapid methods of testing may make identification of the virus in genital secretions of women in labour possible. Along with serology to establish recent versus past infection, this may enable targeted care for neonates at risk. However, this has not yet been evaluated for clinical use.

BOX 5.9 ISSUES TO BE DISCUSSED AT TIME OF INITIAL DIAGNOSIS

- Information about the nature of the infection and how it can be acquired and transmitted. The complex nature of herpes in relation to recurrence and asymptomatic infection will mean identification of source of infection may not be clear.
- Partner notification*
- Risk reduction for transmission – condom use
- Risk of maternal transmission to fetus and the need to inform midwife, obstetrician

* In cases of positive diagnosis in a male partner but where the woman is uninfected, transmission during pregnancy would be a particular concern

(McMillan & Ogilvie 2002a)

Management in pregnancy

Management in pregnancy is complex and should be coordinated between the obstetric and midwifery team and the GUM clinicians. First episode genital herpes in early pregnancy is associated with miscarriage, although it is thought not to cause any developmental abnormality if the pregnancy continues. The main aim of management is to prevent transmission to the fetus or newborn.

Box 5.10 summarises the principles of management for women who have a *recurrence* of herpes in pregnancy. Box 5.11 summarises the care if it is thought the woman is experiencing a *primary* HSV infection in pregnancy. As discussed in the earlier section 'Complications related to pregnancy', the greatest risk to the neonate is when the mother has a primary HSV infection around the time of delivery. The management of this situation is summarised in Box 5.12. BASHH provides detailed clinical guidance including the management in preterm delivery and in those with HIV (BASHH 2014a).

BOX 5.10 PRINCIPLES OF MANAGEMENT FOR PREGNANT WOMEN WITH KNOWN *RECURRENT* GENITAL HERPES

- Recurrent episodes of genital herpes usually resolve without treatment within 7–10 days. Saline baths and analgesia may be helpful to alleviate symptoms.
- When a recurrent episode occurs at the time of delivery, the mode of delivery needs to be discussed with the woman. Caesarean section may be considered but as the risk of neonatal transmission during vaginal delivery is so low (0%–3%), this needs to be balanced against the risk of complications of caesarean section for the mother. Clinical circumstances will also dictate decisions regarding mode of delivery. The woman will be given the choice based on discussion of the balance of risks and individual circumstances.
- Those having a vaginal delivery should avoid prolonged rupture of membranes, fetal scalp electrode and fetal blood sampling (Stamm *et al.* 2008).
- Referral to the paediatrician should be made of babies born to mothers with recurrent HSV at the time of delivery.

(BASHH 2014a, Wilson 2011)

BOX 5.11 PRINCIPLES OF MANAGEMENT WHEN A WOMAN HAS A *PRIMARY* (FIRST) EPISODE OF GENITAL HERPES *DURING PREGNANCY*

FIRST AND SECOND TRIMESTER (UNTIL 27 COMPLETED WEEKS OF PREGNANCY)
- Refer to GUM clinic for diagnosis and treatment that will include a screen for other STIs and partner testing. It is important to determine whether the infection is a primary episode or not.
- A specialist GUM physician or obstetrician should discuss the potential risks and benefits of antiviral treatment with the woman. Medication may reduce the duration and severity of symptoms and decrease in viral shedding (BASHH 2014a).
- Women with suspected genital herpes who are having midwifery-led care should be

referred for review both to the GUM specialist and to an obstetrician and a clear plan of care documented in the notes.

- Provided delivery is not premature, vaginal delivery can be anticipated, although treatment with antiviral medication may be prescribed from 36 weeks' gestation.

THIRD TRIMESTER ACQUISITION (FROM THE 28TH WEEK OF PREGNANCY)

- Urgent referral should be made to the GUM specialist and obstetrician for diagnosis and treatment. Treatment with antiviral medication is recommended and will be continued until delivery.
- It is important to determine whether a presentation of genital herpes in pregnancy is a primary or non-primary infection. As primary infection is often asymptomatic, clinical history is unreliable. Serological tests can determine primary infection by using IgG and IgM type-specific antibody testing. This is particularly important in late pregnancy, as this will influence decisions regarding the need for caesarean section (Wilson 2011).
- Delivery by caesarean section is recommended when primary infection occurs within 6 weeks of delivery.

BOX 5.12 PRINCIPLES OF MANAGEMENT WHEN A WOMAN HAS AN EPISODE OF *PRIMARY* GENITAL HERPES AT THE *TIME OF DELIVERY*

- The midwife will need to refer to the obstetrician to make a clinical assessment of the lesions and take a history in order to ascertain whether this is likely to be a primary or recurrent episode.
- Although the results of tests will not be available in time, taking a viral swab from the lesion(s) is recommended, as the result may influence management of the neonate.
- The neonatologist should be informed.
- Caesarean section delivery is recommended to all women with a primary genital herpes lesion at, or within, 6 weeks of birth.
- Although vaginal birth is not recommended for those with primary infection, for those women who opt for vaginal birth, aim to keep the membranes intact and avoid invasive procedures such as application of fetal scalp electrode and fetal blood sampling
- Intravenous antiviral medication may be considered
- Women with HIV may have more severe and frequent episodes of HSV during pregnancy and be more likely to shed HSV at term. Co-infection of these two viruses increases the replication of both and thus increases the risk of perinatal transmission of both HSV and HIV.

(BASHH 2014a)

PREVENTION OF HERPES SIMPLEX VIRUS INFECTION

UK surveillance data demonstrate a low incidence of neonatal herpes, and screening to determine those at risk of primary HSV infection in pregnancy is not currently advocated. Women without a history of genital herpes who have partners known to have genital herpes should be advised to use condoms and/or consider abstaining from sexual intercourse during the third trimester. Condoms do not provide complete protection, as the condom may not cover the herpetic lesion and viral shedding is unpredictable (Roos & Baker 2011). Women can acquire genital herpes through the oral–genital route if their partners have oral herpes (Roos & Baker 2011)

Postnatal transmission of HSV to infants may also occur via cold sores (BASHH 2014a). Family members and healthcare workers should take measures to avoid contact with young infants when they have a cold sore until the lesion has completely healed over and disappeared.

SYPHILIS

EPIDEMIOLOGY

There has been a steady increase in the rates of syphilis diagnoses in England over the last 10 years, although the majority of cases are attributed to men having sex with men. However, there remains concern over rates among women, which had increased rapidly in the period 1999–2008. In 2012 there was a 96% uptake of antenatal screening for syphilis and 0.15% of tests had an initial positive result (PHE 2013). Diagnosis of congenital syphilis remains low due to the effectiveness of this screening programme (UK NSC 2013).

Syphilis is a worldwide problem, especially in resource-poor countries where the incidence is as high as 20% among African women of reproductive age (Goldenberg *et al.* 2010). When a mother is infected but untreated, up to 40% of fetuses will die in utero and another 40% will be born alive but have congenital syphilis. Each year more than 1 million babies are born with congenital syphilis. Russia, Asia and South America also have high rates of syphilis (Goldenberg *et al.* 2010). Treatment is easy and inexpensive and the WHO has instigated a programme to try to eliminate this distressing but preventable condition (WHO 2007).

CAUSATIVE ORGANISM

Syphilis is caused by the bacterium *Treponema pallidum*.

CLINICAL FEATURES AND COURSE OF THE DISEASE

After initial infection *T. pallidum* reproduces locally and then disseminates via the lymphatic system, causing a systemic disease that can lead to a variety of clinical manifestations. Features will vary from no symptoms to a wide spectrum once there is multisystem involvement. Table 5.2 provides an overview of the course of the disease.

TABLE 5.2 Pathogenesis of syphilis

Stage of disease	Signs and symptoms	Pathogenesis
2–10 weeks (average 3 weeks) after initial contact		
↓ **Primary syphilis** Symptoms last 3–6 weeks ↓	**Chancre**, begins as small papule; develops into painless, raised well-defined ulcer Enlarged lymph nodes in the groin Spontaneous recovery	Multiplication of treponemas at site of infection Highly infectious Proliferation of treponemas in lymph nodes
2–6 weeks after disappearance of chancre ↓ **Secondary syphilis** Symptoms may disappear within a few weeks or come and go over months	Multisystem involvement; flu-like illness: muscle pain, fever, headache Non-itchy maculopapular rash involving palms and soles Perianal warty lesions (condylomata lata) Any organ can be affected Spontaneous recovery	Multiplication and production of lesions in lymph nodes, liver, joints, muscles, skin and mucous membranes causing a variety of systemic reactions and symptoms
Latent syphilis 3–30 years	No signs and symptoms but may be diagnosed on serological testing	Treponemas dormant Evades recognition and elimination by host immune response
Tertiary syphilis	Neurosyphilis – dementia and episodes of psychosis Cardiac syphilis – aortic lesions, heart failure Ophthalmic symptoms	Reawakening and multiplication of treponemas Further dissemination Gummas (lesions with necrotic centre that vary in size from microscopic to tumour-like) in skin and bone

(Goering *et al.* 2013, Bannister *et al.* 2006, Khare & Khare 2007)

TRANSMISSION

When syphilitic lesions are present in mucosa, sexual transmission occurs via minor abrasions during sexual intercourse. Close contact is required because the organism doesn't survive well outside the body and is very sensitive to drying, heat and disinfectants (Goering *et al.* 2013). Vertical transmission from mother to fetus can occur via the placenta during pregnancy (Goering *et al.* 2013).

If pregnancy occurs in the early stages of untreated syphilis, fetal transmission is nearly 100%. Even 4 years after the initial infection, the rate of transmission is still around 70%, although it will be low (10%) in women with latent syphilis (Khare & Khare 2007, UK NSC 2010).

INCUBATION PERIOD

The average time between initial infection and the appearance of the chancre is about 21 days, but it can be up to 90 days.

COMPLICATIONS RELATED TO PREGNANCY

Congenital syphilis is a preventable condition but this depends on timely diagnosis and treatment of the mother (UK NSC 2010). When the mother is not treated, the fetus or newborn may develop a number of features indicative of congenital syphilis. This may manifest as:

- serious infection causing intrauterine death
- hydrops
- low birthweight and premature delivery
- congenital infection in the newborn that may not become apparent until the infant is about 2 years of age and may include abnormal skeletal and tooth development, enlarged lymph nodes, hepatosplenomegaly and glomerulonephritis; neurological damage, including visual and hearing impairment may occur.

(Goering *et al.* 2013, Stamm *et al.* 2008, Wilson 2011)

SCREENING AND DIAGNOSIS

Screening for syphilis in pregnancy is part of the Infectious Diseases in Pregnancy Screening Programme (UK NSC 2010). The high uptake of this screening (>95%), early identification and treatment of those found to have the infection have ensured that rates of congenital syphilis remain low (Goering *et al.* 2013, PHE 2013).

Specific tests for syphilis include treponemal enzyme immunoassay, *T. pallidum* particle agglutination assay and *T. pallidum* haemagglutination assay. Non-specific serology tests for syphilis may also be useful and include the Venereal Disease Research Laboratory test, also known as the rapid plasma reagin test (Kingston *et al.* 2008). Newer, rapid 'point of care' tests have been evaluated and may prove useful for use in resource-poor settings (Jafari *et al.* 2013).

MANAGEMENT

Guidelines for the assessment and management of syphilis in pregnancy and infancy are provided by BASHH and these represent best practice (Kingston *et al.* 2008). Any woman with a positive screening test for syphilis needs prompt referral. Midwives should be aware that less than a third of women who screened positive for syphilis actually had an active infection that required treatment (PHE 2013).

A multidisciplinary approach is advised and the specialist midwife often coord-inates this. Further specialist tests are arranged to confirm diagnosis and referral made to the GUM clinic where investigation for other STIs, partner screening and treatment will be undertaken. Treatment of sexual partners is essential to prevent rein-fection, and evaluation of HIV status is recommended (Stamm *et al.* 2008, Kingston *et al.* 2008).

Discussion with the woman will include the need to confirm the diagnosis, the significance of syphilis to her and her baby's health and the details of the practical arrangements for multidisciplinary care (UK NSC 2010). Referral to the fetal medi-cine unit is advised. Serial scans are recommended to assess for signs of fetal infection and to monitor fetal growth (Khare & Khare 2007, Kingston *et al.* 2008).

Benzathine penicillin G is the drug of choice for treating syphilis. Penicillin reli-ably treats the fetus when administered to the pregnant mother (Goering *et al.* 2013).

BASHH guidelines provide details of treatment regimens for pregnancy as well as alternatives for those known to be allergic to penicillin (Kingston *et al.* 2008). There is a possibility of an anaphylactic reaction to penicillin. For this reason facilities for resuscitation should be available in treatment areas. Women need to wait on the premises for at least 15 minutes after their first injection and should be advised to seek urgent medical treatment should they experience any signs of an allergic reac-tion (Kingston *et al.* 2008).

The Jarisch–Herxheimer reaction can follow initial treatment of syphilis in about 40% of cases. It is characterised by a flu-like illness with headache, muscle and joint pain and fever that lasts 12–24 hours. It is thought to be due to the breaking up of the dying bacteria, which release inflammatory substances into the bloodstream. It occurs more frequently following treatment of the early stages of syphilis (Barlow 2006). In pregnancy, the fever of this reaction may cause uterine contractions, along with fetal heart decelerations and may result in preterm delivery and fetal demise. Therefore, women experiencing a fever related to this reaction need to be given medication to bring down their temperature. Liaison between the obstetric team, midwives, paedi-atrics and fetal medicine unit is advised (Kingston & McAuliffe 2011).

A plan of care for mother and baby should be clearly documented in the notes. Liaison with the paediatric team is essential following a diagnosis of syphilis in preg-nancy, to establish a plan of care for the baby following delivery. The neonatal team should be informed during labour to ensure prompt transfer of care (UK NSC 2010).

TRICHOMONAS VAGINALIS

EPIDEMIOLOGY

T. vaginalis was diagnosed in 6002 women in England in 2013 (PHE 2014b). It is reported that up to 30% of pregnant women in resource-poor countries have this infection (Khare & Khare 2007).

CAUSATIVE ORGANISM

T. vaginalis is a flagellated protozoan parasite found in the vagina and urethra.

CLINICAL FEATURES IN WOMEN

- Vaginal discharge: this varies in consistency and amount, and it may be frothy and yellow or green and have a foul-smelling, fishy odour
- Vulval itching
- Cervix appears red with multiple small lesions (strawberry-like appearance); this is seen in only 2% of those with trichomonas
- Dysuria
- Vague low abdominal discomfort
- Discomfort and bleeding during sexual intercourse
- May be asymptomatic (10%–50%).

(Schwebke 2007, BASHH 2014b, Lazaro 2013)

TRANSMISSION

T. vaginalis is a sexually transmitted infection but it can be transmitted to the fetus during vaginal delivery. It is thought to infect only about 5% of babies born to infected mothers and the infection is rarely severe (BASHH 2014b, McMillan 2002).

INCUBATION PERIOD

The incubation period for *T. vaginalis* is 1–21 days.

COMPLICATIONS RELATED TO PREGNANCY

T. vaginalis infection is associated with premature rupture of membranes, preterm delivery, low birthweight and post-partum maternal sepsis (Bannister *et al.* 2006, BASHH 2014b, Lazaro 2013). However, in a randomised controlled trial, treatment of asymptomatic trichomonias did not reduce the risk of premature birth (Klebanoff *et al.* 2001). Screening for asymptomatic *T. vaginalis infection* is therefore not currently recommended (BASHH 2014b). It may be that the link between *T. vaginalis* and premature labour relates to other co-existing genital infections including BV. Further research is required to establish or refute *T. vaginalis* as a direct cause of premature birth (Clutterbuck 2004).

DIAGNOSIS AND MANAGEMENT

Midwives should ensure appropriate referral to GUM clinic for diagnosis and treatment of trichomonas. Women with characteristic lower genital tract symptoms should be tested for *T. vaginalis*. Direct microscopy of vaginal discharge from a high vaginal swab is recommended. Microscopy shows the flagellated organism. This test is commonly carried out immediately in most GUM clinics, as the organism will die within a few hours of the sample being taken.

Sexual partner(s) should be treated simultaneously and sexual abstinence is advised until treatment is complete. Screening of other STIs should be undertaken at the same time. The *T. vaginalis* parasite causes damage to the vaginal lining, with a breakdown of the epithelial cells and increased inflammation. Therefore, in common with other STIs, trichomonas increases the risk of HIV transmission. Women and their partners should be given clear verbal information backed up by detailed written material on trichomonas that includes the risk of premature birth and other long-term complications (BASHH 2014b).

The recommended treatment is a course of the antibiotic metronidazole. A meta-analysis of the safety of metronidazole in pregnancy concluded it is safe for use in pregnancy, even in the first trimester (Burtin *et al.* 1995). Metronidazole can cause nausea and vomiting and leave a slight metallic taste in the mouth. Alcohol is not advised when taking this medication, as it can cause more severe side effects. It is also thought to affect the taste of breast milk and manufacturers thus recommend to avoid high doses if breastfeeding (BASHH 2014b). BASHH (2014b) guidelines provide information on treatment regimens in pregnancy and advise avoiding a high-dose regimen.

GENITAL WARTS AND HUMAN PAPILLOMA VIRUS
INTRODUCTION
There are over 100 distinct types of HPV, of which about 40 infect the genital tract. The clinical lesions of HPV are warts (Bannister *et al.* 2006). Although most HPV infections are asymptomatic and self-limiting, some types of HPV cause genital warts and others are associated with cervical cancer (McCance 2009, McMillan & Ogilvie 2002b).

EPIDEMIOLOGY
It is difficult to ascertain the true prevalence of HPV genital infection. Many people with genital warts do not seek medical advice or have no obvious symptoms (McMillan & Ogilvie 2002b). Genital warts are common among men and women attending GUM clinics and are the most common viral STI in the UK (Fenton and Lowndes 2004). Over 70 000 new cases were diagnosed in those attending GUM clinics in England in 2013, and 32 614 of these were in women (PHE 2014b). However, there has been a decline in cases of genital warts in women aged 15–19. It is thought that HPV vaccination programmes have had an impact on the rate (PHE 2014a, Howell-Jones 2013).

CAUSATIVE ORGANISM

The HPV serotypes 6 and 11 are the more common types found in genital warts. These are considered 'low risk' HPV types. HPV-16, 18, 31, 33 and 45 are the HPV types associated with cervical cancer and are thus termed 'high risk' (McMillan & Ogilvie 2002b, Hay & Kieran 2009).

CLINICAL FEATURES IN WOMEN

It is common not to have any symptoms of HPV infection (McMillan & Ogilvie 2002b). When genital warts surface as an indication of HPV infection they usually don't cause physical discomfort but they are generally considered unsightly and embarrassing (Barlow 2006, Lazaro 2013).

Most often, warts first appear near the posterior part of the vaginal introitus and on the adjacent labia majora and minora (McMillan & Ogilvie 2002b). Warts can look different depending on where they are situated. In moist areas such as the vulva, they have a softer surface and if situated on harder skin that is exposed to the air, they have a more callous appearance (Barlow 2006). They can be as small as a pinhead and rarely can grow very large (Barlow 2006). In some locations they can cause soreness, anal irritation or bleeding. They can be single or multiple, broad based or on a stem (pedunculated) (BASHH 2007a).

TRANSMISSION

Genital warts have high prevalence, high infectivity, a long period between initial infection and presentation of symptoms, and have a poor response to treatment. These factors make the infection more likely to be passed on (McMillan & Ogilvie 2002b). Primarily, transmission is through sexual intercourse, although it may be transmitted from digital lesions. The risk of transmission increases with the number of sexual partners and the use of condoms reduces but does not eliminate the risk of sexual transmission (BASHH 2007a). HPV infection can be present without genital warts being evident and therefore people pass on the virus unwittingly.

Mother-to-newborn transmission can occur by passage through the birth canal, although the rate of transmission is low (only 1 in 80) (Allstaff & Wilson 2012), and rarely does this cause any complications (McMillan & Ogilvie 2002b).

INCUBATION

Genital warts may appear from 3 weeks to 8 months after primary infection, although with an asymptomatic HPV infection, genital warts may not appear until much later and can sometimes surface for the first time in pregnancy (McMillan & Ogilvie 2002b, Barlow 2006).

COMPLICATIONS RELATED TO PREGNANCY

Genital warts may appear for the first time during pregnancy either as a result of recent infection or due to reactivation of latent HPV infection (McMillan & Ogilvie 2002b). It appears the relative suppression of the immune system during pregnancy allows the warts to appear (Barlow 2006).

In pregnancy, genital warts can become large but tend to regress after pregnancy, even without treatment (McMillan & Ogilvie 2002b, Barlow 2006). However, treatment may be considered to minimise the number of lesions present at delivery, as this may reduce neonatal exposure to the virus (BASHH 2007a).

A rare complication for the newborn is the development of laryngeal papillomatosis (warts in the larynx) (BASHH 2007a). The newborn may also develop genital warts, and, extremely rarely, a HPV respiratory complication (Allstaff & Wilson 2012).

MANAGEMENT

For the majority of women, information and reassurance should be given that lesions are unlikely to cause any problems and will regress after delivery (Ooi & Dayan 2004). Most clinicians prefer to adopt a non-interventionist approach, particularly where the lesions are small (McMillan & Ogilvie 2002b). The perinatal transmission rate is low and there is no evidence that removing the warts during pregnancy changes the rate of transmission, although treatment may be offered to alleviate anxiety (McMillan & Ogilvie 2002b).

Options for treatment include cryotherapy, electrocautery, surgical excision and chemical treatment. Chemical applications for treatment of warts are contraindicated in pregnancy (BASHH 2007a, Ooi & Dayan 2004). Cryotherapy is considered a safe, cheap, effective method of treatment (Ooi & Dayan 2004) although warts may return after treatment (Barlow 2006, BASHH 2007a).

In extremely rare circumstances, where bulky warts obstruct the vaginal passage, or cause extensive cervical disease, caesarean section may be indicated (BASHH 2007a, Allstaff & Wilson 2012).

In common with all STIs exclusion, detection and, if required, treatment of other STIs should be undertaken. It is important any other local infections are treated before any wart therapy is commenced (McMillan & Ogilvie 2002b). Current sexual partners may be offered examination and treatment (Bannister *et al.* 2006). Women with genital warts should follow normal cervical screening intervals (BASHH 2007a). As with all management of STIs, midwives will need to be sensitive to women when discussing genital warts. Clear, detailed information backed up by written information should be given.

HUMAN PAPILLOMA VIRUS VACCINATION

An extensive HPV vaccination programme for 12- to 13-year-old girls began in the UK in 2008. Box 5.13 gives further information on the HPV vaccination programme, which may be of interest to midwives as part of their wider public health education role. Vaccination during pregnancy is not advised, although there is no known risk associated with inadvertent vaccination. HPV vaccine is not a live vaccine and thus cannot replicate and cause any disease in mother or fetus. However, data are limited to support its safety in pregnancy. TOP following inadvertent immunisation is not advocated. If a woman starts the vaccination schedule and then discovers she is pregnant the remaining doses should be withheld until after the pregnancy (DH 2012).

BOX 5.13 HUMAN PAPILLOMA VIRUS VACCINATION

The main purpose of the HPV vaccination programme for girls aged 12–13 years is to reduce the burden of cervical cancer (Ault & Future 11 Study Group 2007). The vaccination schedule requires three doses, ideally given at 0, 1- to 2-, and 6-month intervals. When the quadrivalent HPV vaccine (protects for serotypes 16, 18, 6 and 11) is used, a further benefit of the vaccination programme is the potential to prevent genital warts. An Australian study reported the near eradication of genital warts among Australian women under 21 years of age attending GUM clinics (Ali *et al.* 2013). The quadrivalent vaccine has been in use in the UK since 2012.

BACTERIAL VAGINOSIS

INTRODUCTION

BV is a frequent cause of abnormal vaginal discharge in women of childbearing age, and yet its cause and progression are poorly understood (BASHH 2012b). BV in pregnant women is associated with a risk for preterm birth (Stamm *et al.* 2008). The 'osis' in vaginosis means 'condition of', as opposed to 'itis' in vaginitis, which means inflammation. In BV there is no inflammation, itching or soreness but just a characteristic 'fishy' smell caused by the bacteria that feature in BV (Barlow 2006).

EPIDEMIOLOGY

BV is the commonest cause of vaginal discharge among women of reproductive age (Yudin 2011, Lazaro 2013). Details of rates of BV in the UK pregnant population are hard to ascertain, although an older study identified a prevalence of 12% among pregnant women attending a UK antenatal clinic (Hay *et al.* 1994) and a higher incidence (30%) was found in women undergoing TOP (BASHH 2012b).

CAUSATIVE ORGANISM

A number of organisms appear to be associated with BV but the key feature of the condition is an imbalance of the cervical and vaginal microflora. In a healthy vagina lactobacilli are the dominant bacteria. The pH is below 4.5 (acidic) and there are low levels of other bacteria. In BV there is an overgrowth of a characteristic 'set' of anaerobic microflora including *Gardnerella vaginalis*, *Prevotella* spp, *Mycoplasma homonis* and *Atopobium vaginalis*. No particular single bacterial type consistently predominates (Khare & Khare 2007). These organisms replace the usually present lactobacilli causing a rise in vaginal pH making it more alkaline (BASHH 2012b).

CLINICAL FEATURES IN WOMEN

- Many women are asymptomatic (approximately 50%)
- Offensive 'fishy' smelling milky-white watery discharge that is not associated with soreness or irritation

TRANSMISSION

There is uncertainty as to whether BV is a mere imbalance of the ecology of the organisms or whether the change is initiated by sexual activity (BASHH 2012b), or perhaps by bathing/douching (Barlow 2006). The imbalance can appear and resolve spontaneously. It is therefore not considered to be a sexually transmitted condition (Bannister *et al.* 2006). Risk factors include vaginal douching, recent change of sex partner, smoking and the presence of another STI, but it has been described in virgins (BASHH 2012b).

COMPLICATIONS RELATED TO PREGNANCY

BV in pregnant women is associated with up to a sevenfold increased risk of preterm birth. It is thought that preterm labour is triggered by the cytokines and prostaglandins produced as a result of the bacterial imbalance (McMillan 2002, Donders *et al.* 2009). It is also associated with an increased risk of preterm rupture of membranes, post-partum endometritis and post-caesarean section infection (Yudin 2011). The microbes associated with BV, along with the host inflammatory response, may influence prostaglandin release and weaken the amniotic membrane (Stamm *et al.* 2008). In common with other genital tract infections, BV may increase susceptibility to acquisition of HIV (Stamm *et al.* 2008). BV is more common in women undergoing TOP and is associated with post-TOP endometritis and PID (BASHH 2012b). Complications for the newborn will include those related to prematurity.

DIAGNOSIS AND MANAGEMENT

Almost half of women carry the organism *G. vaginalis* normally (Lazaro 2013).

Diagnosis is therefore based on characteristic signs and symptoms, a pH vaginal fluid greater than 4.5, few or absent lactobacilli and the presence of large numbers of other characteristic organisms such as *Gardnerella* spp in vaginal fluid (Khare & Khare 2007, Bannister *et al.* 2006, BASHH 2012b).

Because of its link with premature labour, screening for BV in pregnancy has been considered. A recent Cochrane review concluded that screening and treating pregnant women who were asymptomatic for BV would not prevent preterm birth. However, for women with additional risk factors for preterm birth, treatment before 20 weeks' gestation may be beneficial (McDonald *et al.* 2007). Pregnant women with symptoms may be treated to relieve those symptoms. However, antibiotic treatment of BV remains debatable and clinicians should refer to guidance provided by BASSH (BASHH 2012b, Lazaro 2013).

To prevent BV, women should be advised against vaginal douching, which involves washing inside the vagina with a showerhead. The water can disturb the vital lactobacilli (Barlow 2006). In addition, the use of shampoos and bath gels in the bath should be discouraged, as they tend to be alkaline, and therefore lower the acidity, allowing the pathogenic bacteria to flourish (BASHH 2012b).

Non-antibiotic-based treatment with probiotic lactobacilli appear interesting, but studies to date have not shown consistency or reproducibility and therefore are not currently advocated as treatment (Senok *et al.* 2009). However, some small studies have shown benefit from these treatments in preventing recurrent lapses of BV (Ya *et al.* 2010, Eriksson *et al.* 2005).

Screening and treatment of other causes of vaginal discharge including candidiasis and trichomoniasis should be undertaken. Screening of sexual partners is not indicated for diagnosis of BV alone and women should be reassured that the diagnosis carries no implication of infidelity in a regular partner (Clutterbuck 2004). It may be helpful to use the analogy that BV is similar to thrush or urinary tract infection in that it occurs 'out of the blue' (Clutterbuck 2004). Backup of verbal discussion with written material is recommended.

VULVOVAGINAL CANDIDIASIS (THRUSH)

EPIDEMIOLOGY

Vulvovaginal candidiasis is the most commonly diagnosed cause of vaginal symptoms in the UK (Clutterbuck 2004). There were 78 512 cases of candidiasis diagnosed in GUM clinics in England in 2013 (PHE 2014b), although this number will under-represent the extent of those affected, as many women treat themselves for thrush with over the counter medication. Clutterbuck (2004) suggests that almost 75% of sexually active women report one or more episodes of thrush at some point.

CAUSATIVE ORGANISM

Candidiasis (also known as candidosis) is a generic term for infections caused by yeasts (McMillan 2002). *Candida albicans* is found to be the cause of thrush in 90% of cases (Lazaro 2013). Up to 20% of non-pregnant and 40% of pregnant women carry *Candida* spp as normal flora in the vagina (BASHH 2007b).

CLINICAL FEATURES IN WOMEN

- Vulval itching that can range from slight to intolerable
- Cheesy, white vaginal discharge with little odour. Discharge is more common in pregnant women
- Redness and oedema of mucosal surfaces (erythema)
- Itching or burning after intercourse or micturition
- Those with severe itching may have excoriations from scratching around the vulval area
- (McMillan 2002, BASHH 2007b, Clutterbuck 2004).

Although considered a minor condition, symptoms can be irritating and distressing. Recurrent vaginal candidiasis can cause considerable disruption to the women's sense of well-being (Clutterbuck 2004). Recurrent thrush is defined as four episodes within 12 months and for most women the cause of this recurrence is unknown (McMillan 2002).

TRANSMISSION AND SUSCEPTIBILITY

C. albicans is an opportunistic pathogen that flourishes when host defences are impaired. Yeasts that normally inhabit the gastrointestinal tract are probably introduced into the vagina from the perianal region. While not considered a sexually transmitted disease, the incidence of thrush increases at the onset of sexual activity (McMillan 2002, Clutterbuck 2004).

Pregnancy, uncontrolled diabetes, HIV, immunosuppressive medication and damage to tissue all predispose a woman to develop thrush (McMillan 2002, Clutterbuck 2004). Colonisation of the genital region by *Lactobacillus acidophilus* raises the pH of the vagina, which protects against thrush. Pregnancy alters this balance and allows *C. albicans* to flourish (Bannister *et al.* 2006). It is commonly thought that antibiotic use increases the incidence of thrush but there has been limited supporting evidence (Clutterbuck 2004, McMillan 2002, Bannister *et al.* 2006).

COMPLICATIONS RELATED TO PREGNANCY

Pregnant women have higher rates of fungal infections, in particular thrush. This is thought to be due to the effects of oestrogen in creating an enhanced nutrient availability (glycogen) in the vaginal mucus and an alteration to the local mucosa barrier in favour of fungal growth (Blackburn 2013). Asymptomatic colonisation with *Candida* spp is thus more prevalent in pregnancy (Bauters *et al.* 2002, Blackburn 2013) and women are also more likely to experience symptoms of thrush when they are pregnant. However, this colonisation by *Candida* spp is not associated with low birthweight or premature delivery (Cotch *et al.* 1998).

Candidiasis in the newborn may involve the umbilicus, mouth and nappy area. Transmission to the neonate may be via the maternal vagina but other sources include the bowel and mouth flora, as well as environmental sources and health professionals. Candida is associated with pain and excoriation of the nipple area during breastfeeding, although incorrect positioning and attachment may cause similar symptoms (Jones *et al.* 2006) (*See* section entitled 'Mastitis' in Chapter 2). Candida is a cause of late-onset sepsis in very low birthweight infants. This is linked to invasive therapies and immunological vulnerability rather than transmission from the mother.

DIAGNOSIS AND MANAGEMENT

Diagnosis of thrush is usually made on clinical characteristics and many women self-diagnose and treat themselves with over-the-counter preparations. However, a number of women when tested after self-diagnosis did not have *C. albicans* and thus laboratory testing is advocated as part of general screening for STIs in those women

---

ROLE OF THE MIDWIFE

- Maintain up-to-date knowledge of symptoms of genital and STIs
- Ask appropriate questions in a sensitive and professional way that will uncover symptoms or history of an STI
- Ensure a private environment and an attitude by the midwife that will encourage disclosure of potentially embarrassing and confidential information.
- Facilitate referral to appropriate specialists, in particular involvement of GUM physicians while providing ongoing care, support and communication with the obstetric team, paediatrician and other members of the multidisciplinary team
- Maintain confidentiality
- Use effective communication and counselling skills to offer help and advice to women who have been affected by STIs
- Promote an awareness of sexual health issues that includes the discussion of safe sex and the use of condoms with all women
- Provide information and access to services such as HIV and STI testing and treatment
- Provide clear, accessible information on STIs

who present themselves (Clutterbuck 2004). When indicated a vaginal swab should be taken from the anterior fornix (BASHH 2007b).

Treatment is only required when the woman experiences symptoms. Anti-fungal medication as topical cream or vaginal pessaries has been widely used in the management of candidiasis in pregnant women without adverse affect. However, oral medication is contraindicated in pregnancy. A longer course (up to 7 days), as opposed to one-dose treatment, is recommended to improve cure rate (BASHH 2007b). Treatment in pregnancy should be directed by a doctor.

Women are advised to avoid wearing tight-fitting synthetic clothing, and the use of perfumed products, which may irritate the vulval region. The use of probiotics, either orally or as topical application has not been supported by evidence although there is anecdotal report of benefit (Falagas *et al.* 2006).

USEFUL RESOURCES

- Barlow D (2006) *Sexually Transmitted Infections: the facts.* 2nd ed. Oxford: Oxford University Press.
- British Association for Sexual Health and HIV (BASHH): www.bashh.org/BASHH/Guidelines/ Guidelines/BASHH/Guidelines/Guidelines.aspx (provides up-to-date evidence based guidelines for the management of a range of STIs discussed in this chapter).
- Family Planning Association: www.fpa.org.uk (provides information for women on a range of STIs).
- Fletcher J, Ball G (2006) Chlamydia screening in pregnancy: a missed opportunity? *Br J Midwifery.* **14**(7): 390–2 (includes a recommended care pathway for screening for chlamydia in pregnancy).
- Herpes Virus Association: www.herpes.org.uk (a charity that aims to improve the lives of people who have herpes simplex).
- Lazaro N (2013) *Sexually Transmitted Infection in Primary Care* (RCGP/BASHH) [online]. 2nd ed. Available at: www.rcgp.org.uk/clinical-and-research/clinical-resources/~/media/Files/ CIRC/RCGP-Sexually-Transmitted-Infections-in-Primary-Care-2013.ashx (concise, accessible and practical guide to STIs).
- National Chlamydia Screening Programme: www.chlamydiascreening.nhs.uk/ps/resources. asp (extensive range of resources for service provision, explanation of tests and information for women available in a variety of languages).
- NHS Infectious Diseases in Pregnancy Screening Programme: http://infectiousdiseases.screen ing.nhs.uk (this government-funded programme publishes a range of useful resources for women and midwives and includes an e-learning package).

REFERENCES

Adams EJ, Charlett A, Edmunds WJ, *et al.* (2004) *Chlamydia trachomatis* in the United Kingdom: a systematic review and analysis of prevalence studies. *Sex Transm Infect.* **80**(5): 354–62.

Ali H, Donovan B, Wand H, *et al.* (2013) Genital warts in young Australians five years into national human papillomavirus vaccination programme: national surveillance data. *BMJ*. **346**: f2032.

Allstaff S, Wilson J (2012) The management of sexually transmitted infections in pregnancy. *Obstet Gynaecol*. **14**: 25–32.

Andrews WW, Goldenberg RL, Mercer B, *et al*. (2000) The Preterm Prediction Study: association of second-trimester genitourinary chlamydia infection with subsequent preterm birth. *Am J Obstet Gynecol*. **183**(3): 662–8.

Ault KA; Future 11 Study Group (2007) Effect of prophylactic human papillomavirus L1 virus-like-particle vaccine on risk of cervical intraepithelial neoplasia grade 2 grade 3 and adenocarcinoma in situ: a combined analysis of four randomised clinical trials. *Lancet*. **369**(9576): 1861–8.

Bakken IJ, Skjeldestad FE, Lydersen S, *et al*. (2007) Births and ectopic pregnancies in a large cohort of women tested for *Chlamydia trachomatis*. *Sex Transm Dis*. **34**(10): 739–43.

Bannister B, Gillespie S, Jones J (2006) *Microbiology and Management*. 3rd ed. Oxford: Blackwell Publishing.

Barlow D (2006) *Sexually Transmitted Infections: the facts*. 2nd ed. Oxford: Oxford University Press.

Bauer HM, Gibson P, Hernandez M, *et al*. (2002) Intimate partner violence and high-risk sexual behaviors among female patients with sexually transmitted diseases. *Sex Trans Dis*. **29**(7): 411–16.

Bauters T, Dhont M, Temmerman M, *et al*. (2002) Prevalence of vulvovaginal candidiasis and susceptibility to fluconazole in women. *Am J Obstet Gynecol*. **187**(3): 569–74.

Bignell C, Fitzgerald M; Guideline Development Group; British Association for Sexual Health and HIV UK (2011) UK national guideline for the management of gonorrhoea in adults, 2011. *Int J STD AIDS*. **22**(10): 541–7.

Blackburn ST (2013) *Maternal, Fetal and Neonatal Physiology*. 4th ed. Philadelphia: Saunders Elsevier.

British Association of Sexual Health and HIV: Clinical Effectiveness Group (BASHH) (2006) *2006 UK National Guideline for the Management of Genital Tract Infection with* Chlamydia trachomatis [online]. Available at: www.bashh.org/documents/65.pdf (accessed 30 April 2014).

British Association of Sexual Health and HIV: Clinical Effectiveness Group (BASHH) (2007a) *United Kingdom National Guideline on the Management of Ano-genital Warts, 2007* [online]. Available at: www.bashh.org/documents/86/86.pdf (accessed 30 April 2014).

British Association of Sexual Health and HIV: Clinical Effectiveness Group (BASHH) (2007b) *United Kingdom National Guideline on the Management of Vulvovaginal Candidiasis (2007)* [online]. Available at: www.bashh.org/documents/1798.pdf (accessed 30 April 2014).

British Association of Sexual Health and HIV: Clinical Effectiveness Group (BASHH) (2010) Chlamydia trachomatis *UK Testing Guidelines* [online]. Available at: www.bashh.org/documents/3352.pdf (accessed 30 April 2014).

British Association of Sexual Health and HIV Clinical Effectiveness Group (BASHH) (2012a) *United Kingdom National Guideline for Gonorrhoea Testing 2012* [online]. Available at: www.bashh.org/documents/4490.pdf (accessed 30 April 2014).

British Association of Sexual Health and HIV: Clinical Effectiveness Group (BASHH) (2012b) *UK National Guideline for the Management of Bacterial Vaginosis 2012* [online]. Available at: www.bashh.org/documents/4413.pdf (accessed 24 August 2013).

British Association for Sexual Health and HIV: Clinical Effectiveness Group (BASHH) (2013a)

2013 UK National Guideline for Consultations Requiring Sexual History Taking [online].
Available at: www.bashh.org/documents/Sexual%20History%20Guidelines%202013%20final.
pdf (accessed 25 August 2014).

British Association for Sexual Health and HIV (BASHH) (2013b) *Re-testing of Young Persons
Diagnosed with Chlamydia Infection* [online]. Available at: www.bashh.org/documents/
Retesting%20of%20young%20peoplediagnosed%20with%20chlamydia%20(Sep%202013).pdf
(accessed 23 November 2013).

British Association for Sexual Health and HIV, Clinical Effectiveness Group (BASHH) (2014a)
UK National Guideline for the Management of Genital Herpes in Pregnancy 2014 (draft) [online].
Available at: www.google.co.uk/?gfe_rd=cr&ei=gcqVU_jNFMmi8gOQ-YHACw&gws_
rd=ssl#q=bashh+genital+herpes (accessed 9 June 2014).

British Association of Sexual Health and HIV: Clinical Effectiveness Group (BASHH) (2014b)
United Kingdom National Guideline on the Management of Trichomonas vaginalis *2014* [online].
Available at: www.bashh.org/documents/UK%20national%20guideline%20on%20the%20
management%20of%20TV%20%202014.pdf (accessed 30 April 2014).

Burtin P, Taddio A, Ariburnu O, *et al.* (1995) Safety of metronidazole in pregnancy: a meta-
analysis. *Am J Obstet Gynecol.* **172**(2 Pt. 1): 525–9.

Clutterbuck D (2004) *Sexually Transmitted Infections and HIV.* Edinburgh: Elsevier Mosby.

Conlon CP, Snydman DR (2004) *Mosby's Color Atlas and Text of Infectious Diseases.* Edinburgh:
Mosby.

Cotch MF, Hillier SL, Gibbs RS, *et al.* (1998) Epidemiology and outcomes associated with moderate to heavy *Candida* colonisation during pregnancy. Vaginal Infections and Prematurity Study
Group. *Am J Obstet Gynecol.* **178**(2): 374–80.

Cowan F, Bell G (2011) STI control and prevention. In: Rogstad KE (editor). *ABC of Sexually
Transmitted Infections.* 6th ed. Oxford: Wiley. pp. 11–15.

Department of Health (DH) (2003) *Effective Sexual Health Promotion: a toolkit for primary care
trusts and others working in the field of promoting good sexual health and HIV prevention.*
London: DH.

Department of Health (DH) (2008) *Teenage Parents: who cares?* London: HSMO.

Department of Health (DH) (2012) Human papillomavirus (HPV). In: *Immunisation against
Infectious Disease (the Green Book)* [online]. Available at: www.gov.uk/government/organisa
tions/public-health-england/series/immunisation-against-infectious-disease-the-green-book
(accessed 24 August 2013).

Department of Health (DH) (2013) *A Framework for Sexual Health Improvement in England.*
London: DH.

Donders GG, Van Calsteren K, Bellen G, *et al.* (2009) Predictive value for preterm birth of
abnormal vaginal flora, bacterial vaginosis and aerobic vaginitis during the first trimester of
pregnancy. *BJOG.* **116**(10): 1315–24.

Eriksson K, Carlsson B, Forsum U, *et al.* (2005) A double-blind treatment study of bacterial vaginosis with normal vaginal lactobacilli after an open treatment with vaginal clindamycin ovules.
Acta Derm Venereol. **85**(1): 42–6.

Falagas ME, Betsi GI, Athanasiou S (2006) Probiotics for prevention of recurrent vulvovaginal
candidiasis: a review. *J Antimicrob Chemother.* **58**(2): 266–72.

Fenton KA, Korovessis C, Johnson AM, *et al.* (2001) Sexual behaviour in Britain: reported sexually transmitted infections and prevalent genital *Chlamydia trachomatis* infection. *Lancet.*
358(9296): 1851–4.

Fenton KA, Lowndes CM (2004) Recent trends in the epidemiology of sexually transmitted infections in the European Union. *Sex Transm Infect.* **80**(4): 255–63.

Fenton KA, Rogstad KE (2011) Sexually transmitted infections: why are they important? In: Rogstad KE (editor). *ABC of Sexually Transmitted Infections.* 6th ed. Oxford: Wiley. pp. 1–10.

Fletcher J, Ball G (2006) Chlamydia screening in pregnancy: a missed opportunity? *Br J Midwifery.* **14**(7): 390–2.

Gardella C, Brown Z (2011) Prevention of neonatal herpes. *BJOG.* **118**(2): 187–92.

Goering RV, Dockrell HM, Zuckerman M, *et al.* (2013) *Mims' Medical Microbiology.* 5th ed. Oxford: Elsevier, Saunders.

Goldenberg RL, McClure EM, Saleem S, *et al.* (2010) Infection-related stillbirths. *Lancet.* **375**(9724): 1482–90.

Gupta R, Warren T, Wald A (2007) Genital herpes. *Lancet.* **370**(9605): 2127–37.

Hay D, Kieran E (2009) Non-HIV sexually transmitted infections. *Obstet Gynaecol Reprod Med.* **19**(8): 210–14.

Hay PE, Lamont RF, Taylor-Robinson D, *et al.* (1994) Abnormal bacterial colonisation of the genital tract and subsequent preterm delivery and late miscarriage. *BMJ.* **308**(6924): 295–8.

Hay S, Oakeshott P (2005) Non-invasive chlamydia testing of pregnant teenagers. *Br J Midwifery.* **13**(7): 434–9.

Health Protection Agency (HPA) (2012) *National Chlamydia Screening Programme Standards.* 6th ed. [online]. Available at: www.chlamydiascreening.nhs.uk/ps/resources/core-requirements/NCSP%20Standards%206th%20Edition_October%202012.pdf (accessed 30 April 2014).

Health Protection Agency (HPA) (2013) *Gonococcal Resistance to Antimicrobials Surveillance Programme (GRASP) Action Plan for England and Wales: informing the public health response* [online]. Available at: http://webarchive.nationalarchives.gov.uk/20140714084352/http://www.hpa.org.uk/Publications/InfectiousDiseases/HIVAndSTIs/1302GonoccocalResistancetoAntimicrobialsSurveillance/ (accessed 18 September 2014).

Howell-Jones R, Soldan K, Wetten S, *et al.* (2013) Declining genital warts in young women in England associated with HPV 16/18 vaccination: an ecological study. *J Infect Dis.* **208**(9): 1397–403.

Jafari Y, Peeling RW, Shivkumar S, *et al.* (2013) Are *Treponema pallidum* specific rapid and point-of-care tests for syphilis accurate enough for screening in resource limited settings? Evidence from a meta-analysis. *PLoS One.* **8**(2): Epub 26 February.

Jones W, Sachs M, Buchanan P (2006) Is candida of the breast being correctly diagnosed and treated? *MIDIRS.* **16**(3): 381–6.

Khare MM, Khare MD (2007) Infections in pregnancy. In: Greer IA, Nelson–Piercy C, Walters BNJ (editors). *Maternal Medicine: medical problems in pregnancy.* Churchill Livingstone Elsevier: Edinburgh pp. 217–35.

Kieran E, Hay D (2006) Sexually transmitted infections. *Curr Obstet Gynaecol.* **16**(4): 218–25.

Kingston M, French P, Goh B, *et al.* (2008) UK national guidelines on the management of syphilis 2008. *Int J STD AIDS.* **19**(11): 729–40.

Kingston M, McAuliffe F (2011) *Update on Management of Syphilis in Pregnancy. BASHH CEG Statement* [online]. Available at: www.bashh.org/documents/3693.pdf (accessed 30 April 2014).

Klebanoff MA, Carey JC, Hauth JC, *et al.* (2001) Failure of metronidazole to prevent preterm delivery among pregnant women with asymptomatic *Trichomonas vaginalis* infection. *N Eng J Med.* **345**(7): 487–93.

Lamontagne DS, Baster K, Emmett L, *et al.* (2007) Incidence and reinfection rates of genital chlamydial infection among women aged 16–24 years attending general practice, family planning and genitourinary medicine clinics in England: a prospective cohort study by the Chlamydia Recall Study Advisory Group. *Sex Transm Infect.* **83**(4): 292–303.

Lazaro N (2013) *Sexually Transmitted Infection in Primary Care* (RCGP/BASHH) [online]. 2nd ed. Available at: www.rcgp.org.uk/clinical-and-research/clinical-resources/~/media/Files/CIRC/RCGP-Sexually-Transmitted-Infections-in-Primary-Care-2013.ashx (accessed 18 September 2014).

Manavi K (2006) A review on infection with *Chlamydia trachomatis. Best Pract Res Clin Obstet Gynaecol.* **20**(6): 941–51.

Mårdh P (2002) Influence of infection with *Chlamydia trachomatis* on pregnancy outcome, infant health and life-long sequelae in infected offspring. *Best Pract Res Clin Obstet Gynaecol.* **16**(6): 847–64.

McCance D (2009) Papillomaviruses. In: Zuckerman AJ, Banatvala JE, Schoub BD, *et al.* (editors). *Principles and Practice of Clinical Virology.* 6th ed. Chichester Wiley & Sons. pp. 807–22.

McCathie R (2006) Vaginal discharge: common causes and management. *Curr Obstet Gynaecol.* **16**(4): 211–17.

McDonald HM, Brockelhurst P, Gordon A (2007) Antibiotics for treating bacterial vaginosis in pregnancy. *Cochrane Database Syst Rev.* (1): CD000262.

McMillan A (2002) Vaginal infections and vulodynia. In: McMillan A, Young H, Ogilvie MM, *et al.* (editors). *Clinical Practice in Sexually Transmissible Infections.* Edinburgh: Saunders. pp. 474–512.

McMillan A, Ballard RC (2002) Non-specific genital tract infection and chlamydial infection, including lymphogranuloma venereum. In: McMillan A, Young H, Ogilvie MM, *et al.* (editors). *Clinical Practice in Sexually Transmissible Infections.* Edinburgh: Saunders. pp. 281–305.

McMillan A, Ogilvie MM (2002a) Herpes simplex virus infection. In: McMillan A, Young H, Ogilvie MM, *et al.* (editors). *Clinical Practice in Sexually Transmissible Infections.* Edinburgh: Saunders. pp. 107–44.

McMillan A, Ogilvie MM (2002b) Human papillomavirus. In: McMillan A, Young H, Ogilvie MM, *et al.* (editors). *Clinical Practice in Sexually Transmissible Infections.* Edinburgh: Saunders. pp. 71–102.

McMunn VA, Caan W (2007) Chlamydia infection, alcohol and sexual behaviour in women. *Br J Midwifery.* **15**(4): 221–4.

Melvin L, Cameron ST, Glasier A, *et al.* (2009) Preferred strategies of men and women for managing chlamydial infection. *BJOG.* **116**(3): 357–65.

National Institute for Health and Care Excellence (NICE) (2010) *Antenatal Care.* NICE Clinical Guideline 62 [online]. Available at: www.nice.org.uk/nicemedia/live/11947/40115/40115.pdf (accessed 18 September 2014).

Oakeshott P, Hay P, Hay S, *et al.* (2002a) Detection of *Chlamydia trachomatis* infection in early pregnancy using self-administered vaginal swabs and first pass urines: a cross-sectional community-based survey. *Br J Gen Pract.* **52**(483): 830–2.

Oakeshott P, Hay P, Hay S, *et al.* (2002b) Association between bacterial vaginosis or chlamydial infection and miscarriage before 16 weeks' gestation: prospective community based cohort study. *BMJ.* **325**(7376): 1334.

Ooi C, Dayan L (2004) STIs in pregnancy: an update for GPs. *Aust Fam Physician.* **33**(9): 723–6.

Peate I (2005) *Manual of Sexually Transmitted Infections.* London: Whurr Publishers.

Pimenta J, Catchpole M, Rogers P, *et al.* (2003) Opportunistic screening for genital chlamydia infection. 1: Acceptability of urine testing in primary and secondary healthcare settings. *Sex Transm Infect.* **79**(1): 16–21.

Public Health England (PHE) (2013) Recent epidemiology of infectious syphilis and congenital syphilis. *Health Protection Report.* **7**(44): 1 November [online]. Available at www.gov.uk/govern ment/uploads/system/uploads/attachment_data/file/336760/hpr4413_sphls.pdf (accessed 18 September 2014).

Public Health England (PHE) (2014a) Sexually transmitted infection and chlamydia screening in England 2012. *Health Protection Report.* **8**(24): 17 June 2014 [online]. Available at: www.gov.uk/ government/uploads/system/uploads/attachment_data/file/345181/Volume_8_number_24_ hpr2414_AA_stis.pdf (accessed 18 September 2014).

Public Health England (PHE) (2014b) *Table 5: Number of STI diagnoses and services in England 2009-2013* [online]. Available at: www.gov.uk/government/uploads/system/uploads/ attachment_data/file/340439/Table_5_All_STI_diagnoses_and_services_by_gender_and_ sexual_risk.pdf (accessed 18 September 2014).

Roos T, Baker DA (2011) Cytomegalovirus, herpes simplex virus, adenovirus, Coxsackievirus, and human papillomavirus. In: James D (editor). *High Risk Pregnancy: management options.* 4th ed. New York: Elsevier Saunders pp. 503–20.

Rours GI, Hammerschlag MR, VanDoornum GJ, *et al.* (2009) *Chlamydia trachomatis* respiratory infection in Dutch infants. *Arch Dis Child.* **94**(9): 705–7.

Schachter J, McCormack WM, Chernesky MA, *et al.* (2003) Vaginal swabs are appropriate spec-imens for diagnosis of genital tract infection with *Chlamydia trachomatis. J Clin Microbiol.* **41**(8): 3784–9.

Schiffer J, Swan D, Magaret A, *et al.* (2011) Rapid spread of herpes simplex virus-2 in the human genital tract. *Sex Transm Infect.* **87**: A84–5.

Schwebke J (2007) Trichomoniasis. In: Klauser JD, Hook EW (editors). *Current Diagnosis and Treatment of Sexually Transmitted Diseases.* New York: McGraw Medical. pp. 116–18.

Scottish Intercollegiate Guidelines Network (SIGN) (2009) *Management of Genital* Chlamydia trachomatis *Infection.* National Clinical Guideline 109 [online]. Available at: www.sign.ac.uk/ pdf/sign109.pdf (accessed 23 November 2013).

Senok AC, Verstraelen H, Temmerman M, *et al.* (2009) Probiotics for the treatment of bacterial vaginosis. *Cochrane Database Syst Rev.* (4): CD 006289.

Sheffield JS, Andrews WW, Klebanoff MA, *et al.* (2005) Spontaneous resolution of asymptomatic *Chlamydia trachomatis* in pregnancy. *Obstet Gynecol.* **105**(3): 557–62.

Stamm CA, McGregor JA, French JI, *et al.* (2008) Other sexually transmitted diseases and geni-tourinary tract infections. In: Rosene-Montella K, Keely E, Barbour LA, *et al.* (editors). *Medical Care of the Pregnant Patient.* 2nd ed. Philadelphia: ACP Press. pp. 672–82.

Stanberry LR (2006) *Understanding Herpes.* Mississippi: University Press of Mississippi.

Tookey P, Peckham C (2006) G192 The epidemiology of neonatal herpes simplex virus infection in the UK and Ireland: surveillance through the BPSU 2004–05 [abstract]. *Arch Dis Child.* **91**(Suppl. 1): A64–70.

UK National Screening Committee (UK NSC) (2010) *Infectious Diseases in Pregnancy Screening Programme: programme standards* [online]. Available at: http://infectiousdiseases.screening. nhs.uk/publications (accessed 18 September 2013).

UK National Screening Committee (UK NSC) (2011) *Screening for Chlamydia Infection in Pregnancy* [online]. Available at: www.screening.nhs.uk/policydb_download.php?doc=125 (accessed 22 August 2013).

UK National Screening Committee (UK NSC) (2013) *Screening for Syphilis in Pregnancy: external review against programme appraisal criteria for the UK national screening Committee (UK NSC)* [online]. Available at: www.screening.nhs.uk/syphilis (accessed 30 April 2014).

Wilson J (2011) Sexually transmitted infections and HIV in pregnancy. In: Rogstad KE (editor). *ABC of Sexually Transmitted Infections*. 6th ed. Oxford: Wiley. pp. 59–63.

World Health Organization (WHO) (2007) *The Global Elimination of Congenital Syphilis: rationale and strategy for action* [online]. Available at: www.who.int/reproductivehealth/publications/rtis/9789241595858/en/ (accessed 22 August 2013).

World Health Organization (WHO) (2010) *Developing Sexual Health Programmes: a framework for action* [online]. Available at: http://whqlibdoc.who.int/hq/2010/WHO_RHR_HRP_10.22_eng.pdf?ua=1 (accessed 18 September 2014).

Ya W, Reifer C, Miller LE (2010) Efficacy of vaginal probiotic capsules for recurrent bacterial vaginosis. *Am J Obstet Gynecol.* **203**(2): 120–6.

Young H, McMillan A (2002) Gonorrhea. In: McMillan A, Young H, Ogilvie MM, *et al.* (editors). *Clinical Practice in Sexually Transmissible Infections*. Edinburgh: Saunders. pp. 313–53.

Yudin MH (2011) Other infectious conditions. In: James D, Steer PJ, Weiner CP, *et al.* (editors). *High Risk Pregnancy: management options*. 4th ed. Edinburgh: Elsevier Saunders. pp. 521–42.

CHAPTER 6

Group B streptococcus

Group B streptococcus (GBS) will rarely cause infection in adults: those at risk are pregnant women, individuals who are immunosuppressed or have serious underlying medical conditions or the elderly, but most commonly, and severely, it occurs in newborn babies, either as early or late onset. In many countries in the world GBS is routinely screened for in pregnancy; however, currently the UK tests and treats only those women with risk factors. This is an area of much controversy at present.

HISTORY AND EPIDEMIOLOGY

Screening during pregnancy is routinely carried out in most of the developed world (Australia and New Zealand, North America and parts of South America, and much of Europe); however, the UK does not undertake this, despite evidence that the rate of GBS-infected neonates is rising, in contrast to a fall in most countries where routine screening takes place (Steer & Plumb 2011). At present in the UK, the National Screening Committee's policy position on GBS is that screening should not be offered routinely (UK NSC 2012) and a risk factor-based approach is used (*see* Box 6.3 for a list of risk factors). However, only about 60% of neonates with early-onset GBS had mothers who demonstrated a risk factor in pregnancy or labour (Heath *et al.* 2004, Daniels *et al.* 2011). A registered charity called Group B Strep Support (GBSS), as well as many practitioners, is campaigning for routine screening, via a vaginal/rectal swab at 35–37 weeks' gestation, to be introduced into antenatal care in the UK. However, at present it seems the rate of GBS infection in the UK has an incidence rate comparable with the US rate despite the US policy of universal screening (Bedford Russell 2010, RCOG 2012).

Group B haemolytic streptococci was first mentioned in 1887 (Heath & Schuchat 2007), but the first description of GBS sepsis in a neonate did not occur until 1964 (Ohlsson & Shah 2013). Since the 1970s GBS has continued to be identified as one of the most common causes of neonatal morbidity and mortality in the developed world (Kaambwa *et al.* 2010). In the UK GBS sepsis is the most common cause of life-threatening infection in the neonate (Edmond *et al.* 2012) and is estimated to be 0.45–0.64 per 1000 live births (RCOG 2012, Steer & Plumb 2011). In the United States, GBS remains a leading cause of neonatal morbidity and mortality (Dermer *et al.* 2004, Steer & Plumb 2011) despite dramatic reductions of about 70%–80% (Jordon *et al.* 2008) since GBS guidelines (involving routine assessment at 35–37 weeks' gestation and intravenous (IV) antibiotic treatment in labour for all high-risk women) were implemented. It is also thought that there is currently an increasing rate of GBS neonatal infection in developing countries (Ohlsson & Shah 2013).

GBS infection in the neonate is divided into 'early onset' (EOGBS), defined as from birth to 3–7 days old (these cut-off days are the most common, although the literature is not consistent, and different countries have various definitions), and 'late onset' (LOGBS – *see* Box 6.1), 3–7 days to 3 months of age. Since LOGBS is frequently outside the remit of the midwife (although she should ensure the mother has a good knowledge of basic hygiene measures and how to recognise a sick baby), only EOGBS will be discussed in this chapter.

BOX 6.1 LATE-ONSET GROUP B STREPTOCOCCUS

LOGBS in the neonate may be the result of infection transmitted from a mother carrying GBS, but it may also come from others – GBS can be transmitted by skin-to-skin contact or via the respiratory system. It has been estimated that a significant number of LOGBS-affected babies have GBS-negative mothers, or those who are colonised with a different serotype (Yudin 2011). The recommended treatments for EOGBS have not been shown to prevent LOGBS (Dermer *et al.* 2004) and there is currently no known prophylaxis. The risk of a baby developing a GBS infection decreases with age; it is rare after 1 month of age and virtually unknown after 3 months.

CLINICAL FEATURES AND TRANSMISSION

Streptococci are divided into at least 20 different types, called Lancefield groups. The main Lancefield types of beta-haemolytic streptococci are group A, group B and groups C–G. Also known as *Streptococcus agalactiae*, GBS is a Gram-positive coccus. It is divided into eight serotypes (I–VIII) and recently a new serotype (IX) was isolated (Slotved *et al.* 2007). Type I is further subclassified (Ia, Ib and Ia/c) (Mullaney 2001), according to the specific capsular polysaccharides (Lachenauer *et al.* 1999), and it is this polysaccharide antiphagocytic capsule that is its main virulence factor. In general, most EOGBS is caused by types Ia, II, III and V, while LOGBS is mainly serotype III (Heath & Schuchat 2007). The predominant serotypes have changed over time and vary in different geographic regions.

In both men and women the normal reservoir for GBS is the gastrointestinal tract, and it is carried by up to 30% of adults. Once colonised, antibiotics are unlikely to completely eradicate it. In the United States, colonisation rates have been shown to vary between ethnic group, geographic locations and by age (Steer & Plumb 2011). Women may develop antibodies against certain types of GBS, and these may offer some protection to the neonate – one reason young women are at higher risk is that they may not have previously been exposed to antigens and therefore have not built up immunity (Bhushan *et al.* 1998).

In women colonisation of the gut commonly leads to transient colonisation of the vagina and urinary tract. Although this may be normal and intermittent, when GBS is found in the urine during pregnancy, the woman will probably receive treatment – and she then may be offered IV antibiotics in labour. Approximately one in three women are carriers of GBS (Dermer *et al.* 2004) and the vast majority will be unaware of this, as GBS will cause no signs or symptoms – or harm. It is estimated that GBS will normally – and intermittently – colonise the lower genital tract of 15%–40% of women at any one time (Woensdregt *et al.* 2008).

GBS is not classified as a sexually transmitted disease, although it can be transferred between partners. However, skin-to-skin or respiratory transmission is possible. GBS is also common in cattle and fish, and it may be acquired through food (Foxman *et al.* 2007). The colonisation, or infection, of the fetus or neonate is usually a result of ascending GBS from the mother's vagina, and many adults will be have been originally colonised, with no ill effects, in this way.

In pregnancy, although the majority of women colonised with GBS are asymptomatic, GBS can cause urinary tract infections, or, more rarely, amnionitis, endometritis, sepsis or meningitis (Woensdregt *et al.* 2008). During pregnancy, despite the ability of GBS to cross intact membranes, it is considered that the vast majority of infections occur during labour and/or after membrane rupture (Steer & Plumb 2011). If caesarean section is undertaken before labour commences or the membranes rupture, the incidence of neonatal GBS is extremely low (Verani *et al.* 2010) and therefore antibiotic prophylaxis is not thought necessary (Steer & Plumb 2011).

Premature babies are most at risk of becoming infected and dying or sustaining long-term damage because of their relatively undeveloped immune system. It is estimated that at least 25% of all cases of GBS infection occur in premature babies (Van Dyke *et al.* 2009), as well as 65% of the deaths (UK NSC 2012). The risk to babies of women who carry GBS has been expressed in several ways. The organisation GBSS (2011) quotes potential outcomes for a baby born to a GBS colonised mother who received no treatment.

If 230 000 babies are born to women who carry GBS each year:

- 88 000 (1:8) become colonised with GBS
- 700 babies develop severe GBS infection
- about 75–100 babies die from GBS infection

- most babies recover from GBS infection with no long-term damage
- up to half of survivors of GBS meningitis suffer permanent (mild to severe) mental and/or physical problems.

Brocklehurst and Kenyon (2008) suggest that for every woman who carries GBS in her genital tract in late pregnancy, the risk of neonatal death from EOGBS is 0.03%. Other sources have estimated that in the absence of medical interventions, approximately 1%–2% of infants whose mothers were colonised by GBS at delivery will develop EOGBS (Clifford *et al.* 2012). It has been estimated that 1000–1191 women would need to be treated to prevent 1–1.4 cases of neonatal infection (McCartney 2012, Angstetra *et al.* 2007).

PREVENTION AND MANAGEMENT

Prevention and/or treatment of GBS for the neonate begins with treatment of the GBS-positive mother and may include:

- antenatal identification of risk factors
- antenatal screening
- identification of risk factors in labour
- antibiotic treatment in labour
- monitoring/care of the neonate.

Antenatal care and identification of risk factors

During booking, the midwife can identify any pre-existing history of GBS. A woman who has had a GBS-infected baby previously will usually be offered IV antibiotics in labour, whether or not she has screened positive herself during the current pregnancy (Steer & Plumb 2011, RCOG 2012).

Routine urinalysis in pregnancy may reveal asymptomatic bacteruria caused by GBS. This will be treated with antibiotics and the woman is now considered at high risk for transmitting GBS to her newborn – she will usually be offered antibiotic therapy in labour (RCOG 2012). The importance of routine screening of pregnant women's urine is underpinned by the increased rate of premature labour or rupture of membranes and associated intrapartum chorioamnionitis, in the presence of GBS colonisation (Yudin 2011).

There is some question about whether it is safe for a woman carrying GBS to have a membrane sweep at term plus. At present there is no evidence or professional guidance, but the GBSS (2011) suggests there is a theoretical risk of GBS in the lower vagina being introduced into the uterus, so perhaps a prostaglandin gel induction may be advisable.

Screening

Many babies who develop early-onset GBS infection are born to women who had no risk factors at delivery apart from carrying GBS (Heath *et al.* 2004, 2009) and if screening is not undertaken, neither they nor their caregivers will be aware of the risk. Although screening swabs are not offered routinely to women in UK practice at present, a swab may be done, according to local guidelines, if there are risk factors present (*see* Box 6.3).

Both rectal and vaginal swabs are recommended (ACOG 2002). A rectal swab will be most likely to show the presence of GBS, as this is the normal site for colonisation. A low vaginal swab is recommended, as this is obviously the vaginal area most likely to be colonised – a high vaginal swab is likely to test negative, even when there is GBS present in the lower vagina.

GBS colonising the vagina is thought to be intermittent in many women. The optimum time for testing for GBS in pregnancy is considered to be between 35 and 37 weeks' gestation. It has been demonstrated that a positive result in this period will indicate an approximately 87% chance she will be positive at delivery, and only about 4% who test negative will be positive at delivery (Yancey *et al.* 1996).

Consideration must be taken as to the method of testing (*see* Box 6.2). One reason for a false negative result could be inappropriate sampling methods, the choice of media the sample was plated on, or suboptimal transport to the laboratory (Towers *et al.* 2010).

There is much work being undertaken towards development of a rapid 'bedside'

BOX 6.2 SCREENING FOR GROUP B STREPTOCOCCUS

- *Rectal and vaginal swab – direct plating method.* This is the normal swab done at present in the National Health Service for most reasons. If the result is positive for GBS it is considered to be very reliable; however, it has been estimated that up to 50% of the negative results are false negatives (Benitz *et al.* 1999) leaving the woman – and her caregivers – with a false sense of security.
- *Rectal and vaginal swab – enriched culture medium.* This is the swab considered to be most effective by the Health Protection Agency (HPA 2006); however, it is not widely available in the National Health Service. Women often access this test privately.
- *Polymerase chain reaction* may be available in the future to provide a 'bedside' test for GBS during labour (Honest *et al.* 2006). Since preterm birth is a high-risk group for EOGBS infection, this would be a particularly useful tool if it were found to be efficient to administer and if the outcome could be available in time for the optimum 4 hours of IV antibiotics to be achieved (Daniels *et al.* 2011).

test that a woman could have when in labour and which would give results in time for sufficient intrapartum antibiotic prophylaxis to be given (Young *et al.* 2011, Honest *et al.* 2006). Although some women labour too quickly for this to be useful, for many women it may be an appropriate choice.

Risk factors

In the UK at present, treatment in labour for GBS is highly dependent on identification of risk factors in the mother. Maternity units will have their own individual protocols concerning risk factors (and what combination of them will trigger which treatment). Box 6.3 lists all risk factors for possible GBS colonisation.

BOX 6.3 RISK FACTORS FOR POSSIBLE GBS COLONISATION AT DELIVERY

- Previous baby with GBS infection
- Teenage mother
- GBS identified during pregnancy (urine specimen and/or vaginal/rectal swab)
- Gestational diabetes
- Gestational age <37 weeks
- Gestational age >42 weeks
- Preterm pre-labour rupture of membranes
- Pre-labour rupture of membranes
- Prolonged membrane rupture (more than 12–18 hours)
- Prolonged labour
- Maternal infection including chorioamnionitis
- Maternal pyrexia (≥37.8°C/38°C) in labour
- Birthweight <2500 g

Labour care and antibiotics

A woman carrying undiagnosed GBS may present with premature labour, preterm pre-labour rupture of membranes or pre-labour rupture of membranes. The Royal College of Obstetricians and Gynaecologists (RCOG 2012) does not recommend routine antibiotic therapy for any of these conditions; however, the existence of other risk factors may trigger routine IV antibiotic administration. Each local area should have established protocols on care of women with GBS risk factors.

A woman with known GBS colonisation and term pre-labour rupture of membranes, may be offered an immediate induction of labour with IV oxytocin. Pre-labour rupture of membranes may be caused by GBS, although opinions vary on this (Kenyon *et al.* 2001a, b, McKenzie *et al.* 1994).

The underlying basis of care for women carrying GBS is IV antibiotics in labour (or from rupture of membranes), as this has been shown to reduce the colonisation of the newborn, and therefore the infection rate (Heath & Schuchat 2007). These will be given according to local protocol, but it usually involves a 'loading' dose and then regular administration every 4 hours until delivery. A minimum amount of antibiotic received by the woman to be effective is not clear: 4 hours (e.g. two doses) has been suggested (GBSS 2011), but others (RCOG 2012) have said one dose a minimum of 2 hours before delivery would be beneficial, if that was all that could be fitted in before an imminent delivery.

Intravenous antibiotic use need not restrict a woman's labour unduly, although it is unlikely a home birth will be possible. The antibiotics may be given as a slow injection through a cannula or, if given via an IV infusion, this can be taken down between doses, allowing the woman increased mobility. The cannula site can be covered with waterproof covering if she wishes to use a birthing pool or take a shower. There is no evidence that access to water birth should be denied because of GBS status (Zanetti-Dällenbach *et al.* 2007, Plumb *et al.* 2007).

Despite evidence of the effectiveness of using IV antibiotics in labour for preventing neonatal GBS infection in women who screened positive in pregnancy to GBS, there are nevertheless potential unintended consequences of antibiotic use. Women can react to the drugs, either with a mild allergic reaction (such as a rash) or with a severe anaphylaxis (Berthier *et al.* 2007). As with antibiotic use for any cause, the risk of a yeast infection is increased (Dinsmoor *et al.* 2005). There is also the risk of the development of resistant strains of any infection (Barcaite *et al.* 2008), and this has been reported to have occurred in the United States, with clindamycin, the antibiotic of choice when the woman is allergic to penicillin (Heath & Schuchat 2007). Manning *et al.* (2003) suggested that even when antibiotics were given to the mother, about 30% of babies were infected, and 10% died, and this may be due to resistant strains of GBS.

Low-dose antibiotics have historically been used as a growth enhancer in farm animals, because of the change in metabolism caused by alteration in intestinal bacteria, and there has also been literature detailing the association of early exposure of antibiotics to infants and increased early-life body mass (Trasande *et al.* 2012). There has been some suggestion, although this is by no means clear, that antibiotics given to the mother may increase the risk of the baby developing allergies (Law *et al.* 2005, Murch 2001), in particular cow's milk intolerance (GBSS 2011) as well as future long-term effects to the baby's immune system (Bedford Russell & Murch 2006). Antibiotic use in the neonate may also lead to an increase in infants developing antibiotic-resistant infections (Daley & Garland 2004). A recent study looking at premature labour, assessing antibiotics (although not those usually used for GBS) demonstrated some increase in long-term functional impairment to children (Kenyon *et al.* 2008). The risks and benefits of any treatment need to be clearly discussed with the woman, so she can make a properly informed choice that is right for her and her baby.

There has been mention of alternative strategies, such as chlorhexidine used as a vaginal disinfectant during labour, or to wash the baby following birth; however, this has not been demonstrated to be effective in reducing infection (Cutland *et al.* 2009).

Assessment and care of neonate

Some units have introduced a single antibiotic intramuscular injection, for babies of mothers who should have received intrapartum antibiotic prophylaxis but did not (usually those who laboured too fast to receive this). This should be given within 1–2 hours of birth (Woodgate *et al.* 2012).

Maternity units will have specific policies in place to deal with individual cases; however, it has been suggested that babies born to mothers carrying GBS, but with no other risk factor, do not necessarily need antibiotics. As 80%–90% of EOGBS infections occur with 12 hours of birth (Heath *et al.* 2009), careful observation of the neonate (*see* Box 6.4) for up to 48 hours should be undertaken. Newborns usually present with signs of respiratory disease, sepsis and/or meningitis (Ohlsson & Shah 2013), although meningitis is more common with LOGBS. In at least 60% of newborn infected babies, there are signs apparent at birth (Faxelius *et al.* 1988) or in the first 90 minutes of life (Yudin 2011). A useful algorithm (*see* Figure 6.1) has been designed by GBSS (2011) and suggests one regimen for these babies at risk.

BOX 6.4 POSSIBLE SIGNS OF NEONATAL GBS INFECTION

- Inability to maintain body temperature
- Inability to maintain blood sugar
- Abnormally high or low temperature, respiratory rate and/or heart rate
- Lethargy
- Poor feeding
- Seizure activity

(Bromberger *et al.* 2000)

GBS infection in the neonate would be diagnosed when the bacteria was grown from usually sterile body fluids – normally blood, urine or spinal fluid. As sometimes these tests are not completely reliable, and as they may take some time to produce a result, attention will also be paid to signs and symptoms (*see* Box 6.4) and general blood tests such as white blood cell count, platelet count and C-reactive protein. If a baby who is one of a multiple birth develops GBS infection, the other baby or babies are at increased risk of also becoming infected and will usually be given antibiotics as prophylaxis (GBSS 2011).

With any policy that involves treating some women with antibiotics following the start of labour to prevent GBS infection, a strategy for the subsequent management of the newborn baby required. Below is GBSS's recommended paediatric prevent on strategy against early-onset GBS infection (reproduced with permission)

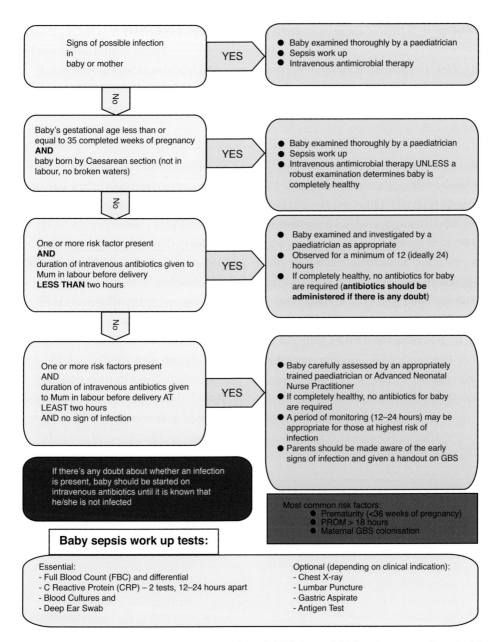

FIGURE 6.1 Suggested care for babies at risk of GBS (from GBSS, 2011, reproduced with permission)

Postnatal care of the mother

Breastfeeding can theoretically transfer GBS to a neonate, but as the bacterium will probably stay within the baby's gastric system, infection is unlikely (Steer & Plumb 2011). The benefits of breastfeeding will far outweigh this very rare risk and there is no evidence to discourage breastfeeding (RCOG 2012).

GBS can cause an antenatal (urinary tract infection or chorionamnionitis) or postnatal infection (wound infection, endometritis, septicaemia or urinary tract infection), but antibiotics usually easily eradicate these. The midwife will be instrumental in identifying these infections and referring for the appropriate treatment.

Long term: mother and baby

Much work is being undertaken to develop a vaccine (Johri *et al.* 2006). A clear advantage of such a vaccine over current practice would be the additional benefit of protection against LOGBS.

There is a small risk (1%–3%) of a baby who has recovered from GBS infection becoming re-infected; long-term antibiotics may be prescribed, although there is no evidence to support this as a routine practice (GBSS 2011).

ROLE OF THE MIDWIFE

- Maintain an up-to-date knowledge of GBS, a frequently changing field, to ensure that all questions from pregnant women can be accurately and comprehensively answered.
- Sustain a good working knowledge of labour ward protocols in individual places of work, in order to determine when antibiotics are to be prescribed in labour.
- Ensure the ability to effectively monitor all newborns, recognise the signs and symptoms of infection, and refer as necessary.
- Teach women about general assessment of well-being of the neonate.

USEFUL RESOURCES

- Group B Strep Support is a national charity offering information and support to parents affected by GBS and to health professionals. GBSS also campaigns to raise awareness of how GBS infections in newborns can be prevented, and supports research into GBS prevention. Information can be obtained from their comprehensive website (www.gbss.org.uk).
- Royal College of Obstetricians and Gynaecologists (RCOG) (2012) *The Prevention of Early-Onset Neonatal Group B Streptococcal Disease.* London, RCOG.

REFERENCES

American College of Obstetricians and Gynecologists (ACOG) (2002) ACOG Committee Opinion: number 279, December 2002. Prevention of early-onset group B streptococcal disease in newborns. *Obstet Gynecol.* **100**(6): 1405–12.

Angstetra D, Ferguson J, Giles W (2007) Institution of universal screening for Group B streptococcus from a risk management protocol results in reduction of early-onset GBS disease in a tertiary obstetric unit. *Aust N Z J Obstet Gynaecol.* **47**(5): 378–82.

Barcaite E, Bartusevicius A, Tameliene R, *et al.* (2008) Prevalence of maternal group B streptococcal colonisation in European countries. *Acta Obstet Gynecol Scand.* **87**(3): 260–71.

Bedford Russell A (2010) Neonatal sepsis. *Paediatr Child Health.* **21**(6): 265–9.

Bedford Russell A, Murch S (2006) Could peripartum antibiotics have delayed health consequences for the infant? *BJOG.* **113**(7): 758–65.

Benitz W, Gould J, Druzin M (1999) Risk factors for early-onset group B streptococcal sepsis: estimation of odds ratios by critical literature review. *Pediatrics.* **103**(6): e77.

Berthier A, Sentilhes L, Hamou L, *et al.* (2007) [Antibiotics at term: questions about five severe allergic accidents] [French]. *Gynecol Obstet Fertil.* **35**(5): 464–72.

Bhushan R, Anthony BF, Frasch CE (1998) Estimation of group B streptococcus type III polysaccharide-specific antibody concentrations in human sera is antigen dependent. *Infect Immun.* **66**(12): 5848–53.

Brocklehurst P, Kenyon S (2008) *Evaluation of Antenatal Screening for Group B Streptococcal (GBS) Carriage against NSC Handbook Criteria* [online]. Available from: www.screening.nhs.uk/policydb_download.php?doc=44 (accessed 14 March 2014).

Bromberger P, Lawrence J, Braun D, *et al.* (2000) The influence of intrapartum antibiotics on the clinical spectrum of early-onset group B streptococcal infection in infants. *Pediatrics.* **106**(2 Pt. 1): 244–50.

Clifford V, Garland S, Grimwood K (2012) Prevention of neonatal group B streptococcus disease in the 21st century. *J Paediatr Child Health.* **48**(9): 808–15.

Cutland C, Madhi S, Zell E, *et al.* PoPS Trial Team (2009) PoPS Trial: Chlorhexidine maternal-vaginal and neonate body wipes in sepsis and vertical transmission of pathogenic bacteria in South Africa: a randomised, controlled trial. *Lancet.* **374**(9705): 1909–16.

Daley A, Garland S (2004) Prevention of neonatal Group B strep disease: progress, challenges and dilemmas. *J Paediatr Child Health.* **40**(12): 664–8.

Daniels J, Gray J, Pattison H, *et al.* GBS Collaborative Group (2011) Intrapartum tests for group B streptococcus: accuracy and acceptability of screening. *BJOG.* **118**(2): 257–65.

Dermer P, Lee C, Eggert M, *et al.* (2004) A history of neonatal group B streptococcus with its related morbidity and mortality rates in the United States. *J Pediatr Nurs.* **19**(5): 357–63.

Dinsmoor M, Viloria R, Leif L, *et al.* (2005) Use of intrapartum antibiotics and the incidence of postnatal maternal and neonatal yeast infections. *Obstet Gynecol.* **106**(1): 19–22.

Edmond K, Kortsalioudaki C, Scott S, *et al.* (2012) GBS disease in infants aged younger than 3 months: systemic review and meta-analysis. *Lancet.* **379**(9815): 547–56.

Faxelius G, Bremme K, Kvist-Christensen, *et al.* (1988) Neonatal septicaemia due to group B streptococci – perinatal risk factors and outcome of subsequent pregnancies. *J Perinat Med.* **16**(5–6): 423–30.

Foxman B, Gillespie B, Manning S, *et al.* (2007) Risk factors for group B streptococcal colonization: potential for different transmission systems by capsular type. *Ann Epidemiol.* **17**(11): 854–62.

Group B Strep Support (GBSS) (2011) *Group B Streptococcus: the facts for health professionals* [online]. Available at: www.gbss.org.uk/filepool/2012_07_13_The_Facts_4_HealthProfessionals.pdf (accessed 18 September 2014).

Health Protection Agency (HPA) (2006) *Processing Swabs for Group B Streptococcal Carriage.* National Standard Method BSOP 58 Issue 2. Available at: www.hpa-standardmethods.org.uk/pdf_sops.asp

Heath P, Balfour G, Tighe H, *et al.* (2009) Group B streptococcal disease in infants: a case control study. *Arch Dis Child.* **94**(9): 674–80.

Heath P, Balfour G, Weisner A, *et al.* (2004) Group B streptococcal disease in UK and Irish infants younger than 90 days. *Lancet.* **363**(9405): 292–4.

Heath P, Schuchat A (2007) Perinatal group B streptococcal disease. *Best Pract Res Clin Obstet Gynaecol.* **21**(3): 411–12.

Honest H, Sharma S, Khan K (2006) Rapid tests for group B streptococcus colonization in laboring women: a systematic review. *Pediatrics.* **117**(4): 1055–66.

Johri A, Paoletti L, Glaser P, *et al.* (2006) Group B streptococcus: global incidence and vaccine development. *Nat Rev Microbiol.* **4**(12): 932–42.

Jordon H, Farley M, Craig A, *et al.* (2008) Revisiting the need for vaccine prevention of late-onset neonatal group B streptococcal disease: a multistate, population-based analysis. *Pediatr Infect Dis J.* **27**(12): 1057–64.

Kaambwa B, Bryan S, Gray J, *et al.* (2010) Cost-effectiveness of rapid tests and other existing strategies for screening and management of early-onset group B streptococcus during labour. *BJOG.* **117**(13): 1616–27.

Kenyon S, Pike K, Jones D, *et al.* (2008) Childhood outcomes following prescription of antibiotics with spontaneous preterm labour: 7-year follow-up of the ORACLE II trial. *Lancet.* **372**(9646): 1319–27.

Kenyon S, Taylor D, Tarnow-Mordi W; ORACLE Collaborative Group (2001a) Broad-spectrum antibiotics for preterm, prelabour rupture of fetal membranes: the ORACLE I randomised trial. *Lancet.* **357**(9261): 979–88.

Kenyon S, Taylor D, Tarnow-Mordi W; ORACLE Collaborative Group (2001b) Broad-spectrum antibiotics for spontaneous preterm labour: the ORACLE ll randomised trial. *Lancet.* **357**(9261): 989–94.

Lachenauer C, Kasper D, Shimada J, *et al.* (1999) Serotypes VI and VIII predominate among group B streptococci isolated from pregnant Japanese women. *J Infect Dis.* **179**(4): 1030–3.

Law M, Palomaki G, Alfirevic Z, *et al.* (2005) The prevention of neonatal group B streptococcal disease: a report by a working group of the Medical Screening Society. *J Med Screen.* **12**(2): 60–8.

Manning SD, Foxman B, Pierson CL, *et al.* (2003) Correlates of antibiotic-resistant group B streptococcus isolated from pregnant women. *Obstet Gynecol.* **101**(1): 74–9.

McCartney M (2012) Streptococcus B in pregnancy: to screen or not to screen? *BMJ.* **344**: e2803.

McKenzie H, Donnet M, Howie P, *et al.* (1994) Risk of preterm delivery in pregnant women with group B streptococcal urinary infections or urinary antibodies to group B streptococcal and *E. coli* antigens. *Br J Obstet Gynaecol.* **101**(2): 107–13.

Mullaney D (2001) Group B streptococcal infections in newborns. *J Obstet Gynecol Neonat Nurs.* **30**(6): 649–58.

Murch S (2001) Toll of allergy reduced by probiotics. *Lancet.* **357**(9262): 1057–9.

Ohlsson A, Shah V (2013) Intrapartum antibiotics for known maternal Group B streptococcal colonization. *Cochrane Database Syst Rev.* (3): CD007467.

Plumb J, Holwell D, Burton R, *et al.* (2007) Waterbirth for women with GBS: a pipe dream? *Pract Midwife.* **10**(4): 25–8.

Royal College of Obstetricians and Gynaecologists (RCOG) (2012) *The Prevention of Early-Onset Neonatal Group B Streptococcal Disease.* London: RCOG.

Slotved H, Kong F, Lambertsen L, *et al.* (2007) Serotype IX, a proposed new *Streptococcus agalactiae* serotype. *J Clin Microbiol.* **45**(9): 2929–36.

Steer P, Plumb J (2011) Myth: group B streptococcal infection in pregnancy; comprehended and conquered. *Semin Fetal Neonatal Med.* **16**(5): 254–8.

Towers C, Rumney P, Asrat T, *et al.* (2010) The accuracy of late third-trimester antenatal screening for group B streptococcus in predicting colonization at delivery. *Am J Perinatol.* **27**(10): 785–90.

Trasande L, Blustein J, Liu M, *et al.* (2012) Infant antibiotic exposure and early-life body mass. *Int J Obes (Lond).* **37**(1): 16–23.

UK National Screening Committee (UK NSC) (2012) *Group B streptococcus: the UK NSC policy on group B streptococcus screening in pregnancy.* London, NSC. Available at: www.screening.nhs.uk/groupbstreptococcus (accessed 18 September 2014).

Van Dyke M, Phares C, Lynfield R, *et al.* (2009) Evaluation of universal antenatal screening for group B streptococcus. *N Engl J Med.* **360**(25): 2626–36.

Verani JR, McGee L, Schrag SJ; Division of Bacterial Diseases, National Center for Immunization and Respiratory Diseases, Centers for Disease Control and Prevention (CDC) (2010) Prevention of perinatal group B streptococcal disease: revised guidelines from CDC, 2010. *MMWR Recomm Rep.* **59**(RR-10): 1–36.

Woensdregt K, Lee H, Norwitz E (2008) Infectious diseases in pregnancy. In: Funai E, Evans M, Lockwood C (editors). *High Risk Obstetrics: the requisites in obstetrics and gynecology.* New York: Mosby, Elsevier. pp. 287–316.

Woodgate P, Flenady V, Steer P (2004) Intramuscular penicillin for the prevention of early onset group B streptococcal infection in newborn infants. *Cochrane Database Syst Rev.* (3): CD003667.

Yancey M, Schuchat A, Brown L, *et al.* (1996) The accuracy of late antenatal screening cultures in predicting genital group B streptococcal colonization at delivery. *Obstet Gynecol.* **88**(5): 811–15.

Young B, Dodge L, Gupta M, *et al.* (2011) Evaluation of a rapid real-time intrapartum group B streptococcus assay. *Am J Obstet Gynecol.* **205**(4): 372.e1–6.

Yudin M (2011) Other infectious conditions. In: James D, Steer P, Winer C, *et al.* (editors). *High Risk Pregnancy: management options.* 4th ed. New York: Elsevier, Saunders. pp. 521–42.

Zanetti-Dällenbach R, Holzgreve W, Hösli I (2007) Neonatal group B streptococcus colonization in water births. *Int J Gynaecol Obstet.* **98**(1): 54–5.

CHAPTER 7

Human immunodeficiency virus

INTRODUCTION

The human immunodeficiency virus (HIV) is a relatively new infection, first being diagnosed in the early 1980s. Initially the condition was seen as a 'gay disease' being mainly identified in homosexual men (or MSM: men who have sex with men); however, very quickly it was discovered that heterosexual transmission was not only possible but also common. It was also initially assumed that once diagnosed with HIV, the acute phase (acquired immune deficiency syndrome: AIDS) followed rapidly, and death would ensue almost immediately. If a woman with HIV were to become pregnant, this prognosis and the assumption that the baby would also be infected, led to many women terminating their pregnancies.

Currently, however, HIV is seen as a chronic medical condition, which, if untreated, is still associated with high morbidity and mortality, but for those having access to knowledgeable medical care and an expensive drug regimen when necessary, a relatively normal life can be enjoyed. This same increase in understanding of the condition, and the development of ever-more effective drugs, has resulted in many babies being born disease-free to HIV-positive women who are healthy enough to enjoy motherhood.

Epidemiology

HIV is broadly divided into HIV-1 and HIV-2, and although distinct biologically, they are morphologically similar (Pratt 2003). HIV-2 is more closely related to the simian immunodeficiency viruses that cause disease in many species of monkeys, and it is less common and thought to be less easily transferable and less virulent (Calles *et al.* 2010). There are various strains and subtypes that have been identified and are generally local to different parts of the world. However, with increasing travel the subtype distribution is changing and mixed. This may have an impact on different rates of disease progression or the response of individuals to drug therapy.

HIV is a disease with radically different outcomes in different parts of the world, and outcomes will be directly related to the resources available to provide expensive drugs and other aspects of specialised care. Since identification of HIV, it is estimated that throughout the world over 25 million people have died, and there were approximately 1.7 million deaths in 2011 (WHO 2012). It is estimated that 34 million people are infected worldwide (Avert 2010); however, the majority of severe illness at present is in resource-poor areas.

In 2011 it was estimated that approximately 96 000 people were HIV positive in the UK, an increase from 91 500 in 2010 (HPA 2012a). Women, mostly of childbearing age, made up about half of this number (HPA 2012a, Nelson-Piercy 2010). At present in England and Scotland it is estimated that the prevalence of HIV infection in those giving birth is 1 in 448, with London the highest area at 1 in 285 (HPA 2012b).

Less than 1% of infants born to women diagnosed with HIV prior to delivery in the UK acquired perinatal infection in 2010–11 (HPA 2012b).

CLINICAL FEATURES

HIV is a blood-borne retrovirus that infects and destroys T-lymphocytes (which play an integral role in cell-mediated immunity, B-cell activation, and antibody production), together with altering macrophage activation and neutrophil function (Woensdregt *et al.* 2008). This leads to the immune suppression that eventually results in AIDS (NHS IDPSP 2010). HIV/AIDS disease progresses through three phases (*see* Box 7.1).

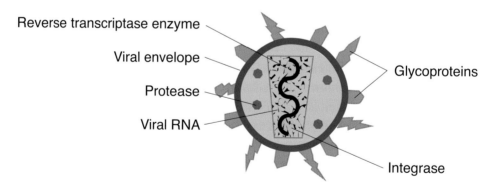

FIGURE 7.1 Human immunodeficiency virus

HIV is in the lentevirus group of retroviruses and is composed of two identical copies of single-stranded RNA plus specific proteins and enzymes necessary for duplication and maturation of the virus (Carter & Hughson 2012). These are attached to an enzyme (reverse transcriptase) that, once the virus is in a cell, allows the virus to transcribe its RNA genome into DNA, which then moves into the host cell DNA (Pratt 2003). When HIV is in the host cell, the virus can replicate itself whenever the cell is

BOX 7.1 PROGRESS OF HIV/AIDS

1. **Seroconvension**: following the first infection, a mild mononucleosis-type or flu-like illness may be experienced, usually with complaints of headache and/or pyrexia (Woensdregt *et al.* 2008). In some cases a maculopapular rash may also occur. HIV viraemia spreads the virus to target cells, and serum antibodies may be detected within a few weeks. This acute infection and rapid widespread viral dissemination is followed by a chronic asymptomatic stage.

2. **Latent (asymptomatic) infection**: viral replication is reduced dependent on the immune response and the woman usually remains well. The duration of this stage is reliant on a number of factors including the viral genotype, host immune response and whether antiretroviral therapy is being used. Infected cells are, however, still present and virus replication continues to destroy CD4 and other cells until the immune system deteriorates.

3. **Symptomatic infection**: the cell-mediated immune responses decline to a level where serious opportunistic diseases occur. The first symptoms a woman with HIV infection may have that lead her to suspect illness and seek medical advice may be relatively vague, such as weight loss, diarrhoea, pyrexia or candidiasis. These may be the initial signs that an opportunistic infection (which may be bacterial, viral, fungal, parasitic and mycobacterial infections and/or certain malignancies) is taking advantage of the woman's damaged immune system. Common bacterial infections, pneumonia, cytomegalovirus, toxoplasmosis, Kaposi's sarcoma and encephalopathy are among the conditions seen most frequently.

stimulated to reproduce. The cell is now acting as a workshop for new viruses and as the virus reproduces within the cell the cell membrane ruptures, releasing progeny viruses, a process known as budding. These progeny viruses can now infect other cells. The rate of replication is immense – billions of new virions may be produced each day, and these will be unique to that person (Pratt 2003).

The ability of the virus to replicate so rapidly, including a high rate of mutation, is one of the virus's strengths, making it able to evolve constantly. This makes it difficult to develop a vaccine to prevent HIV, and contributes to growing drug resistance.

The body's initial response to the infection is to activate the immune system to reduce the HIV viraemia (viral load). Virus-specific CD8-positive T-cells and neutralising antibodies are formed. However, infectious virus particles and infected lymphocytes continue to be produced and reduce the effectiveness of the immune system leading to its eventual failure.

HIV preferentially targets lymphocytes that express CD4 molecules (CD4 lymphocytes). CD4 is a protein on the surface of T-lymphocytes and some other immune system cells such as macrophages. Without antiretroviral drug therapy, the virus can cause progressive immune-suppression by selectively destroying the CD4 lymphocytes.

The normal CD4 'count' varies but is usually between 400 and 1600 cells/mm^3. When CD4 lymphocytes fall below a critical level (usually suggested to be <200 cells/mm^3), infected individuals become very susceptible to opportunistic infections and malignancies (RCOG 2010).

Transmission

Transmission of HIV can be:

- blood-borne via infected blood, organs or contaminated medical (or drug using, or recreational, such as tattooing) equipment
- horizontal: sexual
- vertical: mother to baby (*see* Box 7.2).

HIV is transmitted sexually and also via blood-to-blood contact, and, to a lesser extent, contact with other body fluids. In the UK it has been reported that about 55% of all people diagnosed with HIV acquired the infection from heterosexual contact. During heterosexual intercourse, there is an increased risk to women if anal sex is undertaken, if lesions are present and when co-infected by a sexually transmitted infection (STI). In pregnancy, while there is some controversy about whether there is an increased risk of vertical transmission in the presence of an STI, the recommendation is that STIs should be routinely screened for and even those infections that are asymptomatic should be treated (de Ruiter *et al.* 2012).

Healthcare workers can be at risk of HIV infection – in particular, following a 'sharps' injury. Midwives are at particular risk because of the nature of their work: unexpected exposure to uncontrolled blood loss is common. *See* Chapter 14 for discussion of avoidance of 'sharps' injury and exposure to high-risk body fluids, as well as possible actions to take if these situations occur.

Risk of vertical (mother-to-child) transmission

BOX 7.2 TRANSMISSION FROM MOTHER TO CHILD

- Via the placenta during pregnancy
- Ascending through the birth canal following rupture of membranes
- During vaginal birth
- Breastfeeding

The risk of maternal transmission of HIV to the unborn or newborn child varies widely throughout the world and is difficult to quantify. It is suggested that for women not receiving treatment it ranges between 15% and 40% in non-breastfeeding women in Europe, and between 25% and 40% for breastfeeding women in Africa (Working Group on Mother-To-Child Transmission of HIV 1995). Avoiding breastfeeding and giving one dose of antiretroviral drug to both mother and child has been shown to reduce the transmission by 47% (Goering *et al.* 2013). These findings can be particularly valuable in resource-poor areas where access to drugs is limited, although obtaining safe feeding substitutes may be problematic. For treated and non-breastfeeding women in resource-rich countries, transmission rates less than 1% have been reported (RCOG 2010).

In untreated women it is considered that the risk of transmission is determined by *maternal health* (specifically her viral load but also associated with nutritional status and concurrent infections), *obstetric factors* (such as length of time of membrane rupture and delivery before 32 weeks) and *method of infant feeding*. The health of the mother during pregnancy and delivery is important, as there is evidence that the greater her viral load, the higher the chance of her baby being infected (Townsend *et al.* 2008, Khan *et al.* 2012), although there have been incidences noted in the literature of transmissions even when the plasma viraemia was less than 50 copies/mL during delivery (Townsend *et al.* 2008, Warszawski *et al.* 2008, RCOG 2010). Those women who are newly infected and seroconverting while pregnant, or who have developed symptomatic disease, are particularly vulnerable to transmitting the virus to their fetus (Pratt 2003).

Screening and diagnosis

Antenatal screening for HIV has been part of the midwife's role in the UK since the 1980s, and recommendations from the Department of Health for good practice have changed several times since then. Currently the latest Royal College of Obstetricians and Gynaecologists guidelines (RCOG 2010) and National Institute for Health and Care Excellence Antenatal Guidelines (NICE 2012) recommend all pregnant women are screened for HIV in every pregnancy at booking. As HIV usually remains symptomless for many years it is an advantage for women to know their diagnosis in order to access medical care early, receive treatment at the optimum time and perhaps then prolong their health and life (May *et al.* 2007). Specifically to antenatal care, screening offers the opportunity to receive interventions that may cut the risk of transmission of the HIV infection to her unborn child to less than 1%.

All midwives should be competent to explain and obtain consent for an HIV test, along with the other tests that are routinely done at booking. The rate of uptake is about 95% at present (RCOG 2010), which demonstrates that midwives are successfully undertaking screening. However, it is noted that approximately 25% of

HIV-infected babies are born to previously diagnosed women (Khan *et al.* 2012). These women may be accessing maternity care late, find treatment challenging or have complex social problems. Since the woman's health may be compromised by lack of care, and there is also a potential risk to the baby, midwives must ensure that those women are effectively targeted so they can access appropriate care.

Testing is normally carried out in early pregnancy at booking. However, if not tested until ≥26 weeks, results should be requested urgently, as it is important to commence drug interventions as soon as possible to be effective.

Recommendations for women who decline the HIV test at booking include re-offering the test at 28 weeks. This may be undertaken by the HIV specialist midwife or other appropriate specialist who may be seen to have the advanced knowledge perhaps required and also, crucially, may have more time for discussion than the midwife undertaking routine antenatal care. If the woman continues to decline (or if a woman arrives unbooked in labour and then consents to a test) then a 'rapid' test may be carried out at this time.

Following infection, there is a time period of up to 3 months (and sometimes, rarely, up to 6 months) – the 'window period' – when HIV antibody testing will not be positive (RCOG 2010), although newer tests now provide a more rapid result. During this period of seroconversion, if the woman is routinely tested her result will be negative, and for this reason an HIV test may be repeated during pregnancy in special situations, such as in those with ongoing risk factors, or perhaps if symptoms arise that may suggest an acute HIV infection (Watts 2011). The Royal College of Obstetricians and Gynaecologists considers high-risk women to include those having unprotected sex with an HIV-positive partner or injecting drug users who share needles (RCOG 2010), but a repeat test can be done for any woman. In an audit on perinatal HIV transmission in England (2002–05) ≥20% of the babies later diagnosed with HIV had mothers who had received a negative HIV test result in early pregnancy (CHIVA 2007).

Tests

Testing is an area that changes frequently as new and more effective tests are developed. At present the recommended screening tests for HIV are 'fourth generation' assays, which detect HIV-1 antibodies, HIV-1, p24 antigen and HIV-2 antibodies (NHS IDPSP 2010). This type of test can reduce the diagnostic window to 1 month, as p24 antigen is detectable during seroconversion (RCOG 2010). It is recommended that for anyone testing positive, a second sample is then taken and tested to confirm the diagnosis (RCOG 2010, Watts 2011).

Test results for the newly diagnosed woman will be given to her according to the local protocol. It is likely that an HIV specialist midwife will be involved, and may then take over the woman's antenatal care, together with the rest of the multidisciplinary team, but it may be appropriate for the midwife who originally booked the woman to be present so the woman does not feel she has been abandoned and 'passed on'.

Rapid HIV tests (also known as 'bedside' or 'point-of-care' tests) can deliver a result within minutes (from a finger-prick or mouth swab). However, most of these tests will only test for antibodies and therefore the woman will have a negative result if she is seroconverting. Midwives or doctors may do these tests if a previously untested woman presents in labour (de Ruiter *et al.* 2012, RCOG 2010) and gives her consent. All positive tests must be followed by laboratory confirmation.

The paediatrician will usually undertake responsibility for the newborn screening, although the midwife may have to collect cord blood at delivery to begin the process. Ideally the woman will have already met the paediatric doctors and/or community nurse specialists in the antenatal period, as they are a vital part of the multidisciplinary team, and will be a valuable resource for the woman in the postnatal period.

Prevention

For the woman

If a woman receives a negative result from her HIV test, 'she should still receive information about safe-sex and high-risk scenarios for HIV transmission' (direct quote from the RCOG 2010 guidelines). This falls into the role of the midwife as a health educator, although it may be a challenge in present-day practices to identify time to do this effectively.

It has long been known that the use of condoms can prevent transmission of HIV (Weller & Davis-Beaty 2002). Since many women associate condoms only with pregnancy prevention, it may be necessary for a midwife to remind women of this fact. It is also recommended that couples who are both HIV positive use condoms, as there is a possibility of a 'superinfection' with unprotected sex (RCOG 2010).

For the fetus or baby

Much of maternity care for the HIV-positive woman is focused on avoiding transmission from the mother to the fetus or baby, as well as maximising the woman's health. The presence of a high viral load and low CD4 count make transmission more likely, as well as concurrent maternal conditions such as tuberculosis, malaria or STIs, so assessment to monitor these is necessary. Areas that the multidisciplinary team will concentrate on include:

- drug treatment for the woman, with frequent blood tests to assess results
- consideration of the best way to deliver the baby
- specific care for the baby post delivery, including drug therapy
- avoidance of breastfeeding.

For the midwife

Midwives, as one of the most vulnerable healthcare groups, need to ensure their practice protects them as much as possible. *See* Chapter 14 for further discussion.

MANAGEMENT ISSUES

Antenatal

Preconception care is important for a woman with HIV, as her drug regimen can be reviewed to ensure it is the best for her – newer drugs may be better tolerated, so it would be ideal to commence them before the potential morning sickness of pregnancy. Blood tests would ensure her viral load was as low as possible when she began trying to conceive. However, as with most other medical conditions, preconception care is often not accessed. A midwife may usefully remind a woman of this in the postnatal period, to ensure the woman knows the importance of preconception care for her next pregnancy.

Attention needs to be paid to nutrition for the HIV-positive woman – it is suggested that her resting energy expenditure is increased by around 10% even while asymptomatic (Hsu *et al.* 2005). It may or may not be appropriate to use nutritional supplements, but great care must be taken that she does not become overloaded with iron: there are some suggestions that larger iron stores result in a faster progression of HIV, probably because it supports viral replication (Montgomery 2003). It would be advisable to seek expert advice.

Care for the HIV-positive woman, whether newly diagnosed or long-standing, will be by a multidisciplinary team. This will usually include an HIV physician, an obstetrician, a specialist midwife, a health advisor and a paediatrician. The general practitioner is not automatically informed, but the woman is encouraged to disclose her results to him or her. If there are other issues, a variety of other professionals may also be involved according to need, such as social workers, clinical psychologists and drug-dependency specialists (de Ruiter *et al.* 2012). It has been suggested that social circumstances may aggravate the delivery of optimal care to many HIV-positive women (Khan *et al.* 2012), and the specialist midwife is well placed to coordinate care to meet the needs of these women.

Confidentiality is a vital part of care of the HIV-positive woman. The stigma of HIV, although perhaps lessening as time goes on, is still evident throughout UK society and may be of extreme concern to the woman. This may be a particular challenge for the midwife if the woman's partner or other close family do not know – and especially if they accompany her to antenatal appointments or labour. It must never be assumed that these individuals know the woman's HIV status, and the midwife must take particular care during general conversation. The midwife's duty of care is to the woman and she owes her total confidentiality (NMC 2008, 2012), but she may be put in a very compromising position if, for example, a partner asks what drug the midwife is administering to his newborn child. The specialist HIV midwife can possibly have anticipated these difficult situations and devised strategies, together with the woman, in the antenatal period. The World Health Organization, the General Medical Council and the British Medical Association consider breaking confidentiality a last resort, and this needs to be discussed and managed by the multidisciplinary team (RCOG 2010). For the midwife undertaking care and distressed by this situation, her Supervisor of Midwives may be of particular help and support. Accurate record keeping is of course essential, but the need for confidentiality may entail keeping a separate set of notes apart from the ones held by the woman. Local policies should allow for this.

Of course women will always be encouraged to disclose their HIV status to their partner, but this will take place with proper discussion and counselling in the antenatal period, and it is not an issue that can be addressed ad hoc by a midwife unknown to the woman. It is particularly important that a woman who is wary of becoming involved with medical interventions and care is well supported and maintains confidence in her caregivers, as there is the possibility of her evading caregivers and therefore both she and her child will be lost to future beneficial care.

Drug therapy

Drug therapy (*see* Box 7.3) is central to treatment of HIV. A woman who has been previously diagnosed with HIV may present for booking already taking combination therapy (HAART: **H**ighly **A**ctive **A**nti**R**etroviral **T**herapy). If this is working well for her

---

BOX 7.3 ANTIRETROVIRAL DRUGS USED COMMONLY IN HIV

HAART uses drug combinations that can target the viral enzyme and protein throughout the HIV life cycle.

- *Nucleoside/nucleotide reverse transcriptase inhibitors*: interfere with the action of reverse transcriptase, which is necessary for the virus to make copies of itself.
- *Non-nucleoside reverse transcriptase inhibitors*: also work to stop the viral cells replicating by inhibiting reverse transcriptase.
- *Viral protease inhibitors*: inhibit protease, which is necessary for HIV to replicate.
- *Fusion or entry inhibitors*: work to prevent HIV binding to or entering cells.
- *Integrase inhibitors*: interfere with the enzyme integrase, which is necessary for the viral DNA to enter host DNA.

Combination regimens are usually given. This may help to avoid drug resistance, mediate side effects and minimise doses of individual drugs, thereby reducing the risk of toxicity – some combinations can also increase the risk of toxicity; therefore all drug changes must be supervised by knowledgeable clinicians.

it is unlikely to be changed for pregnancy, but her response to it will be monitored, and since some of the drugs may have adverse effects in pregnancy, these may be altered. If she is not taking any drugs for her own health, or she is newly diagnosed in pregnancy, she may be offered HAART, or a regimen of a single drug only. These may commence between 20 and 28 weeks, but timing varies depending on her viral load, medical and obstetric history and the presence of any other conditions such as hepatitis C.

Antiretroviral drugs have many potential side effects and may not be easy to tolerate, especially during pregnancy. It is particularly important that her drug regimen is followed with complete adherence, as missing doses may lead to increased drug resistance (US DHHS 2012). A guide from HIV i-Base called *Avoiding and Managing Side Effects* (*see* Useful Resources section at the end of this chapter) may be very helpful for the woman, and for the midwife offering support.

It should be noted the common side effects associated with HAART drugs – such as nausea, vomiting, fatigue, tachycardia, dyspnoea, abdominal pain – may not only mimic normal pregnancy symptoms but also be indistinguishable from symptoms of pre-eclampsia or other liver involvements such as cholestasis. Any symptoms reported by the woman need to be assessed by the multidisciplinary team, considering both her pregnancy and her HIV status.

All drugs used for HAART have the potential of toxicity and damage to the mother and/or the fetus and therefore drug treatment may be a cause of anxiety for both the woman and her caregivers. The British HIV Association has excluded many concerns of teratogenicity (de Ruiter *et al.* 2012), but ongoing research continues, especially as new drugs are introduced. During pregnancy the healthcare team may notify the pregnancy (and later the birth and outcome) to the Antiretroviral Pregnancy Registry (www.apregistry.com). This registry is an international collection of information relating to births to women with HIV and has been tracking birth defects in babies exposed to antiretroviral drugs since 1989. The data obtained allow clinicians to base their prescriptions for drugs on the best available information to maximise benefit and avoid harm to both the woman and the fetus or infant.

For those women taking HAART medication, there is a suggestion both gestational diabetes and pre-eclampsia may be more common (Hitti *et al.* 2007, Wimalasundera *et al.* 2002, Mattar *et al.* 2004, RCOG 2010). The midwife should undertake appropriate screening for both these common conditions.

There has also been a suggested association between HAART and preterm delivery (Thorne *et al.* 2004, Townsend *et al.* 2007), and the midwife should ensure the woman has a knowledge of early signs of labour and what to do if they occur.

Additional screening

Part of routine care of women with HIV involves monitoring the disease via blood tests. Blood tests will be done on a frequency based on individual needs, but they are usually about every 4 weeks throughout the antenatal period.

- *Viral load assays*: HIV RNA polymerase chain reaction (PCR). The aim is for these to be below 50 copies/mL. It has been suggested that if the viral load is less than 50 copies/mL at the time of delivery, this reduces the transmission rate to 0.1% (Townsend *et al.* 2008). The previous term of 'undetectable viral load' is no longer recommended, as in the past this has meant several different values (RCOG 2010).
- *CD4 counts* should not fall below 350 cells/mm³. A level below 350 cells/mm³ is considered to leave a woman vulnerable to opportunistic infection, and below 200 cells/mm³ is particularly serious.

Supplementary blood tests to monitor antiretroviral drugs may also be undertaken, such as a resistance test to assess whether the infection is resistant to the drug being given, or therapeutic drug monitoring, to ensure the correct dose is being used. Depending on the drug regimen she is taking, regular full blood counts, urea and electrolytes, and liver function tests may be undertaken to monitor for drug toxicities.

In addition to the routine blood tests undertaken at booking, it is suggested women who are known to have HIV also are tested for hepatitis C, varicella zoster, measles and toxoplasmosis (RCOG 2010). Recommendations for immunisations may be made depending on these results, although some vaccines will have to be offered postnatally as they are contraindicated in pregnancy. The Royal College of Obstetricians and Gynaecologists (RCOG 2010) also recommends that women who are HIV positive are screened for genital infections, so these can be identified and treated promptly (*see* Chapter 5). A tuberculin skin test may also be offered, as co-infection of tuberculosis and HIV is relatively common (*see* section on tuberculosis in Chapter 9).

Although non-invasive antenatal screening for aneuploidy can be offered to the woman with HIV as normal, it should be noted that HIV may increase the assessed hormone levels, and false positive results may occur (de Ruiter *et al.* 2012). Diagnostic testing may carry a small risk of transmission to the fetus. Amniocentesis should not be carried out without discussion between the fetal medicine unit and the specialist obstetrician and HIV physicians, enabling counselling specific to her condition to be offered to the woman. The midwife can play an important part in ensuring the woman obtains all the information she needs to make a properly informed choice.

It is recommended that all HIV pregnancies are notified to the National Study of HIV in Pregnancy and Childhood (www.nshpc.ucl.ac.uk). This is a surveillance programme that is used to monitor many outcomes of HIV and its treatment in pregnancy, including the prevalence of diagnosed HIV infection in pregnant women and children, exploring the natural history of paediatric HIV, monitoring the health of uninfected children born to infected women and providing data to Public Health England, and Health Protection Scotland, where it is combined with other national surveillance data on HIV.

Labour and delivery

The mode of delivery of the baby must be discussed during the antenatal period, and a plan should be in place by 36 weeks' gestation, when the woman's blood results at this time will contribute to decision-making. This plan will not only consider the mode of delivery but also the drugs prescribed for labour, or prior to caesarean section, and for the postnatal period, for both mother and baby. It should also include actions to be taken if the woman presents in advanced labour, as to what drugs may be relevant that will rapidly cross the placenta if appropriate.

For some time it has been known that pre-labour caesarean section can reduce the risk of viral transmission to the baby (EMDC 1999), and this is still recommended in many cases, in particular for those whose viral load is >50 copies/mL at 36 weeks or later, who are not taking HAART or who have a co-infection such as hepatitis C (RCOG 2010). However, more recent studies have shown that if the woman's viral load is <50 copies/mL and she is taking HAART, the mode of delivery does not appear to affect the transmission rate (Warszawski et al. 2008, Townsend et al. 2008). If a woman has had a previous caesarean section, she may wish to have a VBAC (vaginal birth after caesarean), and her individual circumstances will be the basis of a discussion to enable a safe and satisfactory plan. If the pregnancy becomes prolonged, induction may be offered in individual cases (RCOG 2010). Again, the multidisciplinary team and the woman need to consider all the circumstances.

The Royal College of Obstetricians and Gynaecologists (2010) recommends that caesarean section for HIV-related reasons should be planned for 38 weeks, and for non-HIV-related reasons, for ≥39 weeks.

For the midwife caring for an HIV-positive woman undertaking a labour, care elements will mostly be as usual, apart from administration of antiretroviral drugs. It is recommended that artificial rupture of membranes should be avoided, although it may be considered, together with the use of oxytocin if augmentation is necessary. Fetal blood sampling and fetal scalp electrodes should be avoided if possible, and if an instrumental delivery is considered, low-cavity forceps are preferable to the use of ventouse (RCOG 2010). Following delivery, the baby should be washed clean of blood and maternal fluids, or specific relevant areas cleaned with alcohol swabs, before any invasive procedures such as vitamin K injections or blood sampling.

Preterm labour or rupture of membranes

Chorioamnionitis, usually caused by bacterial infection, has been shown to be associated with increased transmission of HIV to the fetus or baby (RCOG 2010) and is also a risk factor for preterm labour (Leitich et al. 2003). As HAART medication has also been shown to predispose to preterm labour (Townsend et al. 2007), a woman with HIV needs to understand that even vague symptoms of possible preterm labour need to be reported to the multidisciplinary team and investigated promptly. Most women that midwives in the UK will see in the labour ward will have been receiving antenatal treatment, and therefore recommendations for their care will be based on known individual circumstances as well as gestation.

Studies have shown that in women without treatment, rupture of membranes for longer than 4 hours resulted in a doubling of transmission risk (IP HIV Group 2001). If pre-labour rupture of membranes occurs before 34 weeks, steroids should be given as normal. Further actions will depend on the woman's individual condition: her viral load, the length of time and type of drugs she has been taking, the condition of the fetus, and the presence of any other conditions or infections will all be taken into account by the multidisciplinary team when making their recommendations. As a very preterm baby may not be able to tolerate oral drugs, it is important that the mother has sufficient medication to 'load' the fetus through the transplacental route (Khan *et al.* 2012). The midwife can be a vital support at this time, as the woman will not only need close observation of both the maternal and the fetal condition but also she will be understandably anxious.

It is recommended that if pre-labour rupture of membranes occurs after 34 weeks, including term, delivery needs to be expedited (RCOG 2010), and if the plasma viral load is <50 copies/mL, labour may be augmented if there is no other indication for caesarean section (RCOG 2010). An infection screen will be carried out, and intravenous antibiotics may be necessary.

If an unknown woman presents in labour, and she is diagnosed at this time, urgent involvement of the multidisciplinary team is necessary. Drugs need to be commenced as soon as possible, and ideally delivery should be delayed for at least 2 hours after drug administration. A caesarean section is likely to be recommended.

Postnatal

Some studies (Duarte *et al.* 2006, Fiore *et al.* 2004) have suggested that there is a higher risk of common complications following caesarean section in women who are HIV positive, although others (Boer *et al.* 2007) have not confirmed this possibility. The normal high standard of midwifery postnatal care should ensure this woman has the least possible risk.

Drugs to suppress lactation may be offered and although the postnatal prescription should have been organised antenatally, the midwife may need to access this. Cabergoline is a commonly used lactation suppress (RCOG 2010) and is usually given within the first 24 hours post-partum.

The woman's drug regimen – whether commenced in pregnancy only or if she had been taking medications previously – needs expert review to ensure her health remains optimum. If the woman was newly diagnosed with HIV in pregnancy, the midwife needs to confirm that the woman knows when and how to access follow-up for her condition.

Childbirth represents a significant change in circumstances for most women, and this change is a factor in social stress. Social stress has been shown in animal studies (Capitanio *et al.* 1998), and research with gay men (Cole *et al.* 1996), to contribute to the rate of progression in HIV-associated disease. This could emphasise the importance of follow-up in the postnatal period for all HIV-positive women, to ensure their medication remains effective for them, and the midwife needs to confirm that the women understand that their health needs to remain a priority despite the time-consuming demands of a newborn.

The importance of pre-conception care for a future pregnancy should be emphasised by the midwife. If the woman has an HIV-negative partner, she needs to know that there are ways that she could become pregnant again but still protect this partner (Moss 2012). In addition, it is important that women with HIV maximise their health, and ensure their drug regimen is the safest and most effective possible, before becoming pregnant. These are all areas of specialist knowledge, and the midwife can make sure the woman knows of the availability of this help, so she can access it when appropriate.

Pre-conception care is dependent on a planned pregnancy, and therefore contraception. The midwife should ensure contraception is discussed early in the postnatal period, as with all women. However, specialist advice should be accessed, especially since there are possible drug interactions between HAART and contraceptive medication.

Care of the baby

Ongoing assessment of the baby will be undertaken. Any birth defects are unlikely to be associated with antiretroviral drugs taken by the mother (*see* previous discussion), although there have been some suggestions of mitochondrial toxicity or anaemia being more common in these babies. Although these are very rare, paediatrician involvement needs to be ensured and easy access to expert practitioners should be available to the woman after she is discharged from hospital.

Infant feeding

Avoidance of breastfeeding is currently one of the key components to reducing the rate of transmission to the baby. Even if there are no other interventions in pregnancy or labour/delivery, international studies have still confirmed that not breastfeeding would reduce the transmission risk by around twofold (RCOG 2010).

In parts of the world where safe artificial feeding may be compromised through contaminated water or lack of resources to buy milk powder, there are many initiatives suggested involving medication for the mother, and emphasising exclusive breastfeeding and early weaning. There may also be a possibility that if the woman has a viral load of <50 copies/mL, transmission during breastfeeding may be restricted, although there may be a wide variation between maternal blood and breast milk viral loads (Khan *et al.* 2012). However, although this subject is receiving increased attention (Morrison *et al.* 2011), at present there is not yet any clear evidence for safe breast-feeding, and current recommendations in the UK are that breastfeeding should be avoided (RCOG 2010).

Although this is a postnatal issue, obviously the discussions concerning methods of feeding would have taken place in the antenatal period, and the midwife is well placed to ensure the mother understands the reasons for and importance of avoiding breastfeeding. It may be necessary to emphasise that even 'occasional' breastfeeding must not be undertaken, as mixed feeding has been shown to probably carry an even higher transmission risk. Many women who are HIV positive come from communities with a strong cultural expectation of breastfeeding, and the midwife can perhaps initiate a discussion with the woman to ensure she has acceptable 'reasons' why she is not breastfeeding – an action that may help protect her confidential status.

The midwife may also take the opportunity during antenatal discussions to advise the woman on what she needs to buy to be ready for the baby, and ensure she can make up artificial feeds correctly. If the woman cannot afford the equipment and supplies, there should be financial help available, and the midwife may need to assist her in accessing this.

Drug therapy

The newborn will be treated with drug therapy, commencing as soon as possible after birth, and at least within the first 4 hours (RCOG 2010), continuing usually for the first 4–6 weeks of life. The choice of drug will depend on the mother's drug regimen and her response to it, and the plan and prescription for the baby should be available from late in the pregnancy, so there is no possible confusion and delay if the baby is born at a time that all members of the HIV specialist multidisciplinary team are not readily available.

Testing

The baby is usually tested on day 1, at 6 weeks of age and 12 weeks of age. The test used currently is the HIV DNA PCR (polymerase chain reaction) or HIV RNA, and this should be conclusive if the baby is not breastfed. IgG antibodies of maternal origin are usually present in the baby's circulation for at least 1 year. Traditionally, an antibody test has been undertaken when the baby is 18 months old, and this may still be carried out, but maternal antibodies may still be detectable after 18 months by the newer, highly sensitive tests (RCOG 2010).

ROLE OF THE MIDWIFE

- Ensure up-to-date knowledge of this fast-changing subject.
- Undertake routine antenatal screening for HIV, enabling informed consent by the woman and know how and when results are given, becoming involved as appropriate.
- Although antenatal care is often undertaken by a specialist midwife, all midwives should be aware of the issues involved during pregnancy to optimise the HIV-positive woman's health and prevent vertical transmission.
- Ensure optimum care is given to mother and baby around delivery, whether by caesarean section or vaginal birth.
- Support the woman in her care of the baby, including safe artificial feeding and drug administration.
- Ascertain that contraception, immunisation and a plan for a further pregnancy, if appropriate, has been addressed before discharge.
- Ensure follow-up and resources available are known to the woman before discharge, especially if she has been newly diagnosed in pregnancy.

USEFUL RESOURCES

- Avert (www.avert.org/treatment.htm): contains useful drug information.
- British HIV Association (www.bhiva.org): this website suggests the best clinical practice in the treatment and management of HIV-positive pregnant women in the UK. They consider the use of antiretroviral therapy, both to prevent HIV mother-to-child transmission and for the welfare of the mother herself, guidance on mode of delivery and recommendations in specific patient populations where other factors need to be taken into consideration, such as co-infection with other agents. The guidelines are aimed at clinical professionals directly involved with, and responsible for, the care of pregnant women with HIV infection.
- HIV i-Base (www.i-base.info): provides many useful information leaflets including *Introduction to Combination Therapy* and *Avoiding and Managing Side Effects*.
- The Terrence Higgins Trust is a charity which was initially set up to support HIV-positive men. It has now vastly expanded its role and includes a website, advice line and moderated forum (which may be useful for newly diagnosed women to hear the personal experiences of others living with HIV). It also has an 'African communities' area. Specific pregnancy information is available at: www.tht.org.uk
- Royal College of Obstetricians and Gynaecologists (2010) *Management of HIV in Pregnancy*: Green-top Guideline No. 39. London, RCOG.

REFERENCES

Avert (2010) Averting HIV and AIDS International HIV and AIDS charity [online] Available at: www.aidsinfonet.org

Boer K, Nellen J, Patel D, *et al.* (2007) The AmRo study: pregnancy outcome in HIV-1 infected women under effective antiretroviral therapy and a policy of vaginal delivery. *BJOG.* **114**(2): 148–55.

Calles N, Evans D, Terlonge D (2010) *Pathophysiology of the Human Immunodeficiency Virus* [online]. Available at: www.bipai.org/hiv-curriculum (accessed 18 September 2014).

Capitanio J, Mendoza S, Lerche N, *et al.* (1998) Social stress results in altered glucocorticoid regulation and shorter survival in simian acquired immune deficiency syndrome. *Proc Natl Acad Sci U S A.* **95**(8): 4714–19.

Carter M, Hughson G (2012) *CD4 Cell Counts* [online]. Available at: www.aidsmap.com/CD4-cell-counts/page/1044596/ (accessed 1 December 2013).

Children's HIV Association (CHIVA) (2007) *Perinatal Transmission of HIV in England 2002–2005*. London: CHIVA.

Cole S, Kemeny M, Taylor S, *et al.* (1996) Accelerated course of human immunodeficiency virus infection in gay men who conceal their homosexual identity. *Psychosom Med.* **58**(3): 219–31.

De Ruiter A, Taylor G, Clayden P, *et al.* (2012) British HIV Association and Children's HIV Association guidelines for the management of HIV infection in pregnant women. *HIV Med.* **13**(Suppl. 2): 87–157.

Duarte G, Read J, Gonin R, *et al.* NISDI Perinatal Study Group (2006) Mode of delivery and post-partum morbidity in Latin American and Caribbean countries among women who are infected with human immunodeficiency virus-1: the NICHD International Site Development Initiative (NISDI) Perinatal Study. *Am J Obstet Gynecol.* **195**(1): 215–29.

European Mode of Delivery Collaboration (EMDC) (1999) Elective caesarean section versus vaginal delivery in prevention of vertical HIV-1 transmission: a randomised clinical trial. *Lancet.* **27**(353): 1035–9.

Fiore S, Newell M, Thorne C (2004) Higher rates of post-partum complications in HIV-infected than in uninfected women irrespective of mode of delivery. *AIDS.* **18**(6): 933–8.

Goering R, Dockrell H, Zuckerman M, *et al.* (2013) *Mims' Medical Microbiology.* 5th ed. Oxford: Elsevier, Saunders.

Health Protection Agency (HPA) (2012a) *HIV in the United Kingdom: 2012 Report*. London: Health Protection Services.

Health Protection Agency (HPA) (2012b) *Data Tables of the Unlinked Anonymous Dried Blood Spot Survey of Newborn Infants: prevalence of HIV in women giving birth*. Surveillance update. Available at: www.gov.uk/hiv-overall-prevalence#unlinked-anonymous-ua-surveys (accessed 5 September 2014).

Hitti J, Andersen J, McComsey G, *et al.* (2007) Protease inhibitor-based antiretroviral therapy and glucose tolerance in pregnancy: AIDS Clinical Trials Group A5084. *Am J Obstet Gynecol.* **196**(4): 331.e1–7.

HIV i-Base (2011) *Guide to HIV, Pregnancy and Women's Health* [online]. Available at: http://i-base.info/guides/files/2011/09/pregnancy-Sep2011e-NEW.pdf (accessed 20 September 2014).

Hsu J, Pencharz P, Macallan D, *et al.* (2005) *Macronutrients and HIV/AIDS: a review of current evidence*. Durban, South Africa: World Health Organization.

International Perinatal HIV Group (IP HIV Group) (2001) Duration of ruptured membranes and vertical transmission of HIV-1: a meta-analysis from 15 prospective cohort studies. *AIDS.* **15**(3): 357–68.

Khan A, Bull L, Barton S (2012) Management of HIV infection in pregnancy. *Obstet Gynaecol Reprod Med.* **23**(1): 1–6.

Leitich H, Bodner-Adler B, Brunbauer M, *et al.* (2003) Bacterial vaginosis as a risk factor for pre-term delivery: a meta-analysis. *Am J Obstet Gynecol.* **189**(1): 139–47.

Mattar R, Amed A, Lindsey P, *et al.* (2004) Preeclampsia and HIV infection. *Eur J Obstet Gynecol Reprod Biol.* **117**(2): 240–1.

May M, Stern J, Sabin C, *et al.* Antiretroviral Therapy (ART) Cohort Collaboration (2007) Prognosis of HIV-1 infected patients up to 5 years after initiation of HAART: collaborative analysis of prospective studies. *AIDS.* **21**(9): 1185–97.

Montgomery K (2003) Nutrition and HIV-positive pregnancy. *J Perinat Educ.* **12**(1): 42–7.

Morrison P, Israel-Ballard K, Greiner T (2011) Informed choice in infant feeding decisions can be supported for HIV-infected women even in industrialized countries. *AIDS.* **25**(15): 1807–11.

Moss J (2012) "How are we going to have a baby? I'm positive and you're not". *HIV Treatment Update.* (213) Autumn: 13–15.

National Institute for Health and Care Excellence (NICE) (2012) *Antenatal Care.* NICE Clinical Guideline 62. London: NICE.

Nelson-Piercy C (2010) *Handbook of Obstetric Medicine.* 4th ed. London: Informa Healthcare.

NHS Infectious Diseases in Pregnancy Screening Programme (NHS IDPSP) (2010) *Handbook for Laboratories.* London: UK National Screening Committee.

Nursing and Midwifery Council (NMC) (2008) *The Code: standards of conduct, performance and ethics for nurses and midwives.* London: NMC.

Nursing and Midwifery Council (NMC) (2012) *Midwives Rules and Standards.* London: NMC.

Pratt R (2003) *HIV & AIDS.* 5th ed. London: Hodder Arnold.

Royal College of Obstetricians and Gynaecologists (RCOG) (2010) *Management of HIV in Pregnancy.* Green-top Guideline 39. London: RCOG.

Thorne C, Patel D, Newell M (2004) Increased risk of adverse pregnancy outcomes in HIV-infected women treated with highly active antiretroviral therapy in Europe. *AIDS.* **18**(17): 2337–9.

Townsend C, Cortina-Borja M, Peckham C, *et al.* (2007) Antiretroviral therapy and premature delivery in diagnosed HIV-infected women in the United Kingdom and Ireland. *AIDS.* **21**(8): 1019–26.

Townsend C, Cortina-Borja M, Peckham C, *et al.* (2008) Low rates of mother-to-child transmission of HIV following effective pregnancy interventions in the United Kingdom and Ireland, 2000–2006. *AIDS.* **22**(8): 973–81.

US Department of Health and Human Services (US DHHS) (2012) *Guidelines for the Use of Antiretroviaral Agents in HIV-1-Infected Adults and Adolescents* [online]. Available at: http:// aidsinfo.nih.gov/guidelines (accessed 24 July 2014).

Warszawski J, Tubiana R, Le Chenadec J, *et al.* ANRS French Perinatal Cohort (2008) Mother-to-child HIV transmission despite antiretroviral therapy in the ANRS French Perinatal Cohort. *AIDS.* **22**(2): 289–99.

Watts H (2011) Human immunodeficiency virus. In: James D, Steer P, Winer C, *et al.* (editors). *High Risk Pregnancy: management options.* 4th ed. New York: Elsevier, Saunders. pp. 479–92.

Weller S, Davis-Beaty K (2002) Condom effectiveness in reducing heterosexual HIV transmission. *Cochrane Database Syst Rev.* (1): CD003255.

Wimalasundera R, Larbalestier N, Smith J, *et al.* (2002) Pre-eclampsia, antiretroviral therapy and immune reconstitution. *Lancet.* **360**(9340): 1152–4.

Woensdregt K, Lee H, Norwitz E (2008) Infectious diseases in pregnancy. In: Funai E, Evans M, Lockwood C (editors). *High Risk Obstetrics: the requisites in obstetrics and gynecology.* New York: Mosby, Elsevier. pp. 287–316.

Working Group on Mother-To-Child Transmission of HIV (1995) Rates of mother-to-child transmission of HIV-1 in Africa, America and Europe: results from 13 perinatal studies. *J Acquir Immune Defic Syndr Hum Retrovirol.* **8**(5): 506–10.

World Health Organization (WHO) (2012) *Use of Antiretroviral Drugs for Treating Pregnant Women and Preventing HIV Infection in Infants – Executive Summary.* Available at: www.who.int/hiv/pub/mtct/programmatic_update2012/en/ (accessed 20 September 2014).

CHAPTER 8

Viral hepatitis

INTRODUCTION

Hepatitis can be defined as inflammation and damage to the liver – this can be caused by many factors, both infectious and non-infectious, including drug toxicity. Viral hepatitis can include other conditions such as cytomegalovirus, human immuno-deficiency virus (HIV), yellow fever and varicella zoster, but hepatotropic viruses are what is usually understood when 'viral hepatitis' or just 'hepatitis' is mentioned, and are commonly defined as hepatitides A through E. Other undefined viral hepatitis agents, often referred to as non-A to non-E hepatitis, have been identified – in particular, hepatitis G, which has been implicated in transmission via a needlestick injury (Shibuya *et al.* 1998) – but at present these are not well established in medical literature. All viral hepatitis can have an adverse effect on the health of both the woman and the fetus or baby, and since it is known that the incidences are rising, it is necessary for the midwife to maintain an up-to-date understanding of these conditions.

All forms of viral hepatitis are considered notifiable diseases under the Public Health (Infectious Diseases) Regulations 1988, and doctors have a statutory duty to notify suspected and confirmed cases. This information is used to monitor the incidence of infections, thereby allowing for preventive action and also identification of local needs.

THE LIVER

The liver is the most important metabolic organ in the body. The hepatic portal system brings venous blood from the intestine where absorbed nutrients are processed, stored and detoxified by the liver. Box 8.1 outlines the numerous functions of the liver in addition to its role in digestion.

Acute viral hepatitis is characterised by the inflammatory process, typically diffuse and patchy hepatocellular necrosis affecting all the functional cells of the liver. Jaundice results from the liver being damaged – the liver can no longer carry bilirubin

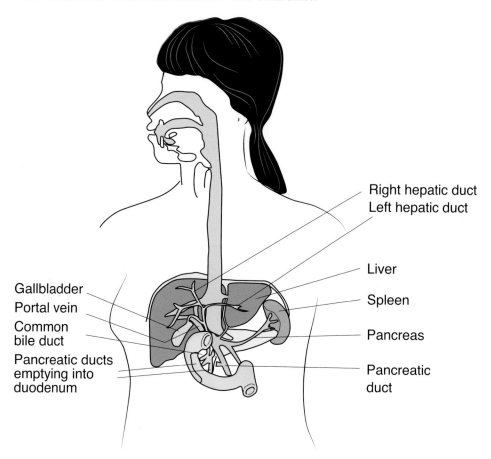

Right hepatic duct
Left hepatic duct

Liver

Spleen

Pancreas

Pancreatic
duct

Gallbladder

Portal vein

Common
bile duct

Pancreatic ducts
emptying into
duodenum

FIGURE 8.1 The liver

BOX 8.1 FUNCTIONS OF THE LIVER

- Metabolic processing of the major nutrients (carbohydrates, proteins, fats) after their absorption from the digestive tract
- Detoxification or degradation of body wastes and hormones as well as drugs. This includes the breakdown of protein, producing waste products urea and uric acid, which are excreted in urine
- Production of plasma proteins including IgA and those essential for blood clotting
- Regulation of blood sugar through storage and release of glycogen
- Removal of bacteria
- Excretion of cholesterol and bilirubin (from breakdown of red blood cells)
- Secretion of bile

into the bile, resulting in increased bilirubin levels in the body fluids. Jaundice is the yellow tinge to the sclera, mucous membranes and skin.

Common signs and symptoms of hepatitis can include general malaise, anorexia, nausea, pyrexia, abdominal pain (in particular right upper quadrant or epigastric) and jaundice. However, for many of those infected, there may be no notable symptoms. The modes of infection and incubation periods differ between classifications (*see* Table 8.1).

TABLE 8.1 Modes of infection and incubation periods

	Mode of infection	**Incubation period**
Hepatitis A	Faecal–oral	2–6 weeks
Hepatitis B	Blood-borne, sexual	6 weeks–6 months
Hepatitis C	Blood-borne	2 months
Hepatitis D	From blood	2–12 weeks
Hepatitis E	Faecal–oral	4–6 weeks

Most of those with acute hepatitis will make a full recovery, but (depending on the classification of the hepatitis) severe morbidity and mortality may occur, and some may develop chronic hepatitis and become a lifelong carrier. Chronic hepatitis encompasses the spectrum of liver disease between acute hepatitis and cirrhosis (*see* Box 8.2). Long-term complications may include cirrhosis and hepatocellular cancer.

BOX 8.2 CIRRHOSIS

Cirrhosis is the result of long-term, continuous damage to the liver. Liver damage leads to scarring (fibrosis) and irregular nodules replace smooth liver tissue. Fibrosis and nodules = cirrhosis. Cirrhosis can lead to complete liver failure. There are few symptoms until the liver disease is very advanced, when pain, general malaise and jaundice may be present.

Risk factors are long-term viral infections (hepatitis B and C), inherited liver disease (e.g. haemochromatosis), alcohol abuse and non-alcoholic fatty liver disease (associated with being overweight and/or diabetes).

Late effects found in cirrhosis:

- oesophageal or gastric varices → internal bleeding
- overload of waste products in blood → hepatic encephalopathy
- fluid retention → ascites
- liver cancer risk.

HEPATITIS A

Epidemiology and pathophysiology

The hepatitis A virus (HAV) was first identified in 1973. The risk of contracting HAV is increased in crowded conditions, with poor hygiene and sanitation. It is endemic worldwide, and in resource-poor areas up to 90% of children have been infected by the time they are 5 years old (Goering *et al.* 2013). It is estimated that every year 10 million people are infected worldwide (Panda *et al.* 2010). In the United States, the incidence of HAV in pregnancy is approximately 1:1000 (Silverman 2008). The clinical disease is usually milder in young children than in adults, and children are often asymptomatic (PHE 2013). In adults, 70%–80% become jaundiced.

HAV is a positive-strand RNA, non-enveloped virus. It is a self-limiting disease with no carrier state. The route of infection is faecal–oral and the incubation period is approximately 2–6 weeks. The severity during the acute phase is related to the viral load.

Transmission

Transmission of HAV is via contaminated water or food, in particular from infected food handlers and shellfish: bivalve molluscs such as oysters, clams and mussels can act as reservoirs for HAV when in contaminated waters (Silverman 2008). There is also a risk from ice or salad vegetables contaminated with infected water (PHE 2013). The virus is excreted in faeces from approximately 1 week before symptoms become apparent, and 1 week after, and maximum infectivity is immediately before and for a few days after the onset of jaundice (Wilson 2006).

Clinical features and diagnosis

Specific signs and symptoms of HAV include general malaise, pyrexia, nausea and vomiting, anorexia and maybe arthralgia. There may also be right upper quadrant pain and hepatosplenomegaly (Panda *et al.* 2010). Adults will commonly become jaundiced, and jaundice appears after about 2 weeks and may last several weeks. Around 5%–10% of those affected may have one or more symptomatic relapses for up to 40 weeks (Panda *et al.* 2010). Fulminating HAV is very rare but can be fatal (Silverman 2008).

Blood tests

Liver function tests will show elevated liver enzymes (aminotransferases) and bilirubin. They may also show elevated bile acids, which, together with itching can lead a midwife to suspect obstetric cholestasis (Grossmith *et al.* 2009). HAV is diagnosed with serum IgM antibody to HAV. Following infection, HAV-specific immunoglobulin G (IgG) is positive for years after infection, demonstrating immunity.

Prevention

There is a vaccine for HAV available and this should be given to travellers to HAV endemic areas and workers whose activities may put them at risk (e.g. sewage workers, laboratory workers). There is also an opinion that midwives, as the care they are giving could lead to accidental contamination, should be vaccinated (Eaton 1996). The vaccine is considered safe for pregnant women travelling (Plotkin & Orenstein 2004).

Care also needs to be taken when in endemic areas to avoid contact with contaminated water, in order to prevent HAV and other common infections (*see* Chapter 12).

Management

HAV should have no effect on pregnancy in a previously well woman (Panda *et al.* 2010), however poor nutritional status in the woman is linked to adverse pregnancy outcome (Silverman 2008). Perinatal transmission is unlikely but immunoglobulin is recommended for the newborn if the mother gives birth within 2 weeks of the acute illness (Panda *et al.* 2010).

Most care is supportive, depending on symptoms. Pre- or post-infection prophylaxis may prevent or lessen the symptoms, although post-exposure treatment is not effective after 2 weeks. This is not contraindicated in pregnancy.

HEPATITIS B

Hepatitis B virus (HBV) is the classification of hepatitis that UK midwives will be most familiar with, as it is screened for routinely at booking, and all midwives must themselves have effective HBV vaccine cover.

Epidemiology and pathophysiology

Although knowledge of HBV had been available previously, hepatitis B was clearly defined in 1964 and at that time was called 'Australia antigen'. It is suggested that a third of the world's population, more than 2 billion people, have been infected with HBV and the number of HBV carriers worldwide is estimated at >350 million, with the highest rates in South East Asia, sub-Saharan Africa and China (Goering *et al.* 2013, PHE 2013). Mother-to-child transmission accounts for up to 50% of carriers (Lee *et al.* 2006).

Mortality from HBV is estimated at 0.5–1.2 million a year (Liaw & Chu 2009) and it is thought that HBV is responsible for up to 80% of all cases of liver cancer. HBV is classified by the World Health Organization as the world's second-greatest carcinogen after tobacco (BLT 2012a).

Approximately 95% of those who become infected as adults will fully recover and develop protective immunity. This drops to 20%–50% for younger children, and only approximately 5% of neonates who acquire the infection from their mother at birth will clear the infection without treatment (Bell & Nguyen 2009, PHE 2013).

In the UK the rate of HBV-positive pregnant women can be >1% in inner-city areas, reflecting the high proportion of those originating from high-endemic areas. Genotypes follow geographical distribution – but in the UK, as the population is from a wide range of areas, all genotypes are represented. Overall the rate in the UK for pregnant women is 0.14% (PHE 2013).

HBV is an enveloped, circular, partially double-stranded DNA virus and is found in blood and body fluids. It is considered to be 50–100 times more infectious than HIV (BLT 2012a). HBV is divided into eight genotypes, and these may influence the outcome of the infection or the response to antiviral treatment, but infection with one strain gives resistance to all strains (Goering *et al.* 2013).

After the virus enters the bloodstream it travels to the liver, resulting in inflammation and necrosis. The incubation period can be from 6 weeks to 6 months. As the first virus-specific antibodies appear, there may be a brief illness (rash, arthralgia), although this is rare. As liver damage increases, clinical symptoms arise (*see* Box 8.3). The immune response increases, causing the virus replication to slow and blood to become non-infectious, but this may take many months. Fulminant HBV occurs in <1% of cases but with a mortality of 70% (Liaw & Chu 2009). About 10% of those infected fail to eliminate the virus completely and so become carriers – their blood remains infectious, usually forever.

Those most at risk of becoming carriers are:

- those who are immunodeficient
- infants infected perinatally
- males more than females.

Approximately 25%–30% of carriers are likely to develop cirrhosis or hepatocellular cancer (Silverman 2008).

Transmission

HBV antigen can be present in all body fluids. Blood is most likely to transmit the virus, but saliva and semen may also be associated with transmission (Silverman 2008). Transmission typically occurs during sexual intercourse or via contaminated blood products or equipment – for example, needles used by injecting drug users, tattooing, or inadequately cleaned medical or dental devices. The virus can remain alive in dried blood for up to 7 days.

In households, sexual transmission is the most common, but other areas may be a risk, such as toothbrushes, razors and eating utensils. Therefore, all those living with HBV carriers should be offered vaccination, and care must be taken.

Those at risk of HBV in the UK include intravenous drug users, sex workers, men who have sex with men, those whose partners are HBV carriers, healthcare workers, immigrants from endemic areas and those in situations where high standards of hygiene are difficult to maintain. There is also a risk in travelling to countries where blood is not screened or medical equipment not adequately sterilised.

Vertical transmission from mother to fetus or baby is also possible, and the risk is dependent on the infectivity status of the woman (*see* Box 8.4). If the mother is hepatitis B surface antigen (HBsAg) positive without treatment, there is estimated to be a 10%–20% risk of passing the infection to her baby, but if the mother is hepatitis B envelope antigen (HBeAg) positive without treatment, it is thought that up to 90% of infants will be infected.

Intrauterine infection of the fetus can occur, probably by transplacental leakage of maternal blood (Collier & Oxford 2006). There is a possibility of these infants becoming infected despite routine treatment at delivery (Lee *et al.* 2006).

Transmission in the healthcare setting

Although percutaneous transmission (e.g. following a needlestick injury) for healthcare workers is the most common risk, contact of infectious material with broken skin or mucous membranes has also been implicated (Silverman 2008). Haemodialysis is a particularly exposure-prone situation, and transmission has been reported both from patient to carer and from hepatitis B carrier carers to a patient (Goering *et al.* 2013). All vulnerable healthcare workers – especially midwives, with their common, and sometimes unexpected and uncontrollable, exposure to blood – should be vaccinated and this is usually a requirement of employment. However, the dangers of hepatitis C and HIV transmission means even immunised healthcare workers must not become complacent in situations of potential risk (*see* Chapter 14 for more information).

Clinical features and diagnosis

Many new infections are subclinical, or perhaps only manifest as flu-like symptoms (*see* Box 8.3 for signs and symptoms that may possibly occur).

BOX 8.3 SIGNS AND SYMPTOMS ASSOCIATED WITH HEPATITIS B VIRUS

- General malaise or feeling of ill health
- Anorexia (loss of appetite)
- Nausea, vomiting
- Mild pyrexia
- Body aches (in particular, tenderness in right upper abdomen)
- Hepatomegaly
- Jaundice (30%–50% of adults)
- Pruritus

Blood tests

The recommended screening test for HBV is an immunoassay to detect HBsAg (NHS IDPSP 2010). Assessing the presence of HBsAg and IgM antibody to hepatitis B core antigen (HBcAg) can be used to make a diagnosis. The main antigens HBsAg, HBcAg and HBeAg all induce their own specific antibodies. These, together with viral DNA polymerase, can be found in the blood during and after the infection.

HBsAg predates clinical signs by about 4 weeks, and titres fall as the symptoms decrease (Panda *et al.* 2010). HBeAg is only present in the blood when infection is active; therefore, it is a marker for infectivity. All these 'markers' (together with polymerase chain reaction (PCR) to assess viral loads) can show how the disease is developing, monitor treatment and identify the degree of infectivity to others (*see* Box 8.4). During the current infection HBsAg is present and if it disappears the woman is not a carrier. Chronic hepatitis B (carrier state) is defined as HBsAg present for longer than 6 months (Panda *et al.* 2010).

BOX 8.4 INFECTIVITY OF HEPATITIS B VIRUS CARRIERS

This indicates the degree of infectivity, based on the characteristics of the woman's individual virus. This information will be necessary when planning care for the newborn.

- *High risk*: HBsAg positive, HBeAg positive, negative hepatitis B surface antibody, negative hepatitis B envelope antibody, positive hepatitis B core antibody
- *Moderate risk*: HBsAg positive, HBeAg negative, negative hepatitis B surface antibody, positive hepatitis B envelope antibody, positive hepatitis B core antibody
- *Low risk*: HBsAg positive, HBeAg negative, positive hepatitis B surface antibody, positive hepatitis B envelope antibody, positive hepatitis B core antibody

High HBV DNA levels (viral load) tested by PCR will indicate high infectivity.

HBsAg negative, positive hepatitis B core antibody, positive hepatitis B surface antibody = evidence of past infection or immunisation.

Management

HBV is usually self-limiting and those with acute HBV are unlikely to need treatment; however, oral antiviral drugs, first used in the late 1990s, can improve outcomes for those who need it, by limiting the replication of the virus and slowing hepatitis activity (Liaw & Chu 2009, Giles *et al.* 2012). Pregnancy is often considered a circumstance where drug treatment may be appropriate, and with an increasing viral load or fulminant infection, the woman can receive treatment to improve maternal and fetal outcomes and reduce the risk of transmission (Panda *et al.* 2010). Early antiviral treatment may also be needed for fulminant hepatitis (<1%). Those with chronic HBV may need treatment to reduce the risk of cirrhosis and cancer (Lai & Yuen 2007). Oral antiviral treatment, often in combinations, is usually offered.

Where a woman is newly diagnosed (or if she has not had care in the UK previously), the multidisciplinary team will assess her, and, if necessary, contacts will need to be traced and immunised. A vaccine has been available since 1981 that involves a series of injections, and protection is estimated at >90%.

Pregnancy

The midwife plays a vital part in caring for a woman with HBV, whether a woman with known carrier status, a newly diagnosed carrier or with acute HBV. The Department of Health has published a document, *Hepatitis B Antenatal Screening and Newborn Immunisation Programme: best practice guidance* (DH 2011), covering areas where the midwife is directly responsible. The midwife is ideally placed to coordinate care for this woman, and this needs to begin at booking or immediately the diagnosis is available.

It has been recommended since the 1990s that all pregnant women be screened for HBV during booking. As in all routine blood tests, the midwife has the responsibility for explaining the test, and the rationale for testing, in order that the woman can make an informed choice to undertake testing. Women booking after 24 weeks' gestation should have their blood samples sent urgently.

If a midwife suspects a woman may have acute hepatitis B, she will obviously refer the woman immediately to the appropriate medical team for diagnosis, treatment and provision of a care plan. However, it is far more likely she will identify a woman with chronic hepatitis B, either one who reveals her status at booking or one who is newly diagnosed from routine booking bloods. These women also need a speedy referral to the appropriate service identified by individual maternity units (this could be a hepatologist, gastroenterologist or infectious diseases specialist). There might also be a specialist antenatal screening midwife or coordinator in post, and she will need to know about this woman. However, the midwife needs to ensure she is still involved in the care of this woman, as it will be her (or her midwifery colleagues) who will be present when labour commences, so record keeping and communication is vital.

The immunisation process for the infant begins in the antenatal period, with the midwife ensuring vaccine, and hepatitis B immunoglobulin (HBIG) if appropriate, is ordered and available for the baby immediately after delivery. It is recommended that these are available from about 32 weeks' gestation (DH 2011). It is also important that the midwife ensures that the mother understands the importance of the complete course of immunisation (lasting until the baby is 1 year old). There has been evidence that most HBV immunisation programmes have failed to provide a full protection for all babies at risk in the past (Giraudon *et al.* 2009, NICE 2009) and to address this, the newest Department of Health guidelines (DH 2011) emphasise the importance of full information being received by the woman, and the DH also provides a leaflet *Hepatitis B: How To Protect Your Baby* in several languages (*see* the 'Useful resources' section at the end of this chapter).

Depending on their condition, women will have their bloods monitored throughout pregnancy. Drug treatment is not usually recommended for women of childbearing age unless absolutely indicated (Liaw *et al.* 2008). However, in mothers with an increased viral load, treatment in late pregnancy may reduce transmission to their infants, although this would not replace the normal neonate HBIG and vaccine (Chang 2007). Acute or exacerbation of chronic HBV may occur during pregnancy (Chang 2007) and may also require treatment. If an acute infection occurs during pregnancy, it may become severe (PHE 2013).

Preterm labour has been reported in acute HBV but other complications of pregnancy seem not to be influenced by HBV status (Chang 2007). If a woman becomes infected while pregnant, the decision on whether to offer an early delivery is one that needs to be made individually, weighing her health and the baby's gestation. There appears to be no effect on the mother's condition from the steroids routinely given before preterm delivery to benefit the baby (Panda *et al.* 2010).

If a woman has the potential of being in a high-risk situation, either visiting areas where HBV is prevalent or her social circumstances increase her risk, there is no recorded adverse effect if vaccination is received during pregnancy or breastfeeding (Plotkin & Orenstein 2004, Dienstag 2008).

Antenatal care by the midwife is summarised as follows.

- Identify HBV-positive woman at booking (if already diagnosed) or from booking bloods.
- Refer to appropriate medical teams plus specialist midwife if available.
- Ensure a multidisciplinary care plan for pregnancy, labour and postnatal care is written, and is available to all relevant staff and amended if necessary during the pregnancy.
- Undertake normal antenatal care, with particular attention to ensuring the woman knows the signs and symptoms of preterm labour.
- Provide all relevant information, underpinning it with written material, to ensure the woman understands the importance of the baby's immunisation programme.
- Ensure vaccine and immunoglobulin (if necessary) is ordered for the baby by about 32 weeks' gestation.

Birth

There is no evidence at present that an elective caesarean section would prevent the baby from becoming infected (Woensdregt *et al.* 2008).

Communication between midwives is essential to ensure that the midwife caring for the HBV-positive woman in labour can provide optimum care. It has been suggested that actions considered high risk for transmission, such as fetal blood sampling or fetal scalp electrodes, should be avoided (DH 2011). The midwife should also ensure that the baby is washed clean of maternal blood and secretions before any injections or blood tests are undertaken.

Some women may present unbooked in labour. An urgent 'rapid test' should be available and recommended to women, in order that, if needed, her baby will be able to have the vaccine (plus probably immunoglobulin) within 24 hours of delivery.

Postnatal and community care

There appears to be no risk of mother-to-child transmission via breastfeeding, provided the baby receives the appropriate immunoprophylaxis (Shi *et al.* 2011).

The community midwife, in her home visits, may become aware of others in the home who would benefit from assessment and immunisation. She may also find it appropriate to reinforce the information on how HBV is spread, the significance of HBV for the woman's own health and the benefit of regular follow-ups, the importance of screening and vaccination for anyone entering the family, and – again – the importance of the baby completing its vaccination schedule (including what to do if moving out of area and so forth).

Some circumstances do not fit easily into the routine screening pathway (e.g. those babies who are fostered or adopted) and the midwife must ensure the communication processes are in place to allow for timely administration of the vaccinations.

Baby

The recommended immunisation schedule for the baby is as follows (DH 2011):

- dose 1 – at birth (plus immunoglobulin* in selected cases)
- dose 2 – 1 month after dose 1
- dose 3 – 2 months after dose 1
- dose 4 – 12 months after dose 1 (plus blood test to check infection or immunity status).

(*According to the HBV status of the mother, some newborns need to receive hepatitis B immunoglobulin (HBIG) within 24 hours of delivery. This is based on the mother's blood results (so therefore can be organised during the antenatal period – ordering HBIG at 32/40 is recommended) apart from one situation: if the baby's birthweight is ≤1500 g. It is likely this baby will be premature, so midwives must ensure when this woman presents in labour that the HBIG – if not already on site – is ordered as a matter of urgency.)

The midwife undertaking postnatal care is responsible for ensuring that the local child health records department is informed of the mother's hepatitis B status, and that the baby had received the first dose of vaccine (plus or minus HBIG) (DH 2011). She needs also to check that the general practitioner and health visitor are aware of the baby's needs for further immunisation. The mother's hepatitis B status and the vaccine (plus HBIG if appropriate) administration need to be included in the baby's personal child health record (DH 2011). A specific insert for 'Hepatitis B infant immunisation programme' is available from the personal child health record supplier (also known as Form 13a).

The response to the vaccine is lower in preterm infants (Losonsky *et al.* 1999), so it is particularly important that full doses of the vaccine are given, plus HBIG if needed. Newborns aged less than 28 weeks need close monitoring of respirations for 72 hours post vaccine, and if the baby reacts to the first vaccine then hospitalisation is needed for later ones to ensure close respiratory monitoring again (PHE 2013).

Fulminant or acute hepatitis can occur in infants, and usually occurs when the HBV is transmitted by a HBsAg-positive and HBeAg-negative woman (Chang 2007).

HEPATITIS C

The hepatitis C virus (HCV) may be the classification of hepatitis that provides the highest risk to UK midwives, as there is an unknown (but possibly substantial) number of women carrying the virus, and there is no immunisation available.

Epidemiology and pathophysiology

HCV (formerly known as non-A, non-B hepatitis) was identified in 1987. The areas of greatest prevalence are East Asia and eastern Europe, but it is found in increasing numbers worldwide. The number of people affected is unknown – estimates range from 170 million to more than 500 million. It is unsurprising that estimates vary so widely, when most cases are in resource-poor areas of the world where assessment would be very difficult, and when the clinical symptoms are usually so mild and uncertain, until the development of complications very much later. The condition has been referred to as 'the silent epidemic'.

In the UK, likewise, there is a wide variation in estimated prevalence, but it has been suggested that numbers of those newly diagnosed with HCV have increased by more than a third recently. However, the British Liver Trust suggests that five out of every six people with chronic hepatitis C are unaware of their infection (BLT 2012b). In the United States it is estimated that up to 1% of pregnant women are HCV positive. The rate of HCV in UK pregnant women varies, but one early study in London reported an incidence of 0.8%, of which 73% had no identified risk factors (Ward *et al.* 2000).

HCV is a single-strand RNA virus, and transmission is blood-borne. There are six identified genotypes and many subtypes. The different types will influence the effectiveness of antiviral treatment (Goering *et al.* 2013) and the rate of disease progression (Silverman 2008). Infection with one genotype does not confer protection against the others and the variety of types, plus a high rate of mutation, makes development of a vaccine a challenge.

The average incubation period is 2–4 months. HCV is more damaging than HBV, as 75%–85% of those affected will go on to develop chronic hepatitis C (carriers), and 10%–15% of these will develop cirrhosis (*see* Box 8.2) and/or liver cancer. The rapidity of development can be influenced by alcohol use or co-infection (especially with HIV or HBV), but the degree of liver injury is not related to the severity of the initial symptoms. HCV is the leading reason for liver transplant in the UK (Goering *et al.* 2013).

In the acute disease, 65%–75% will be asymptomatic, 25% jaundiced and 10% will have acute symptoms. The symptoms appear 4–12 weeks after the infection (Panda *et al.* 2010).

Transmission

HCV is transmitted in the same way as HBV but is less common vertically and sexually. Although sexual transmission is rare, the risk is increased if sexually transmitted infections are present or trauma caused. Social contact transmission via shared toothbrushes, razors, and so forth, is possible. Skin piercing and tattooing have also been associated with transmission (Wilson 2006). It is estimated that 50% of active drug injectors are HCV positive, and this is obviously a very high-risk activity (BLT 2009). Blood transfusion and blood products before 1991 were a potential source of infection, but since then screening in the UK has become routine. The route of infection is unknown in up to 40% of those diagnosed (Goering *et al.* 2013).

Vertical transmission is estimated at about 5%–10%, and this will be increased if the woman is also HIV positive or has a high viral load (BLT 2009, McMenamin *et al.* 2008). If the woman is co-infected with HIV but is not receiving antiretroviral therapy, a meta-analysis demonstrated a threefold increased risk in mother-to-child transmission of HCV (Pappalardo 2003). Most consider that the mode of delivery does not affect this risk (RCOG 2010).

HCV is also a risk to healthcare workers – in particular, midwives, where most women (and their carers) will not know their status. Besides the more common transmission to a carer through a needlestick injury, there are also reports of blood splashes in the eye transmitting the disease (Hosoglu *et al.* 2003). There is also the possibility of transmission from an HCV-positive midwife to her client, as was recently detailed in the media (Muir *et al.* 2014) and it is the midwife's responsibility to ensure her employers have full knowledge of any disease or condition that could potentially put her clients at risk.

Clinical features and diagnosis

In most cases of HCV infection, no symptoms are reported. When there are symptoms, these tend to be non-specific: fatigue, weight loss, loss of appetite, joint pains, nausea, flu-like symptoms and some report a pain in the liver area. Jaundice is uncommon (BLT 2012b).

Blood tests

Past or present infection will be indicated by a positive test for HCV antibodies by enzyme immunoassay (EIA) or enzyme-linked immunosorbent assay (ELISA). A PCR test for HCV RNA can also be used and this will detect the presence or absence in blood, the viral load and the genotype (RANZCOG 2013).

Liver enzymes will be assessed and a liver biopsy may be carried out.

Management

Specialist care is needed, and assessment by a hepatologist or gastroenterologist with an understanding of liver disease is vital. Knowledge and experience of the disease is increasing all the time, so regular assessments are needed to assess the progress of disease and evaluate liver damage.

Treatments will vary depending on duration of the infection, strain of the virus and whether the woman is pregnant. Recent introduction of direct-acting antiviral protease inhibitors appears to have improved care considerably (BLT 2012b) and early treatment may clear the virus, or suppress it and delay progress. The concept of a cure for HCV is being discussed currently in the literature.

Pregnancy

In some countries (i.e. Australia and New Zealand) and in some UK trusts, all pregnant women are screened for HCV. In other UK trusts (and in the United States) screening is done on a 'risk' basis. Risk criteria vary but always include a history of intravenous drug use (in the mother or partner) and place of origin (McMenamin *et al.* 2008, Panda *et al.* 2010).

It is controversial whether women should be routinely screened for HCV at booking. There is no known way at present to prevent vertical transmission, and even if diagnosed there is no guaranteed treatment available. On the other hand, there is some belief that a high viral load in late pregnancy may increase the rate of transmission (Silverman 2008) and therefore an attempt to reduce this load with antivirals may benefit the baby. Diagnosis where it was previously unknown may also act as a public health benefit to enable any modification of the woman's behaviour to reduce transmission to others.

Acute HCV during pregnancy increases the risk of preterm delivery (Gonzalez *et al.* 2006) but those with a chronic state usually show no increased rate of complications

(Kumar *et al.* 2007). Apart from the potential of transmission to the baby, it appears that there are no pregnancy complications associated with HCV for women who are generally well (Panda *et al.* 2010).

Factors affecting transmission to the baby include a high viral load in the mother and co-infection with HIV. There is no known association with the gestational age at delivery or normal steroids given to the mother to enhance the baby's lung function when a preterm delivery is expected (Panda *et al.* 2010). Evidence from some minimal studies (Minola *et al.* 2001) does not demonstrate a risk of transmission via amniocentesis, but expert counselling would be recommended.

There is no evidence showing any protective effect of elective caesarean section in reducing the transmission to the baby (Ghamar Chehreh *et al.* 2011, McMenamin *et al.* 2008). However, it would be common sense to avoid any potentially harmful invasive interventions such as fetal scalp electrodes. The role of the duration of ruptured membranes is unknown (European Paediatric Hepatitis C Virus Network 2001).

The midwife should ensure any injection or blood sampling from the baby is preceded by cleansing of the area with an alcohol swab to remove maternal blood and secretions. Breastfeeding is considered to be safe (Panda *et al.* 2010). These babies are frequently given HBV vaccination. Babies born to mothers with HCV will need follow-up, and tests are usually undertaken after 12 months (HCV antibodies test) or two tests 6 months apart (HCV RNA tests) to determine the baby's HCV status (Arshad *et al.* 2011).

HEPATITIS D (DELTA)
Epidemiology and pathophysiology
The hepatitis D virus (HDV), also known as the hepatitis delta virus, is a very small circular single-strand RNA genome and is an incomplete virus. It can only multiply in a cell infected with the HBV and it exists in about 5% of HBV carriers. HDV is commonly found in South America, Africa and Mediterranean areas, and it is suggested that it affects approximately 15 million people worldwide (BLT 2008).

There is no specific vaccine, but obviously, successful vaccination for HBV will also prevent HDV.

Transmission
HDV infection may occur at the same time as HBV, called 'co-infection', and usually occurs during a more severe disease episode. If it occurs in a HBV carrier it is called 'superinfection' and this may accelerate the course of chronic hepatitis B-related diseases (BLT 2008).

The route of infection is via percutaneous exposure and exposure to blood products. Intravenous drug users are at high risk, but sexual transmission is less efficient than for HBV. Mother-to-child transmission is rare.

Diagnosis

Blood tests

- IgM antibody to HDV in the serum is usually diagnostic.
- A liver biopsy for the HDV antigen may be undertaken.

HEPATITIS E

Epidemiology and pathophysiology

The hepatitis E virus (HEV) occurs mainly in resource-poor areas, commonly in South Asia, Africa and Central America, in particular where there is limited availability of safe drinking water. It is a particular risk to pregnant women, as cases of fulminant disease or abnormality of coagulation occur (Hossain *et al.* 2009).

HEV is also known as enteric non-A, non-B hepatitis. The virus causing hepatitis E is small, single-stranded and non-enveloped with an RNA genome. The incubation period is 4–6 weeks. There is no chronic form of HEV. It has four different genotypes, and several subtypes, and these are associated with variations of transmission and clinical consequences (Pratt 2013).

The virus persists in stools for at least 2 weeks after the onset of jaundice (Wilson 2006).

Transmission

Transmission is faecal–oral, and there is an association with pigs or other foods such as shellfish and venison (Dalton *et al.* 2007). It has been suggested that pigs or other pets may act as a reservoir for infection (Pratt 2013). There can be widespread outbreaks in areas where flooding or monsoons contaminate the water supply with sewage.

Clinical features and diagnosis

Symptoms of HEV are usually non-specific and may include abdominal pain, nausea, vomiting and diarrhoea. Jaundice is not always present. A history of travel to an area where HEV was present will prompt relevant investigations and aid diagnosis.

Blood tests

- IgG and IgM antibodies are present in serum.

Management in pregnancy

Severe fulminant HEV may occur in 10%–20% of pregnancies complicated with HEV and put the lives of both the mother and fetus at risk. Although general mortality in endemic countries is similar to that for HAV, the greatest severity is among pregnant women (Kumar *et al.* 2004). In one study in Pakistan, HEV was found to be the most common cause (63%) of hepatic failure and death in women presenting in pregnancy with liver dysfunction. The incidence of HEV during the second and third trimesters is higher than in the first, or in non-pregnant women (Begum *et al.* 2010), and in comparison with non-pregnant women, HEV symptoms appear to be significantly prolonged (Begum *et al.* 2010). A mortality rate of 80% from fulminant hepatic failure caused by HEV during the third trimester has been suggested (Mamun-al-Mahtab *et al.* 2009). However, others have quoted figures less than this. HEV has also been suggested to be a cause of miscarriage, intrauterine death and preterm labour (Dahiya *et al.* 2005). Immunological and hormonal changes in pregnancy may explain the severity of HEV in pregnancy (Navaneethan *et al.* 2008).

HEV has also been reported in the UK, even in those who have not recently travelled abroad (Ijaz *et al.* 2005). One recent case study (Andersson *et al.* 2008) details a woman without risk factors developing abnormal liver function results (initially referred by her midwife for excessive itching), and being diagnosed with HEV. Following close monitoring and treatment with steroids, the pregnancy ended with a healthy baby, albeit at 34 weeks following prolonged rupture of membranes.

THE ROLE OF THE MIDWIFE

- Maintain up-to-date knowledge of all hepatitis classifications, with particular reference to their effects in pregnancy.
- Be able to give all information necessary to women regarding testing for HBV at booking interviews.
- When caring for a woman with HBV carrier status, ensure all procedures are followed in care of her baby to prevent her child becoming HBV positive.
- Maintain strict infection control principles during care with all women, to protect the women, colleagues and yourself.
- Ensure your hepatitis B vaccine is current.

FURTHER RESOURCES

- The British Liver Trust publishes many useful documents concerning all classifications of hepatitis, some targeted specifically for healthcare professionals. These can be accessed through the British Liver Trust website (www.britishlivertrust.org.uk).
- Department of Health (2011) *Hepatitis B Antenatal Screening and Newborn Immunisation Programme: best practice guidance.* Available through www.dh.gov.uk/publications.
- The Department of Health's leaflet *Hepatitis B: How To Protect Your Baby* is provided in several languages and can be given to the woman by the midwife. Available through www.nric.org.uk.

REFERENCES

Andersson M, Hughes J, Gordon F, *et al.* (2008) Of pigs and pregnancy. *Lancet.* **372**(9644): 1192.

Arshad M, El-Kamary S, Jhaveri R (2011) Hepatitis C virus infection during pregnancy and the newborn period: are they opportunities for treatment? *J Viral Hepat.* **18**(4): 229–36.

Begum N, Polipalli S, Husain S, *et al.* (2010) Duration of hepatitis E viremia in pregnancy. *Int J Gynaecol Obstet.* **108**(3): 207–10.

Bell S, Nguyen T (2009) The management of hepatitis B. *Aust Prescr.* **32**(4): 99–104.

British Liver Trust (BLT) (2008) *Hepatitis D and E.* Ringwood, UK: BLT.

British Liver Trust (BLT) (2009) *A Professional's Guide to Hepatitis C and Injecting Drug Use.* Ringwood, UK: BLT.

British Liver Trust (BLT) (2012a) *Hepatitis B.* Ringwood, UK: BLT.

British Liver Trust (BLT) (2012b) *Hepatitis C.* Ringwood, UK: BLT.

Chang M (2007) Hepatitis B virus infection. *Semin Fetal Neonatal Med.* **12**(3): 160–7.

Collier L, Oxford J (2006) *Human Virology.* 3rd ed. Oxford: Oxford University Press.

Dahiya M, Kumar A, Kar P, *et al.* (2005) Acute viral hepatitis in third trimester of pregnancy. *Indian J Gastroenterol.* **24**(3): 128–9.

Dalton H, Thurairajah R, Fellows H, *et al.* (2007) Autochthonous hepatitis E in southwest England. *J Viral Hepat.* **14**(5): 304–9.

Department of Health (DH) (2011) *Hepatitis B Antenatal Screening and Newborn Immunisation Programme: best practice guidance.* Available at: www.dh.gov.uk/publications/hepatitis-b-antenatal-screening-and-newborn-immunisation-programme-best-practice-guidance (accessed 8 August 2014).

Dienstag J (2008) Hepatitis B virus infection. *N Engl J Med.* **359**(14): 1486–500.

Eaton L (1996) Case notes – subject: Marilyn Smith. *Nurs Times.* **92**(24): 10.

European Paediatric Hepatitis C Virus Network (2001) Effects of mode of delivery and infant feeding on the risk of mother-to-child transmission of hepatitis C virus. *BJOG.* **108**(4): 371–7.

Ghamar Chehreh M, Tabatabaei S, Khazanehdari S, *et al.* (2011) Effect of caesarean section on the risk of perinatal transmission of hepatitis C virus from HCV-RNA+/HIV- mothers: a meta-analysis. *Arch Gynecol Obstet.* **283**(2): 255–60.

Giles M, Visvanathan K, Lewin S, *et al.* (2012) Chronic hepatitis B infection and pregnancy. *Obstet Gynecol Survey.* **67**(1): 37–44.

Giraudon I, Permalloo N, Nixon G, *et al.* (2009) Factors associated with incomplete vaccination of babies at risk of perinatal hepatitis B transmission: a London study in 2006. *Vaccine.* **27**(14): 2016–22.

Goering R, Dockrell H, Zuckerman M, *et al.* (2013) *Mims' Medical Microbiology.* 5th ed. Oxford: Elsevier, Saunders.

Gonzalez F, Medam-Djomo M, Lucidarme D, *et al.* (2006) Acute hepatitis C during the third trimester of pregnancy. *Gastroenterol Clin Biol.* **30**(5): 786–9.

Grossmith A, Bhatia K, Heazell A (2009) Elevated bile acids associated with acute hepatitis A infection in the third trimester of pregnancy. *J Obstet Gynaecol.* **29**(1): 54–5.

Hosoglu S, Celen M, Akalin S, *et al.* (2003) Transmission of hepatitis C by blood splash into conjunctiva in a nurse. *Am J Infect Control.* **31**(8): 502–4.

Hossain N, Shamsi T, Kuczynski E, *et al.* (2009) Liver dysfunction in pregnancy: an important cause of maternal and perinatal morbidity and mortality in Pakistan. *Obstet Med.* **2**(1): 17–20.

Ijaz S, Arnold E, Banks M, *et al.* (2005) Non-travel-associated hepatitis E in England and Wales:

demographic, clinical, and molecular epidemiological characteristics. *J Infect Dis.* **192**(7): 1166–72.

Kumar A, Beniwai M, Kar P, *et al.* (2004) Hepatitis E in pregnancy. *Int J Gynecol Obstet.* **85**(3): 240–4.

Kumar A, Sharma K, Gupta R, *et al.* (2007) Pregnancy outcome in hepatitis C virus infection. *Int J Gynecol Obstet.* **98**(2): 155–6.

Lai C, Yuen C (2007) The natural history and treatment of chronic hepatitis B: a critical evaluation of standard treatment criteria and end points. *Ann Intern Med.* **147**(1): 58–61.

Lee C, Gong Y, Brok J, *et al.* (2006) Effect of hepatitis B immunisation in newborn infants of mothers positive for hepatitis B surface antigen: systematic review and metal-analysis. *BMJ.* **332**(7537): 328–31.

Liaw Y, Chu C (2009) Hepatitis B virus infection. *Lancet.* **373**(9663): 582–92.

Liaw Y, Leung N, Kao J, *et al.* (2008) Asian-Pacific consensus statement on the management of chronic hepatitis B: 2008 update. *Hepatol Int.* **2**(3): 263–83.

Losonsky G, Wassermann S, Stellhens I, *et al.* (1999) Hepatitis B vaccination of premature infants. *Pediatrics.* **103**(2): E14.

Mamun-al-Mahtab S, Rahman S, Khan M, *et al.* (2009) HEV infection as an aetiologic factor for acute hepatitis: experience from a tertiary hospital in Bangladesh. *J Health Popul Nutr.* **27**(1): 14–19.

McMenamin M, Jackson A, Lambert J, *et al.* (2008) Obstetric management of hepatitis C-positive mother-infant pairs. *Am J Obstet Gynecol.* **199**(3): 315. e1–5.

Minola E, Maccabruni A, Pacati I, *et al.* (2001) Amniocentesis as a possible risk factor for mother-to-infant transmission of HCV. *Hepatology.* **33**(5): 1341–2.

Muir D, Chow Y, Tedder R, *et al.* (2014) Transmission of hepatitis C from a midwife to a patient through non-exposure prone procedures. *J Med Virol.* **86**(2): 235–40.

Navaneethan U, Al Mohajer M, Shata M (2008) Hepatitis E and pregnancy: understanding the pathogenesis. *Liver Int.* **28**(9): 1190–9.

National Institute for Health and Care Excellence (NICE) (2009) *Reducing Differences in the Uptake of Immunisations.* NICE Public Health Guidance 21. Available at: http://guidance.nice.org.uk/PH21/Guidance/pdf/English (accessed 14 March 2014).

NHS Infectious Diseases in Pregnancy Screening Programme (NHS IDPSP) (2010) *Handbook for Laboratories.* London: UK National Screening Committee.

Panda B, Panda A, Riley L (2010) Selected viral infections in pregnancy. *Obstet Gynecol Clin North Am.* **37**(2): 321–31.

Pappalardo B (2003) Influence of maternal human immunodeficiency virus (HIV) co-infection on vertical transmission of hepatitis C virus (HCV): a meta-analysis. *Int J Epidemiol.* **32**(5): 727–34.

Plotkin S, Orenstein W (editors) (2004) *Vaccines.* 4th ed. Philadelphia: WB Saunders.

Pratt R (2013) Hepatitis E virus infection. *Nurs Stand.* **27**(39): 43–7.

Public Health England (PHE) (2013) *Immunisation against Infectious Diseases: the Green Book.* 3rd ed. London: The Stationery Office.

Royal Australian and New Zealand College of Obstetricians and Gynaecologists (RANZCOG) (2013) *Management of Hepatitis C in Pregnancy.* C-Obs51. Available through www.ranzcog.edu.au (accessed 9 September 2014).

Royal College of Obstetricians and Gynaecologists (RCOG) (2010) *Management of HIV in Pregnancy.* Green-top Guideline 39. London: RCOG.

Shi Z, Yang Y, Wang H, *et al.* (2011) Breastfeeding of newborns by mothers carrying hepatitis B virus: a meta-analysis and systematic review. *Arch Pediatr Adolesc Med.* **165**(9): 837–46.

Shibuya A, Takeuchi A, Sakurai K, *et al.* (1998) Hepatitis G virus infection from needlestick injuries in hospital employees. *J Hosp Infect.* **40**(4): 287–90.

Silverman N (2008) Hepatitis virus infections during pregnancy. *Glob Libr Women's Med.* Available at: www.glowm.com/section_view/heading/Hepatitis%20Virus%20Infections%20During%20Pregnancy/item/181 (accessed 20 September 2014).

Ward C, Tudor-Williams G, Cotzias T, *et al.* (2000) Prevalence of hepatitis C among pregnant women attending an inner London obstetric department: uptake and acceptability of named antenatal testing. *Gut.* **47**(2): 277–80.

Wilson J (2006) *Infection Control in Clinical Practice.* 3rd ed. Edinburgh: Baillière Tindall, Elsevier.

Woensdregt K, Lee H, Norwitz E (2008) Infectious diseases in pregnancy. In: Funai E, Evans M, Lockwood C (editors). *High Risk Obstetrics: the requisites in obstetrics and gynecology.* New York: Mosby, Elsevier. pp. 287–316.

CHAPTER 9

Serious respiratory infections

→ Overview
→ Influenza
→ Pneumonia
→ Tuberculosis

OVERVIEW

Pregnant women are not more likely than non-pregnant women to contract a respiratory infection but when they do it is more likely to lead to serious complications including pneumonia. This is due to a number of anatomical, physiological and immune changes of pregnancy, but in particular, it is due to fluid shifts that increase pulmonary oedema and restriction to the ventilation of the lungs. The swine flu outbreak in 2009 highlighted this problem. For most, swine flu was a relatively mild illness; however, 13 pregnant women in the UK and Ireland died as a result of complications from swine flu (Modder 2010). Those women with underlying health problems are more at risk of respiratory complications of infections in pregnancy (*see* Box 9.1), but problems can occur in previously healthy women. Midwives have been urged to improve their basic assessment of women, both to identify early those with deteriorating health (*see* also Chapter 4) and to enable ongoing evaluation when caring for women at the time of illness.

Midwives have a role in health education, particularly in relation to reducing the spread of infectious respiratory diseases such as tuberculosis (TB) and influenza through vaccination, early recognition of symptoms, appropriate isolation, public education and support with treatment.

BOX 9.1 HIGHEST-RISK CATEGORIES FOR COMPLICATIONS OF RESPIRATORY INFECTION

- Smoking
- Substance abuse
- Poor nutrition
- Pre-existing conditions including asthma, diabetes, cardiac disease, anaemia, and renal disease
- Morbid obesity
- Those with immune suppression including HIV
- Pregnancy

(Lim & Mahmood 2010)

CHANGES THAT MAKE PREGNANT WOMEN MORE VULNERABLE TO SERIOUS COMPLICATIONS OF RESPIRATORY INFECTIONS

Physiological changes during pregnancy such as changes in the immune system, increased cardiac output, decreased lung capacity and greater oxygen (O_2) demand are believed to contribute to more serious complications of influenza, including pneumonia and adult respiratory distress syndrome (Hegewald & Crapo 2011). This risk seems more pronounced in the second and third trimester (Louie *et al.* 2010). The gravid uterus displaces the diaphragm upwards and the thoracic rib cage splays out. This may make it more difficult for the pregnant woman to clear secretions. Alterations to respiratory function including a reduction in functional residual capacity, increased O_2 capacity and increased pulmonary fluid add to the vulnerability of pregnant women's lungs to injury from infection (Hegewald & Crapo 2011)

Increased permeability of the endothelial linings of capillary blood vessels in the lungs results in fluid moving more easily into the interstitial tissue of the lungs, creating an increase in extravascular lung water. Pregnancy is also known to reduce the colloid oncotic pressure of blood and this further exacerbates the leakage of fluid from the circulation. It is much the same mechanism that results in women having oedema around their ankles but in a more serious location. The oedema in the lung tissue results in alveolar collapse, causing a mismatch of ventilation and perfusion and the lowering of arterial oxygenation (Clutton-Brock 2011). Pre-eclampsia is known to exacerbate this problem. This potential for fluid overload underpins the need for fluid restriction and careful monitoring of fluid balance in pregnant women when they are unwell.

The changes in pregnancy and vulnerability to serious complications may persist into the immediate postnatal period and the concern applied in pregnancy will apply for at least 2 weeks postnatally (Ramussen *et al.* 2011).

ASSESSMENT OF THE RESPIRATORY SYSTEM

Midwifery assessment to detect signs of ill health is included in Chapter 4 and should be read in conjunction with this section. Some key points with regard to specific assessment of the respiratory system are summarised here. A systematic approach that involves the midwife assessing and documenting both subjective and objective data is advocated. The use of modified early obstetric warning system (MEOWS) charts is recommended (Centre for Maternal and Child Enquiries (CMACE) 2011), and has been widely adopted in practice as an aid to ensure timely referral. Observations of respiratory rate, pulse, blood pressure, temperature and O_2 saturations need to be put in context and interpreted as part of a more detailed assessment of mother and fetus. Compensatory mechanisms will attempt to maintain homeostasis in the presence of disease. Breathlessness (increased respiratory rate), tachycardia and changes in blood pressure all indicate deteriorating respiratory function. Box 9.2 lists some specific features the midwife may note in her assessment of respiratory function. The doctor or midwife with advanced practitioner skills will also perform a chest examination involving percussion and auscultation. A chest X-ray will provide valuable information for respiratory assessment and should be arranged without delay. Chest X-rays are not contraindicated in pregnancy, although shielding of the uterus is still advised (Brent 2011). Women may be concerned about having an X-ray and midwives can provide reassurance regarding the safety of a normal X-ray.

BOX 9.2 ASSESSMENT OF RESPIRATORY FUNCTION BY THE MIDWIFE

In addition to the usual set of basic observations the midwife should observe for the following features.

- Stridor, cough, wheeze
- Level of consciousness and degree of orientation
- Verbal response – is the woman able to complete a sentence in one breath?
- Central or peripheral cyanosis
- Decreased capillary refill
- Signs of respiratory distress such as; sitting upright and leaning forward, use of accessory muscles when breathing
- Production of sputum – blood-stained sputum, green
- Change to the rate, depth and symmetry of breathing

(Margereson & Withey 2012, Hunter & Rawlings-Anderson 2008)

Box 9.3 lists the features of deteriorating respiratory function. One of the challenges of assessment of the respiratory system in pregnancy is distinguishing between the physiological breathlessness experienced by up to 75% of pregnant women and breathlessness of a more serious cause. Normal breathlessness comes on gradually over a number of weeks and is not associated with other adverse signs or symptoms. The woman may notice it when she is talking and it can get worse with exercise. The CMACE report (2011) identified 'red flag' features useful in identifying a more serious cause of breathlessness (*see* Box 9.4). The report also recommended that pulmonary oedema be considered as a possible cause of a 'wheeze' in pregnant women, especially in those not known to have asthma.

BOX 9.3 FEATURES OF DETERIORATING RESPIRATORY FUNCTION

- Increased respiratory rate (above 20 breaths per minute – time for a full minute following pulse assessment)
- Decreased O_2 saturation
- Increased supplemental O_2 required to keep O_2 saturation within normal range
- Increased MEOWS chart score
- Carbon dioxide (CO_2) retention (as indicated by arterial blood gas levels)
- Abnormalities of the CTG may reflect deterioration in the mother
- Drowsiness
- Headache
- Flushed face
- Tremor

(O'Driscoll *et al.* 2008)

BOX 9.4 'RED FLAG' FEATURES OF SERIOUS BREATHLESSNESS IN PREGNANCY

- Breathlessness of sudden onset
- Breathlessness associated with chest pain
- Orthopnoea (difficulty breathing when lying flat) or paroxysmal nocturnal dyspnoea (a sensation of shortness of breath that wakes the woman up at night)

(CMACE 2011)

Pulse oximetry

Measurement of O_2 saturation using a probe attached to the finger or toe provides a useful assessment of respiratory function. A healthy O_2 saturation reading is between 95% and 100%. When recording the O_2 saturation it is important to note whether the measurement is taken in room air or with supplemental O_2. O_2 saturation levels need to be considered in the context of other assessments of pulse, blood pressure, the level of haemoglobin and where indicated, compared with arterial blood gas (ABG) estimation (Margereson & Withey 2012). Oxygen is predominantly carried by haemoglobin and so when haemoglobin levels are low the blood will be delivering less total O_2, despite normal saturation levels. Oximetry does not provide information on the partial pressure of carbon dioxide ($PaCO_2$) and therefore ABG analysis is indicated when impairment of ventilation is noted. Box 9.5 lists factors that may affect pulse oximetry readings.

BOX 9.5 FACTORS AFFECTING PULSE OXIMETRY READINGS

- Poor perfusion of extremities (e.g. cold limbs or shock)
- Movement (shivering)
- Carbon monoxide (smokers)
- Dark nail varnish or false nails

(Margereson & Withey 2012, Booker 2008)

Arterial blood gases

A test of ABG will be ordered where there is concern about deteriorating respiratory status. This will provide an assessment of levels of O_2, carbon dioxide (CO2) and any acid–base disturbance. It is assessing the effectiveness of gaseous exchange and ventilation. If the pH of the blood falls outside the normal range of 7.35–7.45 it will affect the release of O_2 from the haemoglobin, depriving the cells of the O_2 required for normal cell metabolism (Margereson & Withey 2012).

A specimen of arterial blood is obtained from either the radial or the femoral artery using a needle and a heparinised syringe. The woman will require a clear explanation of the test and her informed consent obtained. The explanation should include that it is quite painful and the midwife can assist the doctor taking the blood by providing support for the woman and applying pressure to the bleeding point following the procedure for at least 5 minutes to prevent bleeding and bruising (Hennessey & Japp 2007). The sample taken needs to be tested quickly, within 10 minutes, although if kept in ice the time can be extended to 60 minutes. In critical care and maternity high dependency settings the woman may have an arterial line inserted to avoid the need for repeated stabs and to guide the effectiveness of treatment (Margereson & Withey 2012). Midwives will be part of a multidisciplinary team and are generally not expected to have specialist knowledge with regard to the interpretation of ABG results. However, it is useful for midwives to have a basic knowledge of the normal parameters (*see* Table 9.1). Further explanation of the physiology that contributes to changes in ABG may be found in Appendix 1.

TABLE 9.1 Normal arterial blood gas values and their significance

	Normal ranges in arterial blood	Significance
pH	7.35–7.45	Low pH: acid High pH: alkaline Small changes to pH outside the normal ranges create significant problems in the body
PO_2	12–14 kPa	The partial pressure of oxygen (PO_2) dissolved in arterial blood
PCO_2	4.5–6.0 kPa	The partial pressure of carbon dioxide (CO_2) dissolved in arterial blood The reading is used to assess the effectiveness of ventilation; increasing the respiratory rate helps blow off CO_2
HCO_3	22–26 mmol/L	HCO_3 is the chemical formula for bicarbonate, which is an alkali; it collects hydrogen ions and neutralises them, thus acting as a 'buffer' for acidosis in the blood; measurement provides a reflection of the health of the body's metabolic status
O_2 saturation	95% and above	Oxygen is carried in the blood attached to haemoglobin molecules; oxygen saturation is a measure of how much O_2 the blood is carrying as a percentage of the maximum it could carry
Base excess	−2 to +2	Measurement of the surplus amount of base (alkaline) within the blood; it essentially reflects the same thing as HCO_3

(Coggins 2008a, Margereson & Withey 2012, Hennessey & Japp 2007)

INFLUENZA

INTRODUCTION

Influenza (flu) is a contagious respiratory illness caused by influenza viruses. Outbreaks of influenza occur seasonally and more serious pandemic flu occurs periodically. Clinical symptoms of influenza are usually mild (most cases of swine flu were mild) but can be severe, as was seen with avian flu in 2004. Influenza can lead to serious complications, the most common being pneumonia. Morbidity and mortality from influenza varies according to the virus strain but with all influenza, pregnant women and their newborn offspring are more vulnerable to serious complications

(Dodds *et al.* 2007, Jamieson *et al.* 2009, Mosby *et al.* 2011). In 2009, the world experienced its first pandemic influenza outbreak in more than 40 years. An outbreak of a new strain of influenza was reported in Mexico City in March 2009. The virus was identified as swine flu (Novel type A/H1N1 2009) in April 2009, and the first cases were reported in the UK that same month. By June 2009, 30 000 cases were confirmed worldwide and the World Health Organization (WHO) declared swine flu had reached pandemic status. A vaccination programme against swine flu commenced in October 2009 and pregnant women were identified as a high-priority group for vaccination, and for treatment with antivirals should they develop symptoms. Cohort studies from that period confirmed increases in admission to intensive care units, serious morbidity and death from swine flu for pregnant women (Jamieson *et al.* 2009, Knight *et al.* 2010, Ellington *et al.* 2011). There were 13 maternal deaths reported to the Centre for Maternal and Child Enquiries (CMACE) in the UK between April 2009 and January 2010 that were attributed to swine flu (Modder 2010). While the impact of swine flu has now passed, lessons learnt from this pandemic will feature in this chapter to inform midwives as to the nature of influenza and provide a framework for care of pregnant women in times of pandemic flu. Historical perspectives, and knowledge of changes to influenza virus structure, confirm that pandemic flu will happen again and that even greater adverse outcomes may occur. Every year there is an outbreak of seasonal flu in winter that affects approximately 5%–15% of the population. Complications and deaths from seasonal flu usually affect the elderly, but more recently pregnant women have been included as an at-risk group. Midwives need to be conversant with the care of women with flu and with public health measures to prevent spread of influenza including the vaccination of pregnant women.

THE INFLUENZA VIRUS

There are three main types of influenza virus: A, B and C. Influenza A was responsible for three global pandemics in the last century and swine flu this century.

Influenza is caused by the orthomyxovirus family of viruses, which normally affect birds and mammals. These viruses have characteristic spike-like glycoproteins on the envelope covering of the virus, called haemagglutinin and neuraminidase, which interact with the host cells. Haemagglutinin (H) enables the virus to bind to the host cell, whereas neuraminidase (N) assists in the mobility of new virus particles (Lim & Mahmood 2010). The presentation of these glycoproteins determines the naming of the virus – hence, for example, H1N1 (swine flu) – although a fuller description of influenza strains includes the type (A, B or C), the host of origin (such as swine), place of original isolation, strain number and year (Pratt 2009a).

Influenza is an RNA virus that has a small unstable genome divided into eight segments. These RNA viruses are prone to mutation whereby small changes occur to the presenting antigen, known as 'antigenic drift' (Helbert 2006). Seasonal flu epidemics occur because of minor changes to these antigens. When a major 'antigenic shift' occurs, a worldwide pandemic is possible. Pandemics occur every 10–40 years (*see* Table 9.2). Often the source of a particular new strain can be traced to infected birds, poultry or pigs in which there has been a genetic reassortment of subtypes of the virus, resulting in transmission from these animals to humans (Gillespie & Bamford 2012). The recent influenza pandemic is widely known as swine flu, although it has been confirmed that the viral strain did not just originate in pigs but was a complex reassortment of human, avian and swine strains (Panda *et al.* 2010).

HISTORY OF PANDEMIC FLU

A pandemic will occur when the influenza virus is sufficiently different from previous prevalent virus strains, is efficiently transmitted, spreads widely across geographical regions, there is little or no pre-existing immunity in the population and the virus causes significant disease (Pratt 2009a).

TABLE 9.2 Characteristics of influenza outbreaks where accurate estimates available

	Seasonal flu	'Spanish flu'	'Asian flu'	'Hong Kong flu'	'Bird flu' (avian flu)	'Swine flu'
Year	Annually	1918–19	1957–58	1968–69	2004	2009–10
Strain	Varies	H1N1	H2N2	H3N2	H5N1	H1N1
Number infected	*	50% of world's population affected	*	*	431 cases	>540 000 cases in England
Origin	Varies	Not known	China	China	Hong Kong	Mexico
Estimated deaths	378 in England Sept 2010– May 2011	20–100 million	1 million	1–4 million	262 deaths	26 per 100 000 in England, 18 000 worldwide
Maternal mortality	*	30%–50% of those pregnant women infected	20% of those pregnant women infected	*	1	13 in UK/ Ireland 2009–10
Groups most affected	Elderly	Age 20– 40 years	School children and elderly	Elderly	Those in contact with infected birds	Age 5–65 years
Pandemic	No	Yes	Yes	Yes	No	Yes

* Indicates that reliable estimates were not available. (Sources: Lim & Mahmood 2010, Pratt 2009a, Uyeki 2009, Donaldson *et al.* 2009, Modder 2010.)

CLINICAL FEATURES AND COMPLICATIONS OF INFLUENZA

Influenza may be confused with the common cold but it is a more serious illness and is caused by a different virus. Cold symptoms come on gradually and include having a stuffy or runny nose and a sore throat. Flu symptoms come on more suddenly and severely (*see* Box 9.6).

BOX 9.6 COMMON SYMPTOMS OF INFLUENZA

- Chills
- Sudden onset of fever (temperature of 38°C or above)
- Cough and sore throat
- Generalised muscle aches and pains (especially back and legs)
- Severe headache
- Weakness or fatigue
- Loss of appetite
- Gastrointestinal disease (nausea, vomiting, diarrhoea and abdominal pain) was a feature of swine flu in children and adults requiring admission to hospital

(DH 2013, Panda *et al.* 2010)

The mean duration of illness is 7 days, although 50% of people take up to 10 days or longer to recover (Lim & Mahmood 2010, DH 2013). The influenza virus has a 1- to 4-day incubation period and a person is infectious for a day preceding and 3 days after symptoms are evident (Gillespie & Bamford 2012). For most, influenza is a relatively mild illness but for some it may cause considerable morbidity and death. Those at higher risk for complications include those with underlying medical conditions, human immunodeficiency virus (HIV) and pregnancy (Lim & Mahmood 2010).

A primary viral or secondary bacterial pneumonia can complicate the recovery from influenza (Gillespie & Bamford 2012). Complications of H1N1 2009 influenza appear similar to seasonal flu. Reviews of pregnant women admitted to hospital with swine flu indicated a rapid progression of illness requiring admission to the intensive care unit (ITU) and ventilation. Complications, in addition to pneumonia, included sepsis, haematological disorders, pneumothorax, cardiac arrhythmias, renal failure and encephalopathy (Lim & Mahmood 2010, Pratt 2009a, Ellington 2011).

TRANSMISSION OF INFLUENZA

Transmission of influenza viruses is via direct contact with respiratory secretions and through airborne droplets generated by coughing, sneezing and talking. Infection can be acquired through contact with contaminated surfaces. The key ways to prevent spread is to use a tissue to cover the nose and mouth when coughing and sneezing, dispose of tissues immediately after use, and frequent handwashing with warm water and soap. Spread by droplet requires close personal contact, as respiratory droplets can only travel short distances (not more than 1 metre) (Pratt 2009b, Pratt 2010, Brankston *et al.* 2007). Sunlight, disinfection and detergents including soap can inactivate influenza viruses. Box 9.7 summarises general advice to prevent the spread of influenza.

BOX 9.7 GENERAL ADVICE TO PREVENT THE SPREAD OF INFLUENZA

- Cover your nose and mouth when you cough or sneeze, using a tissue where possible
- Dispose of used tissues quickly and sensibly (i.e. bag and bin them)
- Wash hands often, with hot water and soap
- Clean frequently touched hard surfaces (e.g. door handles and kitchen surfaces) frequently using normal cleaning products
- Make sure children follow these hygiene rules

(Pratt 2010)

The wearing of face masks by the general public was not advocated during the swine flu pandemic but was of benefit when used in hospital settings (Lim & Mahmood 2010). Those with swine flu were advised to stay at home for at least 7 days or for 24 hours after symptoms had gone, avoid contact with others, be vigilant in handwashing and wear a mask or cover their nose and mouth when other people were around.

A systematic review by Jefferson *et al.* (2009) of interventions to reduce the spread of respiratory viruses in healthcare settings showed that wearing masks, gloves, gowns and frequent handwashing were all beneficial in minimising the spread of infection associated with flu.

PREGNANT WOMEN AND INFLUENZA

Pregnant women are not thought more likely to be at risk of contracting influenza (DH & RCOG 2009), and for most people, including pregnant women, swine flu was a mild illness. However, as discussed at the beginning of this chapter, pregnancy is considered an independent risk factor for the development of serious complications of influenza. Many pregnant women died during influenza pandemics of the twentieth century (Pratt 2010) and during the 2009 swine flu pandemic, pregnant women were four to seven times more likely to be admitted to hospital with complications of swine flu compared to the non-pregnant population (Jamieson *et al.* 2009, Jain *et al.* 2009, Jalfari *et al.* 2010, Creanga *et al.* 2010, Louie *et al.* 2010). They were also more likely to require admission to intensive care units (Mosby *et al.* 2011, Knight *et al.*

2010) and there were 13 maternal deaths in the UK (Modder 2010). Pregnant women with pre-existing conditions including diabetes, heart disease, respiratory disorders including asthma, obesity, possibly multiple pregnancies and those who smoke are more likely to have severe complications of influenza (Mosby *et al.* 2011, Varner *et al.* 2011). However, a systematic review of studies of swine flu, found that many pregnant women (almost 70%) who were admitted to hospital with swine flu did not have any other high-risk pre-existing factors, apart from pregnancy, that would have complicated their recovery (Mosby *et al.* 2011). The physiological changes of pregnancy that affect respiratory function are thought to account for this. (*See* explanation at beginning of this chapter in section entitled 'Changes that make pregnant women more vulnerable to serious complications of respiratory infections'.)

THE BABIES OF MOTHERS WITH INFLUENZA

The babies of mothers with serious complications of swine flu were much more likely to be delivered prematurely, although very few of them tested positive for swine flu (Mosby *et al.* 2011, Mendez-Figueroa *et al.* 2011). It is generally thought that seasonal flu virus does not affect the fetus. However, a severe or sustained pyrexia during pregnancy has been associated with an increased risk for certain birth defects, including neural tube defects (Moretti *et al.* 2005), and for this reason the midwife should advise measures to ensure women do not develop a high temperature.

RECOMMENDATIONS FOR THE MANAGEMENT OF INFLUENZA IN PREGNANCY

At the time of swine flu outbreak, the Department of Health and Royal College of Obstetricians and Gynaecologists published joint guidelines on the management of pregnant women entitled *Pandemic H1N1 2009 Influenza: Clinical Management Guidelines for Pregnancy* (DH & RCOG 2009). They were published only in an electronic version, with the intention to update them online as any new information emerged. They were only for use during the pandemic and clinicians were urged to keep up to date with emerging information. They have now been archived. Similarly, the Royal College of Midwives published guidance for midwives (RCOG & RCM 2009) and information for the public was provided by the Department of Health. In the event of another pandemic, readers should access information provided by these organisations. Midwives will have a key role in keeping up to date with such recommendations and providing information to women. The guidance here is also useful in outlining principles of care during the annual flu season. Box 9.8 provides general information for the care of women in the community at the time of a flu outbreak. It will be important that women know when they should seek additional advice (*see* Box 9.9). Midwives will need to identify features of deteriorating health and ensure prompt referral and admission to hospital (*see* Box 9.10).

BOX 9.8 INFLUENZA – SUMMARY OF KEY RECOMMENDATIONS FOR CARE OF WOMEN IN THE COMMUNITY

- Women who think they have flu are advised to stay at home and phone their general practitioner, midwife or helpline for advice. Midwives may arrange home visits, where required.
- Pregnant women with uncomplicated influenza should be expected to make a full recovery.
- Women should be given clear information about when to re-consult their general practitioner or midwife and when to seek emergency medical help (*see* Box 9.9).
- Women with flu should stay at home, drink plenty of fluids and use Paracetamol to control high temperature.
- Antibiotics may be prescribed as indicated for secondary bacterial infection.

(DH & RCOG 2009, Modder 2010, RCOG & RCM 2009)

BOX 9.9 INFLUENZA – WHEN WOMEN SHOULD SEEK FURTHER MEDICAL HELP

Women should be advised to seek emergency medical help should they experience any of the following factors.
- Difficulty breathing
- Pain or pressure in chest or abdomen
- Sudden dizziness or confusion
- Severe or long-lasting vomiting
- Bloodstained sputum
- Decreased fetal movements
- High temperature not controlled by paracetamol

(DH & RCOG 2009, Modder 2010)

In cases where a woman does become critically ill, involvement of a wider multi-disciplinary team is vital and will include consultant level obstetrician, respiratory physician, obstetric anaesthetist, haematologist, the intensive care team and the infection prevention and control team. The midwife should remain involved providing an important link for ongoing psychological support for the woman and her family alongside physical care.

BOX 9.10 CRITERIA FOR URGENT HOSPITAL REFERRAL OF SUSPECTED SWINE FLU IN A PREGNANT WOMAN ACCORDING TO GUIDANCE GIVEN AT TIME OF THE 2009 SWINE FLU OUTBREAK (LIST IS NOT EXCLUSIVE)

- Signs of respiratory distress – dyspnoea, tachypnoea (respiratory rate >30 breaths per minute)
- Peripheral O_2 saturation ≤94% in air
- Dehydration or shock
- Any signs of sepsis
- Altered conscious level
- Seizures

(DH & RCOG 2009)

A summary of recommendations for the management of a woman with influenza based on guidance given at the time of the 2009 swine flu pandemic (DH & RCOG 2009, Modder 2010) included the following points.

- Admission to a single room with respiratory isolation.
- A multidisciplinary decision needs to be made with regard to the best place to manage women admitted with influenza. Intensive care unit admission will be indicated if there are signs of respiratory distress, pneumonia, persistent tachycardia (>100 beats per minute) or altered level of consciousness.
- Multidisciplinary assessment for exclusion of other pathology or obstetric complications including pre-eclampsia, chorioamnionitis, urinary tract infection and pulmonary embolism.
- Use of early warning tool (MEOWS chart) to facilitate identification of deteriorating women. Tachycardia and hypoxia were clear signs of severe disease as identified in the CMACE report (Modder 2010).
- Appropriate bacteriological investigations including blood and sputum cultures.
- Chest X-ray is a useful diagnostic test and should be used when indicated to aid diagnosis of respiratory disorders in pregnant women (Modder 2010).
- Possible use of antiviral medication (evidence of benefit under review).
- Careful fluid monitoring and assessment.
- Pulse oximetry and arterial blood gas monitoring (*see* 'Assessment of the respiratory system' section earlier in chapter)
- Control of maternal pyrexia to prevent complications including fetal abnormality and preterm delivery
- Corticosteroids to promote fetal lung maturity may be used with caution. Specialist guidance should be sought.

- Multidisciplinary decision regarding timing and mode of delivery. Preterm delivery may be indicated to improve ventilation of a very ill mother.
- Assessment by the medical team regarding the need for antibiotics.
- Awareness of potential complications including disseminated intravascular coagulation, cognitive impairment, venous thromboembolism and psychological morbidity.
- Appropriate infection control measures: notify infection prevention and control team, handwashing, women cared for in isolation, women should wear a surgical mask and staff should wear surgical mask, plastic apron, gloves and eye protection (where risk of eye splash).
- Women should be offered appropriate psychological support.

Antiviral drugs

In the 2009 swine flu outbreak, pregnant women who received antiviral medication within 2 days of developing symptoms appeared to have a shorter recovery time and fewer complications (Knight *et al.* 2010, Mosby *et al.* 2011). Newer antiviral drugs are neuraminidase inhibitors that work by preventing the virus from budding and escaping from the host cell. Data to support the safety of antiviral medication, and specific guidance regarding those recommended in pregnancy should be sought by the prescribing doctor and discussed with the woman. However, it should be noted that there was some controversy over the transparency of clinical trials for some antiviral medication around the time of the swine flu outbreak and caution is advised when evaluating evidence with regard conflicts of interest (Godlee & Clarke 2009). Sickness and vomiting have been reported side effects of some antiviral medication.

Midwives and other healthcare providers need to educate women about the symptoms of influenza (*see* Box 9.6) and advise them to seek medical advice promptly so that antiviral treatment (if indicated) can be started as early as possible. Ideally this would be within 48 hours of the onset of symptoms (Ramussen *et al.* 2011).

Keeping mother and baby together: breastfeeding and infection control measures

All women with influenza need to be isolated. However, national guidance recommends keeping mother and baby together where possible. Where the baby is premature or has other risk factors this may not be advised, and the neonatal team will have to weigh up the risks involved against the disadvantages of separation.

Women with flu should aim to continue to breastfeed even if they are unwell (if they can). It is not known whether influenza viruses can be passed from mother to baby through breast milk. However, breastfeeding is recommended, as it provides a wealth of anti-infective benefits (Tanaka *et al.* 2009). If possible, additional formula milk should not be given to babies whose mothers are taking antiviral treatment.

This will maximise transfer of the largest amount possible of maternal antibody in the breast milk (Modder 2010). If the mother is too ill to feed, feeding the baby with expressed milk should be considered. Women will need to be careful not to cough or sneeze into their baby's face. It may be useful for mothers with symptoms to wear a face mask when feeding. Vigilant handwashing will also be required.

VACCINATION

Influenza vaccination is the best way to prevent the spread of influenza. It is recommended to reduce the possibility of complications of flu in the mother with the added benefit of providing immunity to the neonate (Benowitz *et al.* 2010, Steinhoff *et al.* 2014, Tamma *et al.* 2009).

In influenza pandemic situations, and periods of vaccine shortage, vaccination of healthy pregnant women and healthcare workers is considered a priority. Influenza vaccinations for pregnant women were first advocated in the late 1950s and seasonal vaccination has been recommended in the United States for all pregnant women, regardless of pregnancy trimester, since 2004 (Jamieson *et al.* 2011). Since 2010, pregnant women in the UK have been included in those recommended to receive seasonal flu vaccination. This is offered to all women regardless of the stage of pregnancy (PHE 2013a).

Seasonal flu vaccines are developed by the WHO Global Surveillance Network, which includes 112 national influenza centres in 83 countries. These centres collect and collate the information required to identify the most virulent strains in circulation that then determine the vaccine 'recipe' for the seasonal flu vaccine. From 2013 a quadrivalent (four strains) vaccine was made available in the UK (DH 2013). Influenza vaccines against a new pandemic virus have to be produced once the specific virus strain has started to circulate and has been identified. In preparation for any new strain, vaccine manufacturers develop and test single strain (monovalent) vaccines that can be quickly manufactured once a new strain is identified (DH 2013).

Influenza vaccines recommended for pregnant women are inactivated, do not contain live viruses and cannot cause flu. Side effects of vaccination are generally mild but may include headache, mild flu-like symptoms such as muscle ache and soreness at the site of injection. The Department of Health (DH 2013) provides detailed guidance on the preparation, storage, administration and contraindications (including allergies) for flu vaccine (*see* contact details in the list of useful resources at the end of this chapter). Data from seasonal influenza vaccination indicates that it takes approximately 2 weeks to acquire immunity once the flu vaccine is given (CDC 2013). A notable benefit of influenza vaccination for pregnant women is the transplacental antibody transfer that provides protection to infants up to 6 months of age. The most benefit for infants is achieved when women have seasonal vaccination in the first 4 weeks of the availability of the vaccine, thus optimising the number of newborns to benefit

(Myers *et al.* 2011). Studies of the effectiveness of flu vaccination programmes for pregnant women have shown benefit (Thompson *et al.* 2014); however, there is some controversy regarding the quality of evidence, given that many, but not all, studies were directed by pharmaceutical companies (Jefferson *et al.* 2010).

There was a widespread recommendation for the uptake of flu vaccination during swine flu pandemic, with directives published from a number of authoritative sources including the Royal College of Midwives, the Royal College of Obstetricians and Gynaecologists, CMACE and the Health Protection Agency. However, there was reticence among women and front-line maternity care providers regarding flu vaccination. Only 37% of those in clinical risk groups, including pregnant women, and 40.3% of health professionals received the vaccination up to March 2010 (DH & HPA 2010a, b). Estimates of the uptake of seasonal flu vaccination by pregnant women in the period 2012–13 across the UK ranged from 40.3% in England to 64.6% in Northern Ireland (DH 2013).

A perceived lack of risk with regard to influenza, general lack of knowledge of the importance of the vaccine and, most commonly, concerns over safety and testing were identified as key areas influencing the uptake of vaccination among health professionals and healthy pregnant women (Broughton *et al.* 2009, Stokes & Ismail 2011 Fisher *et al.* 2011, Goldfarb *et al.* 2011).

There have been a number of cohort studies of seasonal influenza vaccine in pregnancy with no evidence of excess adverse outcomes for mother and fetus (Panda *et al.* 2010). More recent programmes monitoring both seasonal and swine flu vaccination have continued to provide reassuring data on the safety of these vaccines (Moro *et al.* 2011a, b, Rubinstein *et al.* 2013, Fell *et al.* 2014).

The recommendation of a healthcare provider has been identified as a key factor in improving the uptake of vaccination by pregnant women (Steelfisher *et al.* 2011). The Royal College of Obstetricians and Gynaecologists and the Royal College of Midwives (RCOG & RCM 2009) suggest midwives facilitate women's decision-making with regard to flu vaccination by informing women of their higher risk of complications from swine flu, that the vaccines have been licensed as safe for use in pregnancy and that side effects are minimal. Safety and benefit to the baby are likely to be key motivating factors in improving rates of uptake of vaccination and therefore midwives need to evaluate and maintain evidence-based knowledge on the safety and effectiveness of influenza vaccination.

Current advice is that midwives and other healthcare professionals working with pregnant women are advised to have seasonal flu vaccination, which should be readily available through occupational health. It is recommended that heads of midwifery arrange vaccination of staff within the workplace to maximise the uptake of vaccination by staff (PHE 2013a).

ROLE OF THE MIDWIFE

Community

- Point of contact for pregnant women with regard to prevention, symptoms and spread of influenza providing written and verbal advice
- Information and administration of flu vaccination
- Provide detailed information on infection control measures including cough etiquette and handwashing (*see* Box 9.7)
- Midwives will need to provide information regarding self-care at home for women with flu symptoms ensuring women know when and how to seek emergency care if required (*see* Box 9.9)
- Identify any women with deteriorating health and instigate appropriate referral
- Facilitate a home visit if indicated during the time the woman needs to avoid contact with other pregnant women, although it may be prudent to postpone regular antenatal care.

Women admitted to hospital with influenza

- Perform and document range of regular observations; record on MEOWS chart and refer any abnormal findings to appropriate medical staff
- Monitor usual signs of maternal and fetal well-being
- O_2 saturation monitoring
- Fluid balance and administration of fluid regimen as per medical instructions
- Administration of prescribed medication, which may include antiviral medication, antibiotics and medication to bring down the maternal temperature
- Observe strict isolation and infection control measures
- Observe for signs of labour
- Provide assistance with the establishment and maintenance of breastfeeding
- Provide psychological support to the woman and her family

PNEUMONIA

INTRODUCTION

Pneumonia is an inflammation of the lungs caused by microorganisms, usually bacteria or viruses. The inflammation produces fluid and the small air sacs (alveoli) of the lungs become filled with fluid exudate, impairing gaseous exchange. The affected area can be confined to one portion of the lungs (lobar pneumonia) or it can be more widespread (bronchopneumonia) (Margereson & Withey 2012). Pneumonia doesn't occur more often in pregnant women than in the non-pregnant population but it can be more virulent and mortality is higher (Stone & Nelson-Piercy 2012). Pneumonia accounts for nearly 20% of admissions to ITU of women who are currently pregnant (ICNARC 2009). The *Saving Mothers' Lives* report for 2006–08 (CMACE 2011) identified four maternal deaths from pneumonia. These women had complex social issues and one of them had HIV. Pneumonia is a known complication of influenza, caused by both the viral influenza microorganism and subsequent bacterial infection. Of the 13 women who died in the UK during the 2009 swine flu outbreak, six of them had developed pneumonia (Modder 2010). Varicella pneumonia is also a known complication of chickenpox in pregnancy. Women with pneumonia are more likely to deliver preterm and have lower-birthweight infants (Lim *et al.* 2001). Anatomical, physiological and immune changes in pregnancy, including increased pulmonary fluid, make pregnant women more vulnerable to infection and the development of pneumonia (Goodnight & Soper 2005). (*See* 'Changes that make pregnant women more vulnerable to serious complications of respiratory infections' section earlier in chapter.) Pneumonia can develop in fit, healthy women but some factors in addition to pregnancy may increase their susceptibility (*see* Box 9.1).

MICROORGANISMS THAT CAUSE PNEUMONIA

Box 9.11 lists some of the organisms associated with the development of pneumonia.

BOX 9.11 MICROORGANISMS THAT CAN CAUSE PNEUMONIA

- *Streptococcus pneumoniae*
- *Mycoplasma pneumoniae*
- Influenza A viruses
- *Haemophilus influenzae*
- *Chlamydia pneumoniae*
- *Legionella pneumoniae*
- *Pneumocystis carinii* (associated with HIV)
- Varicella zoster virus

(Lim *et al.* 2001, Laibl & Sheffield 2005, Goodnight & Soper 2005)

DIFFERENT TYPES OF PNEUMONIA THAT COMMONLY AFFECT PREGNANT WOMEN

Bacterial pneumonia	Community-acquired pneumonia is most commonly caused by *S. pneumoniae*, *H. influenzae* and *M. pneumoniae* Oral and possibly intravenous antibiotics are recommended

Viral pneumonia	Experience from pandemic flu outbreaks (including A H1N1 2009 swine flu) and seasonal flu epidemics have shown that pregnant women and their offspring are at higher risk of complications of these viral infections including pneumonia
Maternal varicella pneumonia	This may occur in up to 10% of pregnant women with chickenpox; the severity of the illness increases in the third trimester; antiviral treatment and effective intensive care has improved outcomes and yet varicella pneumonia remains a cause of maternal death (*see* Chapter 11 for further details)
P. carinii pneumonia (the causative organism has been renamed *Pneumocystis jiroveci*)	This infection occurs in association with HIV and is the most common opportunistic infection in those with acquired immunodeficiency syndrome
Aspiration pneumonia	This can occur as a result of gastric regurgitation during a general anaesthetic in late pregnancy; factors predisposing pregnant women to this risk include increased intra-abdominal pressure due to the enlarged uterus, relaxation of the gastro-oesophageal sphincter due to progesterone and delayed gastric emptying; the risk is increased in obese women

(Laibl & Sheffield 2005, Stone & Nelson-Piercy 2012, Goodnight & Soper 2005)

CLINICAL FEATURES OF PNEUMONIA

The classic features of pneumonia include a dry cough, breathlessness (increased respiratory rate) and chest pain. There may also be fever, agitation and confusion (Goodnight & Soper 2005). Ventilation and perfusion are likely to be compromised, resulting in reduced O_2 saturation. An examination of the chest may note that lung expansion is reduced on the affected side. Percussion will note dullness over the consolidated area and bronchial breathing may be heard. There may be production of purulent or rusty sputum as the pneumonia clears (Margereson & Withey 2012, Laibl & Sheffield 2005).

Blood cultures should be taken and a chest X-ray will confirm diagnosis (Stone & Nelson-Piercy 2012). There may be a delay in the diagnosis of pneumonia in pregnancy and this may contribute to increased morbidity. The normal breathlessness of pregnancy may mask developing disease. Breathlessness is experienced by nearly 75% of women in the third trimester. The feature of this 'physiological' breathlessness is that it does not interfere with daily activity and rarely occurs at rest (*see* Box 9.4). A woman may also normally experience a degree of chest discomfort due to the mechanical effects of the enlarged uterus on the diaphragm (Lim *et al.* 2001, CMACE 2011). A distinction between these normal findings and disease can be made by detailed assessment and a chest X-ray as indicated. The radiation dose with a chest X-ray is considered minimal (Lim *et al.* 2001), although covering the abdomen with a lead apron would still be advised. Alternative diagnosis includes asthma, pulmonary embolism and spontaneous pneumothorax (Lim *et al.* 2001).

MANAGEMENT OF PNEUMONIA IN PREGNANCY

Key elements of the treatment for pneumonia will include O_2 therapy, rehydration, and antibiotic therapy and/or antiviral medication as indicated. It is important to remember the fetus and to include monitoring of the fetus when treating pregnant women. Blood flow and oxygenation to the placenta is entirely dependent on the mother's haemodynamic state and thus fetal well-being requires effective treatment of the mother (Paruk 2008). The woman may be cared for in a high dependency unit maternity care setting, but if her condition is poor or deteriorating and/or she requires ventilation, she is likely to be transferred into a critical care setting. The consultant anaesthetist and/or the critical outreach team will facilitate and monitor the transfer.

When the woman is being cared for in a maternity setting the midwifery responsibilities will include basic observations and respiratory assessment, positioning, O_2 therapy, monitoring, fluid balance, fetal assessment, administration of medication, effective infection control measures and psychological care. When a woman is experiencing difficulty in breathing it will help to maximise ventilation by encouraging her to adopt a high side-lying position (*see* Figure 9.1). This promotes aeration and perfusion of any healthy lung tissue (Margereson and Withey 2012). This position also avoids any aortocaval compression by the uterus, which is beneficial to mother and baby (Bamber & Dresner 2003). Continuous CTG monitoring may be indicated. O_2 therapy is recommended when there is evidence of hypoxaemia. The aim of O_2 therapy is to maintain O_2 saturation levels at or above 95%. In cases of severe

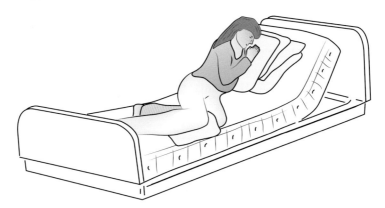

- Sitting upright and on the side, supported by raised backrest and pillows

- Lower shoulder can be brought slightly forwards

- Head and neck should be supported on a pillow

- Knees slightly bent with pillow between the knees

FIGURE 9.1 High side lying

hypoxaemia, high-concentration O_2 (15 L per minute) via a non-rebreathing reservoir mask should be commenced. For those with milder hypoxaemia, O_2 can be administered via nasal cannulae at 2–6 L per minute or via a simple face mask at 5–10 L per minute (O'Driscoll *et al.* 2008). Humidification is not required for low-flow O_2 therapy but may be required when using high-flow O_2 for longer than 24 hours (Margereson & Withey 2012).

Fluid replacement may be indicated. An increase in insensible water loss associated with an increased respiratory rate and fever may lead to dehydration, which can cause secretions to become stickier. Regular sips of water where possible is advocated. A fluid balance chart should be used (Margereson & Withey 2012).

Any critical illness will be a frightening time for a woman and her family. Anxiety and stress will increase the demand for O_2 and the midwife will be required to use excellent communications skills and a sense of calm to support the women and her family. If the woman is transferred to a critical care setting it is important that the midwife provides some continuity and visits to the ITU may be beneficial in meeting both short- and longer-term psychological needs.

ROLE OF THE MIDWIFE

- Effective assessment of respiratory function to enable early detection and prompt referral of women developing critical illness
- Interventions to maximise respiratory function that will include upright positions to expand the chest, and avoidance of aortocaval compression
- Timely and appropriate use of supplemental O_2 therapy when indicated
- Ongoing assessment of mother and fetus, clear documentation including accurate fluid balance and clear communication with appropriate members of the multidisciplinary team
- Timely administration of prescribed medication
- Psychological support to the woman and her family

TUBERCULOSIS

INTRODUCTION

TB is an infectious disease caused by the bacterium *Mycobacterium tuberculosis*. It is a major cause of morbidity and death worldwide. TB is transmitted by coughing and therefore is more easily spread where there is overcrowding, poor natural light and poor ventilation (Bothamley 2012). TB is a notifiable disease in the UK and there have been almost 9000 cases of TB reported each year over the last 5 years. Immigration and travel to and from countries with high prevalence, reduced immunity for those infected with HIV and complex social factors have contributed to the spread of TB in parts of London, West Midlands and other inner-city areas (PHE 2013b).

Although quite rare among pregnant women in the UK overall, midwives working in inner-city urban areas need to recognise possible symptoms of TB and initiate appropriate referral for diagnosis and treatment. Babies and young children are most at risk of serious complications of TB including TB meningitis. Women with TB will need the support of midwives with regard to adherence to treatment regimens. Prevention of the spread of TB through infection control, health promotion, contact tracing and bacillus Calmette–Guérin (BCG) immunisation of the newborn has become part of the role of midwives (Bothamley 2006).

EPIDEMIOLOGY AND RISK FACTORS

The WHO estimates that 8.8 million people worldwide are infected with TB. In 2012, 2.9 million new infections occurred in women. More than a million people die each year due to TB (WHO 2013). An estimated one-third of deaths due to TB occurred in women of childbearing age and it is one of the leading non-obstetric causes of maternal death in resource-poor countries, mainly in the context of HIV (Black *et al.* 2009, Grange *et al.* 2010). In resource-poor settings, where the incidence of HIV is high, women aged 15–24 years have a relatively higher proportion of TB (Mnyani & McIntyre 2010).

Maternal immunological changes, which protect the fetus, reduce cell-mediated immunity and may increase the risk of TB in pregnancy (Bothamley 2012). The symptoms of pregnancy, such as fatigue, may mask some of the characteristic features of TB, and delays in diagnosis may occur. One cohort study in the UK found an increase in the diagnosis of TB in the post-partum period (Zenner *et al.* 2012). When TB is prevalent in the general population there will be a corresponding increase in TB infection among pregnant women. Information on the numbers of women in maternity care settings with TB in the UK is limited. A retrospective review of hospital records over a 5-year period (1997–2001) in a high-prevalence area of London identified 32 women with TB in pregnancy. All these women were from ethnic minorities, the majority of them had not been born in the UK and many had arrived in the UK relatively recently (Kothari *et al.* 2006). The UK Obstetric Surveillance System (Knight *et al.* 2009) collected data on all women who were diagnosed with TB in the UK between August 2005 and August 2006, during which time 33 cases were identified and data analysed for 32 women. All were non-white and only one woman had been born in the UK. The mean time since arrival to the UK was 4.5 years (range 2 months–11 years). The Confidential Enquiry into Maternal Deaths report for 2006–08 stated that two women had died of complications of tuberculosis in pregnancy (CMACE 2011). These small data sets reflect the demographic features found in data from notifications and show that recent immigration from a high-burden country and co-infection with HIV are the most significant risk factors for TB in pregnancy. TB is associated with poverty, poor nutrition – in particular, lack of vitamin D in the non-white population – and complex social factors (PHE 2013b). Overcrowded accommodation makes the passing on of the infection more likely (Bothamley 2006).

Box 9.12 lists areas of high prevalence worldwide and Box 9.13 lists risk factors for TB.

BOX 9.12 AREAS WITH HIGH PREVALENCE OF TUBERCULOSIS

- Sub-Saharan Africa
- Indian subcontinent
- South Asia
- Eastern Europe and Baltic states
- Russian Federation and former Soviet Union states

The WHO provides a more detailed list of high-prevalence countries (2013).

BOX 9.13 LIST OF RISK FACTORS FOR TUBERCULOSIS

LIKELIHOOD OF INFECTION
- Close contact with persons known to have or suspected of having TB
- Self or relatives from area of high prevalence (*see* Box 9.12)
- Coexisting HIV infection
- Overcrowding

LIKELIHOOD OF REACTIVATION
- Poor nutrition – low vitamin D
- Alcohol or intravenous drug abuse

(Maddineni & Panda 2008, Bothamley 2012)

FEATURES OF TUBERCULOSIS INFECTION AND COURSE OF THE DISEASE

TB commonly affects the lungs (pulmonary TB) but other parts of the body such as lymph glands, intestines, meninges, pericardium, bones, joints and kidneys can become infected when the tubercle bacilli spreads via the lymphatic system and bloodstream to more distant sites (extrapulmonary TB) (Mathad & Gupta 2012). *M. tuberculosis* is spread by airborne droplet nuclei that contain the bacilli (Maddineni & Panda 2008). When an infected person with pulmonary TB coughs, aerosol particles travel through the air. The particles are small and can remain airborne for a period of time, particularly where there is poor ventilation. However, TB is not highly contagious and prolonged close contact (>8 hours in a small room) is usually required for the infection to be passed on (Pratt 2007). Although infection is common, not everyone who inhales the TB bacilli will go on to develop active disease (Bothamley 2012). The initial infection may be eliminated by the body, remain latent, or progress to active TB (DH 2011).

Latent tuberculosis

When respiratory droplets containing the bacilli are inhaled, the external defences provided by the sticky mucous membrane will often entrap the bacilli, preventing it from establishing infection. However, some of the droplet nuclei containing *M. tuberculosis* may travel down the bronchial tree and settle in the alveoli where they start to multiply. The body's immune system then activates macrophages in the alveoli of the lungs, which engulf the TB bacillus (Franco & Ernest 2011). As the person's cellular immunity is activated, an immune response can now be detected if the person has a tuberculin skin test. More macrophages and other defensive cells then accumulate at the infection site and form a protective wall around the tubercle bacillus. Within this 'granuloma', the tubercle bacilli do not grow well and may remain dormant for years. This is known as inactive, non-infective or latent TB. People with latent TB feel well and don't have any symptoms of TB but 10% of those people with latent TB will go on to develop active TB (DH 2011). Reactivation of latent TB is more common in those with HIV, soon after seroconversion and anyone diagnosed with TB should be offered an HIV test (BHIVA 2008).

Latent TB is usually diagnosed using a tuberculin skin test or a blood test (*see* 'Diagnosis of tuberculosis' section later in this chapter). Women may choose to have preventive treatment for latent TB while pregnant or delay treatment until the postnatal period (NICE 2011). For those women with HIV infection, treatment of latent TB is advocated in pregnancy, as there is a greater risk of reactivation (Mnyani & McIntyre 2010, WHO 2011).

Primary tuberculosis

This type of TB occurs in those who have not been exposed to TB before, or those who have lost their immune memory for TB (e.g. HIV infection). Primary TB can progress in the very young and others with reduced immunity, causing serious complications including miliary TB and TB meningitis. Midwives need to be aware of these potential complications for the newborn infant (Bothamley 2006).

In post-primary TB the tubercle lesion (granuloma) in the lung slowly enlarges and the centre becomes cheese-like and liquefies. These cavities may join to the air passages and the material can be coughed up, releasing thousands of actively dividing tubercle bacilli. This is when the disease becomes infectious and is known as smear-positive pulmonary TB.

SCREENING FOR TUBERCULOSIS

Symptom questionnaires have been found to be efficient and effective at identifying new cases of TB in primary healthcare settings (Griffiths *et al.* 2007). It takes less that a minute to enquire about the four key symptoms of TB: (1) cough, (2) fever, (3) night sweats and (4) weight loss (*see* Box 9.14). Kothari *et al.* (2006) advocate the use of a similar symptom questionnaire at the booking visit for women at high risk for TB (*see* Box 9.13) and/or recent arrival from high prevalence area (*see* Box 9.12). They propose this would aid early diagnosis as well as raise awareness of TB symptoms for women and health professionals generally. Routine screening for TB using tuberculin skin testing or use of the newer blood tests is not currently advocated in the UK, although it would be used where there is an indication of exposure to TB (Bothamley 2012).

DIAGNOSIS OF TUBERCULOSIS

Diagnostic tests for TB include microscopy and culture of sputum and a chest X-ray. A blood test for inflammatory markers may be useful. Pregnancy is a time that brings women into regular contact with healthcare thus increasing potential for early diagnosis, and yet delayed diagnosis, both in and outside of pregnancy, remains a problem. About 50% of pregnant women with TB have extrapulmonary TB, which will feature atypical symptoms (Knight *et al.* 2009, Kothari *et al.* 2006). In the review of TB cases in London the median delay in diagnosis was 90 days, being longer (180 days) for women with extrapulmonary TB but shorter (45 days) for pulmonary

---

BOX 9.14 SYMPTOMS OF ACTIVE TUBERCULOSIS

- Fever – most often at night and can result in drenching night sweats
- Unexplained weight loss or poor weight gain in pregnancy
- Poor appetite
- Unusual tiredness

In pulmonary TB:

- persistent productive cough that gets progressively worse over several weeks
- coughing up blood.

TB. Late initial attendance for antenatal care and poor attendance for follow-up appointments hampered diagnosis (Kothari *et al.* 2006). Language barriers, wariness of health professionals and social factors may make it difficult for women to access advice (Bothamley 2006).

Sputum is first examined by microscopy to detect the presence of acid-fast bacilli, which are the rod-shaped bacteria that can be identified on a specially stained prepared slide and are members of the genus *Mycobacterium*, of which *M. tuberculosis* is the most common. If extrapulmonary TB is suspected, samples of body fluids and/ or tissue from likely affected areas including lymph nodes and spinal fluid can also be tested. If acid-fast bacilli are present on a sample, the result is termed 'smear positive'. A presumptive diagnosis of TB can be made and treatment is usually initiated. Sputum samples are then placed in culture and incubated to see if the mycobacterium is TB and to determine drug sensitivities. However, results from sputum samples are not always conclusive. The culture of TB from samples usually takes 5–14 days in liquid culture, but it can take up to 2 months, as the bacteria tend to grow slowly in culture (Jarvis 2010a).

A chest X-ray should be performed, if indicated by clinical history, to aid diagnosis. The uterus can be shielded with a lead apron, which minimises radiation exposure to the fetus (Knight *et al.* 2009, Bothamley 2012).

Tuberculin skin testing can detect latent TB infection in those considered high risk. Tuberculin skin testing is considered safe in pregnancy and can be interpreted in the same way as in the non-pregnant population (Bothamley 2012). The test will determine if the immune system already recognises TB. Skin testing involves introducing a small amount of tuberculin, a solution of purified proteins from *M. tuberculosis* into the skin and observing the reaction after 48–72 hours. There were two methods used in skin testing, the multiple puncture Heaf method or the intradermal Mantoux test. A change to the supplies of tuberculin in the UK meant that the Heaf method is no longer used (Pratt 2007).

A new blood test to aid diagnosis is now available. These tests (QuantiFERON-TB Gold, T-SPOT.*TB*) are based on the detection of interferon-gamma released by T-cells after exposure to *M. tuberculosis*. The advantages of these new tests is that the result is available within 24 hours, it does not require a second visit to read the skin test and cross-reactivity with BCG doesn't occur, making it more specific (Bothamley 2007, Pratt 2007).

TREATMENT OF TUBERCULOSIS IN PREGNANCY

A respiratory physician will direct treatment with support from TB nurses. Good outcomes for mother and baby can be expected if anti-tuberculosis treatment regimens are followed (Bothamley 2006). There is reassuring evidence that the most commonly used drug treatments for TB – rifampicin, isoniazid, pyrazinamide and ethambutol – are suitable for use in pregnancy and breastfeeding (Bothamley 2001). Streptomycin, however, is contraindicated in pregnancy, as it causes damage to hearing during fetal development (NICE 2011, WHO 2010). There can be some complications of treatment and close monitoring of liver function and supplements of pyridoxine (vitamin B$_6$) are recommended. The usual treatment for TB requires a 6-month course of medication.

Multi-drug-resistant tuberculosis

Multi-drug-resistant tuberculosis (MDR TB) and extensively drug-resistant TB complicate the effectiveness of anti-tuberculosis treatment and pose considerable threat to the spread of and the ability to treat TB. The most common reason for the development of drug resistance is poor adherence to the long treatment that is required for TB. In resource-poor settings, counterfeit or unreliable supply of medication and inadequate education and support are also problems (Pratt 2007). There are limited data on second-line drug management for MDR TB in pregnancy. However, a small number of cases of successful treatment with good maternal and neonatal outcomes have been reported (Palacios *et al.* 2009, Lessnau & Qarah 2003). The management of MDR TB and co-infection with HIV is complex because of drug interaction between antiretroviral therapy and TB medication and outcomes for mother and infant are worse (Mnyani & McIntyre 2010). Extensively drug-resistant TB is difficult to treat and current treatment options are limited (Pratt 2007).

Tuberculosis and HIV

The suppression of cell-mediated immune response as a result of HIV infection increases the risk and severity of TB. Conversely, TB accelerates the progression of HIV disease (Pratt 2007). The combination of TB and HIV contributes to a higher rate of maternal mortality, which is most strikingly seen in resource-poor settings. The drug management of TB with HIV is complex, with drug interactions a problem (Adhikari & Jeena 2009).

Adherence to treatment

Completion of the full course of drug treatment is the key to optimum outcomes for mother and baby. The woman's motivation to take the medication regularly and over the extended period of time required will be improved if she understands the nature of the infection and the benefits and relative risks of the treatment for her and her baby. A woman-centred approach, free of stigmatisation, supported by motivated health professionals, including TB nurses and continuity of midwifery care, will build the trust and understanding required to support the woman to complete her treatment (Bothamley 2006, Jarvis 2010a, Loveday 2005). Support will include a personal approach, access to information in her own language and help with social factors such as housing and finance. Adherence to medication may be assessed through tablet counts and urine checks, although less confrontational methods such as treatment diaries, home visits and effective education is usually sufficient (Jarvis 2010b). For some pregnant women with TB, directly observed therapy will be recommended (NICE 2011).

EFFECT OF TUBERCULOSIS ON PREGNANCY, FETUS AND NEONATE

There are conflicting data on the effects of TB on outcomes for mother and neonate. Generally, timely and appropriately treated uncomplicated TB in pregnancy results in good outcomes for mother and baby (Mnyani & McIntyre 2010). When TB is diagnosed late in pregnancy, when adherence to treatment is poor and for those women with HIV the outcomes for the neonate are understandably worse, with reduced birthweight and a higher perinatal mortality (Lin et al. 2010). It may be that part of the increased risk for women with TB is associated with confounding risks for poverty and other factors known to increase vulnerability to TB infection (Bothamley 2006, 2009).

Mother-to-child transmission of TB may occur in utero but this is very rare and it is unlikely to occur if the mother is receiving effective treatment (Smith 2002). The neonate is at risk of postnatally acquired infection if the mother, or close contacts of the mother, still have active TB at the time of delivery. The aim will be to try to keep mother and baby together through commencement of effective treatment in the antenatal period. After 2 weeks of medication the woman with active pulmonary TB should not be infectious (Ross & Furrows 2014) unless she has MDR TB or doesn't continue her medication. Non-pulmonary TB is not infectious.

The baby of an infected mother will need to be screened for TB and appropriately treated if found to be infected with TB. Signs and symptoms of TB in the newborn infant tend to be non-specific and include lethargy, poor feeding, poor weight gain and enlarged liver, spleen and lymph nodes (Adhikari & Jeena 2009). Characteristic abnormal findings on chest X-ray can support the diagnosis of TB. Fever, ear discharge and skin lesions have been described in infected neonates (Maddineni & Panda 2008). If active disease is found, full treatment for the neonate is required.

For infants found not to be infected, prophylactic treatment with isoniazid for 6 months is recommended (NICE 2011, Mnyani & McIntyre 2010). Skin testing after about 3 months is recommended and treatment may be stopped if the skin test is negative, provided the infant is no longer in contact with infectious TB (DH 2011). Liaison between the paediatric team and the team supervising the mother's care will be required.

PREVENTING THE SPREAD OF TUBERCULOSIS

Midwives need to acknowledge the fear and stigmatisation associated with a diagnosis of TB, and they should seek to individualise care for the woman that attempts not to ostracise her but rather to build self-worth and dignity. Box 9.15 identifies the key components of effective infection control to prevent the spread of TB.

BOX 9.15 KEY COMPONENTS OF INFECTION CONTROL TO PREVENT THE SPREAD OF TUBERCULOSIS

- Health promotion and awareness that TB is spread by coughing from a person with TB in the lungs
- Teaching cough hygiene – covering the mouth with a hand or tissue when coughing
- Prompt diagnosis and treatment of those affected
- Coordinated services among the multidisciplinary team
- Isolation of individuals while infectious
- Support of adherence to drug therapy
- Protection through BCG vaccination of those at risk

(Jarvis 2010b, Pratt *et al.* 2005, NICE 2011)

Early diagnosis and effective treatment is the key to preventing the spread of TB. This includes the identification, assessment and treatment (if required) of any close contacts, and commitment to the long-term treatment required to remain non-infectious.

When a diagnosis of TB is suspected or confirmed, admission to hospital should be avoided. Where hospital care is required, this needs to be in an area away from other mothers and babies. A single room with an open window to encourage airflow works well to minimise airborne droplet spread. Where there are facilities for negative-pressure respiratory isolation (air mechanically pulled into ducts from the room and moved to outside vents via a filter) these should be used, especially in cases of MDR TB (NICE 2011, Bothamley 2006, Ross & Furrows 2014).

The NICE guidelines on the management of TB (NICE 2011) state that healthcare workers are not usually required to wear face masks, gowns or practise strict barrier nursing unless the women is thought to have MDR TB or is undergoing an aerosol-generating procedure. Covering of the face with a mask increases the stigmatisation of individuals and reduces communication. However, women with active pulmonary TB should be educated in cough etiquette for the protection of the woman's family and friends as well as healthcare workers and other contacts. This involves covering the mouth and nose when coughing and preferably using a tissue that can be thrown away. If they don't have a tissue they should cough into their elbow rather than their hand. Masks may provide short-term protection and may be helpful in cases of MDR TB (Dharmadhikari *et al.* 2012), although they should be changed when damp.

Some authors question the distinction with regard to personal respiratory protection between drug-sensitive and drug-resistant TB and therefore a common-sense approach that looks at an individual assessment of the risk of transmission should be made (Pratt & Curran 2006). Midwives should notify the local infection prevention and control team for specific advice.

Bacillus Calmette–Guérin vaccination

BCG vaccination is named after the two scientists who developed it in the early 1900s (Pratt *et al.* 2005). It is a live but weakened (attenuated) culture of *Mycobacterium bovis*, the bacterium that causes TB in cattle. BCG is most effective for the prevention of TB meningitis and miliary TB in young children (Maddineni & Panda 2008, DH 2011).

Since its introduction in 1953, the BCG vaccination programme in the UK has undergone several changes. Initially, BCG was given to all 13-year-olds at school. In 2005, the schools BCG vaccination programme was replaced by a risk-based approach. Current recommendations for newborn BCG vaccination includes vaccination of those living in areas with a high rate of TB, those whose parents or grandparents were born in a country with a high prevalence of TB, or those with a family history of TB in the last 5 years (NICE 2011). Midwives need to identify those infants who would benefit from BCG vaccination in the antenatal period and provide information to the parents. Ideally, the baby will be vaccinated prior to discharge. The intradermal injection is the same technique used for tuberculin skin testing and training is required to develop the skill for newborn vaccination. Information on the storage and administration of BCG vaccination can be found in the Green Book (DH 2011).

Although no harmful effects to the fetus have been associated with BCG vaccination, live vaccinations are not recommended in pregnancy, although they may be used when breastfeeding (DH 2011). It is recommended that healthcare workers who have not been vaccinated and are tuberculin skin test negative should be assessed for vaccination as part of occupational health screening (DH 2011).

SUMMARY OF CARE OF PREGNANT WOMAN WITH TUBERCULOSIS
Pre-pregnancy

- Avoid pregnancy while being treated for TB, although for those receiving standard medication regimens, pregnancy is not contraindicated and it is vital women continue their medication.
- Women being treated for MDR TB are advised not to conceive, as there is limited data on the safety of second-line drug treatment.
- Oral contraception may be affected by TB medication and barrier methods of contraception are advised.
- HIV testing should be offered.

Antenatal

- Ensure antenatal care is accessible for vulnerable women from ethnic minority groups.
- Use of professional interpreters and symptom questionnaire may be necessary to enable signs and symptoms of ill health to be recognised.
- Coordinated multidisciplinary team service including respiratory physician and TB nurses.
- Liaison with the wider multidisciplinary team with regard to contact tracing and adherence to treatment. There is a risk of infection of the newborn through other family contacts who may have TB and are not being treated.
- Home visits by a known midwife coordinated with TB nurses would be beneficial for antenatal care, alongside regular monitoring for adherence and side effects of treatment. Antenatal care will best be provided away from other pregnant women if the woman has just started treatment, when adherence to treatment is questionable, or when the woman has MDR TB.
- Advice, education and support that empowers the woman, reduces stigma and facilitates reduction in the spread of TB to others. Instruction in cough etiquette, use and disposal of tissues and regular handwashing.

Labour and delivery

- Most women with TB will have been diagnosed antenatally and have completed at least 2 weeks of treatment, making them non-infectious. However, it would be prudent to keep them separate from other mothers and babies. If a negative-pressure room is available it should be used, otherwise care in a single room with an open window is advised.
- As labour will be a high-risk time for aerosol spread, consider use of masks.
- Seek advice from the hospital infection control team.

Postpartum

- Inform the respiratory physician and TB nurses of the delivery.
- Separation of mother and baby is not normally required.
- Promote breastfeeding.
- Continue isolation for mother and baby in a single room with an open window away from the maternity unit.
- Liaise with neonatal team regarding mother's history of TB to ensure appropriate screening, treatment and prophylaxis for the newborn.
- Advise women to discourage visiting from any family contact who may have symptoms of TB (part of contact tracing).
- Continue regular TB medication.
- Advise use of barrier contraception while on TB medication.

ROLE OF THE MIDWIFE

- Recognise risk factors and common symptoms of TB and initiate appropriate referral to specialist respiratory physician for diagnosis and treatment.
- Provide information and encouragement to support women to take their TB medication regularly and complete the course
- Ensure sensible isolation measures are taken to protect other mothers and babies while maintaining dignity and respect for the woman who has TB
- Provide adequate translation services and other support that addresses the complex social factors that often accompanies infection with TB
- Carry out requirements of the newborn BCG vaccination programme

---

USEFUL RESOURCES

- In the event of an influenza outbreak, midwives should seek advice published by the Royal College of Midwives (www.rcm.org.uk), the Royal College of Obstetricians and Gynaecologists (www.rcog.org.uk) and Public Health England (www.gov.uk/government/organisations/public-health-england).
- Department of Health (2013) Influenza. Chapter 19. In: *Immunisation Against Infectious Diseases: The Green Book* [online] available at www.gov.uk/government/uploads/system/uploads/attachment_data/file/239268/Green_Book_Chapter_19_v5_2_final.pdf
- Department of Health (2011) Tuberculosis Chapter 32. In *Immunisation against Infectious Diseases: The Green Book.* London DH [online] available at www.gov.uk/government/publications/tuberculosis-the-green-book-chapter-32
- National Health Service (NHS) Choices (2012) *The Flu Jab in Pregnancy* [online]. Available at: www.nhs.uk/Conditions/pregnancy-and-baby/Pages/flu-jab-vaccine-pregnant.aspx (accessed 1 April 2014).
- National Health Service (2013) *TB, BCG Vaccination and Your Baby* [online]. Available at: www.gov.uk/government/uploads/system/uploads/attachment_data/file/342347/TB_BCG_leaflet_2014_06_.pdf

REFERENCES

Adhikari M, Jeena PM (2009) Tuberculosis in pregnancy and in the neonate. In: Schaaf S, Zumla A, Grange JM, *et al.* (editors). *Tuberculosis: a comprehensive clinical reference.* London: Elsevier. pp. 572–80.

Bamber JH, Dresner M (2003) Aortocaval compression in pregnancy: the effect of changing the degree and direction of lateral tilt on maternal cardiac output. *Anesth Analg.* **97**(1): 256–8.

Benowitz I, Esposito DB, Gracey KD, *et al.* (2010) Influenza vaccine given to pregnant women reduces hospitalization due to influenza in their infants. *Clin Infect Dis.* **51**(12): 1355–61.

Black V, Brooke S, Cherisch MF (2009) Effects of human immunodeficiency virus treatment on maternal mortality at a tertiary center in South Africa: a 5-year audit. *Obstet Gynecol.* **114**(2 Pt. 1): 292–9.

Booker R (2008) Pulse oximetry. *Nurs Stand.* **22**(30): 39–41.

Bothamley G (2001) Drug treatment for tuberculosis during pregnancy: safety considerations. *Drug Saf.* **24**(7): 553–65.

Bothamley G (2007) IFN-γ-release assays in the management of tuberculosis. *Expert Rev Resp Med.* **1**(3): 365–75.

Bothamley G (2009) Management of TB during pregnancy, especially in high-risk communities. *Expert Rev Obstet Gynecol.* **4**(5): 555–63.

Bothamley G (2012) Screening for tuberculosis in pregnancy. *Expert Rev Obstet Gynecol.* **7**(4): 387–95.

Bothamley J (2006) Tuberculosis in pregnancy: the role for midwives in diagnosis and treatment. *Br J Midwifery.* **14**(4): 182–5.

Brankston G, Giterman L, Hirji Z, *et al.* (2007) Transmission of influenza A in human beings. *Lancet Infect Dis.* **7**(4): 257–65.

Brent R (2011) The pulmonologist's role in caring for pregnant women with regard to the reproductive risks of diagnostic radiological studies or radiation therapy. *Clin Chest Med.* **32**(1): 33–42.

British HIV Association (BHIVA) (2008) *UK Guidelines for HIV Testing 2008.* London: BHIVA.

Broughton DE, Beigi RH, Switzer GE, *et al.* (2009) Obstetric health care workers' attitudes and beliefs regarding influenza vaccination in pregnancy. *Obstet Gynecol.* **114**(5): 981–7.

Centers for Disease Control and Prevention (CDC) (2013) *Influenza (Flu) vaccine (Inactivated): What you need to know 2013–14.* Vaccine information statement [online]. Available at: www. cdc.gov/vaccines/hcp/vis/vis-statements/flu.html (accessed 1 April 2014).

Centre for Maternal and Child Enquiries (CMACE) (2011). Saving Mothers' Lives: reviewing maternal deaths to make motherhood safer: 2006–08. The Eighth Report on Confidential Enquiries into Maternal Deaths in the United Kingdom. *BJOG.* **118**(Suppl. 1): 1–203.

Clutton-Brock T (2011) Critical care. In: Saving Mothers' Lives: reviewing maternal deaths to make motherhood safer: 2006–2008. The Eighth Report of the Confidential Enquiries into Maternal Deaths in the United Kingdom. *BJOG.* **118**(Suppl. 1): 173–80.

Coggins JM (2008a) Arterial blood gas analysis 1: understanding ABG reports. *Nurs Times.* **104**(18): 28–9.

Coggins JM (2008b) Arterial blood gas analysis 2: compensatory mechanisms. *Nurs Times.* **104**(19): 24–5.

Creanga AA, Johnson TF, Graiter SB, *et al.* (2010) Severity of 2009 Pandemic Influenza A (H1N1) virus infection in pregnant women. *Obstet Gynecol.* **115**(4): 717–26.

Department of Health (DH) (2011) Tuberculosis. In: *Immunisation against Infectious Disease: the Green Book* [online]. Available at: www.gov.uk/government/publications/tuberculosis-the-green-book-chapter-32 (accessed 4 March 2014).

Department of Health (DH) (2013) Influenza. In: *Immunisation against Infectious Disease: the Green Book* [online]. Available at: www.gov.uk/government/uploads/system/uploads/attach ment_data/file/239268/Green_Book_Chapter_19_v5_2_final.pdf (accessed 23 November 2013).

Department of Health (DH), Health Protection Agency (HPA) (2010a) *Pandemic H1N1 (Swine Flu) and Seasonal Influenza Vaccine Uptake amongst Frontline Healthcare Workers in England 2009/10* [online]. Available at: www.gov.uk/government/uploads/system/uploads/attachment_ data/file/215976/dh_121015.pdf (accessed 23 November 2013).

Department of Health (DH), Health Protection Agency (HPA) (2010b) *Pandemic H1N1 (Swine*

Flu) and Seasonal Influenza Vaccine Uptake amongst Patient Groups in Primary Care in England 2009/10 [online]. Available at: www.gov.uk/government/uploads/system/uploads/attachment_data/file/215977/dh_121014.pdf (accessed 23 November 2013).

Department of Health (DH), Royal College of Obstetricians and Gynaecologists (RCOG) (2009) *Pandemic H1N1 2009 Influenza: clinical management guidelines for pregnancy.* Updated 10 December 2009; now archived. Available at: http://webarchive.nationalarchives.gov.uk/20130107105354/http://www.dh.gov.uk/prod_consum_dh/groups/dh_digitalassets/@dh/@en/documents/digitalasset/dh_107840.pdf (accessed 28 September 2014).

Dharmadhikari AS, Mphahlele M, Stoltz A, *et al.* (2012) Surgical face masks worn by patients with multidrug-resistant tuberculosis: impact on infectivity of air on a hospital ward. *Am J Respir Crit Care Med.* **185**(10): 1104–9.

Dodds L, McNeil SA, Fell DB, *et al.* (2007) Impact of influenza exposure on rates of hospital admissions and physician visits because of respiratory illness among pregnant women. *CMAJ.* **176**(4): 463–8.

Donaldson LJ, Rutter PD, Ellis BM, *et al.* (2009) Mortality from pandemic A/H1N1 2009 influenza in England: public health surveillance study. *BMJ.* **339**: b5213.

Ellington S, Hartman LK, Acosta M, *et al.* (2011) Pandemic 2009 influenza A (H1N1) in 71 critically ill women in California. *Am J Obstet Gynecol.* **204**(6): S21–9.

Fell D, Dodds L, McNeil S, *et al.* (2014) H1N1 influenza vaccination during pregnancy [editorial]. *BMJ.* **348**: g3500.

Fisher BM, Scott J, Hart J, *et al.* (2011) Behaviors and perceptions regarding seasonal and H1N1 influenza vaccination during pregnancy. *Am J Obstet Gynecol.* **204**(6): S107–11.

Franco A, Ernest JM (2011) Parasitic infections. In: James D (editor). *High Risk Pregnancy: management options.* 4th ed. London: Elsevier. pp. 543–62.

Gillespie S, Bamford K (2012) *Medical Microbiology and Infection at a Glance.* 4th ed. Oxford: Wiley.

Godlee F, Clarke M (2009) Why don't we have all the evidence on oseltamivir? *BMJ.* **339**: b5351.

Goldfarb I, Panda B, Wylie B, *et al.* (2011) Uptake of influenza vaccine in pregnant women during the 2009 H1N1 influenza pandemic. *Am J Obstet Gynecol.* **204**(6): S112–15.

Goodnight WH, Soper DE (2005) Pneumonia in pregnancy. *Crit Care Med.* **33**(10 Suppl.): S390–7.

Grange J, Adhikari M, Ahmed Y, *et al.* (2010) Tuberculosis in association with HIV/AIDS emerges as a major nonobstetric cause of maternal mortality in sub-Saharan Africa. *Int J Gynaecol Obstet.* **108**(3): 181–3.

Griffiths C, Sturdy P, Brewin P, *et al.* (2007) Educational outreach to promote screening for tuberculosis in primary care: a cluster randomised controlled trial. *Lancet.* **369**(9572): 1528–34.

Hegewald M, Crapo R (2011) Respiratory physiology in pregnancy. *Clin Chest Med.* **32**(1): 1–13.

Helbert M (2006) *Flesh and Bones of Immunology.* Edinburgh: Elsevier.

Hennessey I, Japp A (2007) *Arterial Blood Gases Made Easy.* London: Elsevier.

Hunter J, Rawlings-Anderson K (2008) Respiratory assessment. *Nurs Stand.* **22**(41): 41–3.

Intensive Care and National Audit Research Centre (ICNARC) (2009) Female admissions (aged 16–50 years) to adult, general critical care units in England, Wales and Northern Ireland, reported as 'currently pregnant' or 'recently pregnant': 1 January 2007 to 31 December 2007. Available at: www.oaa-anaes.ac.uk/assets/_managed/editor/File/Reports/ICNARC_obs_report_Oct2009.pdf (accessed 19 February 2013).

Jain S, Kamimoto L, Bramley AM, *et al.* (2009) Hosptalized patients with 2009 H1N1 influenza in the United States, April-June 2009. *N Engl J Med.* **361**(20): 1935–44.

Jalfari A, Langen ES, Aziz N, *et al.* (2010) The effects of respiratory failure on delivery in pregnant patients with H1N1 2009 influenza. *Obstet Gynecol.* **115**(5): 1033–5.

Jamieson DJ, Honein MA, Rasmussen SA, *et al.* (2009) H1N1 2009 Influenza virus infection during pregnancy in the USA. *Lancet.* **374**(9688): 451–8.

Jarvis M (2010a) Tuberculosis 2: exploring methods of diagnosis, treatment regimens and concordance. *Nurs Times.* **106**(2): 22–4 [online]. Available at: www.nursingtimes.net/tuber culosis-2-exploring-methods-of-diagnosis-treatment-regimens-and-concordance/5010493. article (accessed 26 March 2014).

Jarvis M (2010b) Tuberculosis 1: exploring the challenges facing its control and how to reduce its spread. *Nurs Times.* **106**(1): 23–5 [online]. Available at: www.nursingtimes.net/nursing-practice/ clinical-zones/respiratory/tuberculosis-1-exploring-the-challenges-facing-its-control-and- how-to-reduce-its-spread/5010311.article (accessed 26 March 2014).

Jefferson T, Del Mar C, Dooley L, *et al.* (2009) Physical interventions to interrupt or reduce the spread of respiratory viruses: systematic review. *BMJ.* **339**: b3675.

Jefferson T, Di Pietrantonj C, Rivetti A, *et al.* (2010) Vaccines for preventing influenza in healthy adults. *Cochrane Database Syst Rev.* (6): CD001269.

Knight M, Kurinczuk JJ, Nelson-Piercy C, *et al.* UK Obstetric Surveillance System (2009) Tuberculosis in pregnancy in the UK. *BJOG.* **116**(4): 584–8.

Knight M, Pierce M, Seppelt I, *et al.* (2010) Critical illness with AH1N1v influenza in pregnancy: a comparison of two population-based cohorts. *BJOG.* **118**(2): 232–9.

Kothari A, Mahadevan N, Girling J (2006) Tuberculosis and pregnancy: results of a study in a high prevalence area in London. *Eur J Obstet Gynecol Reprod Biol.* **126**(1): 48–55.

Laibl VR, Sheffield JS (2005) Influenza and pneumonia in pregnancy. *Clin Perinatol.* **32**(3): 727–38.

Lessnau KD, Qarah S (2003) Multidrug-resistant tuberculosis in pregnancy: case report and review of literature. *Chest.* **123**(3): 953–6.

Lim BH, Mahmood TA (2010) Pandemic H1N1 2009 (swine flu) and pregnancy. *Obstet Gynaecol Reprod Med.* **20**(4): 101–6.

Lim WS, Macfarlane JT, Colthorpe CI (2001) Pneumonia and pregnancy. *Thorax.* **56**(5): 398–405.

Lin HC, Lin HC, Chen SF *et al.* (2010) Increased risk of low birth weight and small for gestational age infants among women with tuberculosis. *BJOG.* **117**(5): 585–90.

Louie J, Acosta M, Jamieson D *et al.* (2010) Severe 2009 H1N1 influenza in pregnant and post-partum women in California. *N Engl J Med.* **362**(1): 27–35.

Loveday H (2005) Adherence to antituberculosis therapy. In: Pratt RJ, Grange JM, Williams VG. *Tuberculosis: a foundation for nursing and healthcare practice.* London: Hodder Arnold. pp. 177–88.

Maddineni M, Panda M (2008) Pulmonary tuberculosis in a young pregnant female: challenges in diagnosis and management. *Infect Dis Obstet Gynecol.* 2008: 628985.

Margereson C, Withey S (2012) The patient with acute respiratory problems. In: Peate I, Dutton H (editors). *Acute Nursing Care: recognising and responding to medical emergencies.* London: Pearson. pp. 81–106.

Mathad JS, Gupta A (2012) Tuberculosis in pregnant and postpartum women: epidemiology, management, and research gaps. *Clin Infect Dis.* **5**(11): 1532–49.

Mendez-Figueroa H, Raker C, Anderson BL (2011) Neonatal characteristics and outcomes of pregnancies complicated by influenza infection during the 2009 pandemic. *Am J Obstet Gynecol.* **204**(6 Suppl. 1): S58–63.

Mnyani CN, McIntyre JA (2010) Tuberculosis in pregnancy. *BJOG.* **118**(2): 226–31.

Modder J (2010) *Review of Maternal Deaths in the United Kingdom related to A/H1N1 2009 Influenza* [online]. Available at: www.hqip.org.uk/assets/NCAPOP-Library/CMACE-Reports/12.-December-2010-Review-of-Maternal-Deaths-in-the-United-Kingdom-related-to-AH1N1-2009-Influenza3.pdf (accessed 1 April 2014).

Moretti ME, Bar-Oz B, Fried S, *et al.* (2005) Maternal hyperthermia and the risk for neural tube defects in offspring: systematic review and meta-analysis. *Epidemiology.* **16**(2): 216–19.

Moro PL, Broder K, Zheteyeva Y, *et al.* (2011a) Adverse events following administration to pregnant women of influenza A (H1N1) 2009 monovalent vaccine reported to the Vaccine Adverse Event Reporting System. *Am J Obstet Gynecol.* **205**(5): 473.e1–9.

Moro PL, Broder K, Zheteyeva Y, *et al.* (2011b) Adverse events in pregnant women following administration of inactivated influenza vaccine and live attenuated vaccine reported to the Vaccine Adverse Event Reporting System, 1990–2009. *Am J Obstet Gynecol.* **204**(2): 146.e1–7.

Mosby LG, Rasmussen SA, Jamieson DJ (2011) 2009 pandemic influenza A (H1N1) in pregnancy: a systematic review of the literature. *Am J Obstet Gynecol.* **205**(1): 10–18.

Myers ER, Misurski DA, Swamy (2011) Influence of timing of seasonal influenza vaccination on effectiveness and cost-effectiveness in pregnancy. *Am J Obstet Gynecol.* **204**(6): S128–40.

National Institute for Health and Care Excellence (NICE) (2011) *Tuberculosis: clinical diagnosis and management of tuberculosis, and measures for its prevention and control.* London: NICE.

O'Driscoll BR, Howard LS, Davidson AG (2008) *BTS Guideline for Emergency Oxygen Use in Adult Patients.* London: British Thoracic Society. Available at: www.brit-thoracic.org.uk/document-library/clinical-information/oxygen/emergency-oxygen-use-in-adult-patients-guideline/emergency-oxygen-use-in-adult-patients-guideline/ (accessed 28 September 2014).

Palacios E, Dallman R, Munoz M *et al.* (2009) Drug resistant tuberculosis and pregnancy: treatment outcomes of 38 cases in Lima, Peru. *Clin Infect Dis.* **48**(10): 1413–19.

Panda B, Panda A, Riley LE (2010) Selected viral infections in pregnancy. *Obstet Gynecol Clin North Am.* **37**(2): 321–31.

Paruk F (2008) Infection in obstetric critical care. *Best Pract Res Clin Obstet Gynaecol.* **22**(5): 865–83.

Pratt R J (2007) Examining tuberculosis trends in the UK. *Nurs Times.* **103**(38): 52–54.

Pratt RJ (2009a) The global swine flu pandemic 1: exploring the background to influenza viruses. *Nurs Times.* **105**(34): 18–21.

Pratt RJ (2009b) The global swine flu pandemic 2: infection control measures and preparedness strategies. *Nurs Times.* **105**(35): 16–18.

Pratt RJ (2010) Pandemic A (H1N1) 2009 influenza: an enhanced hazard during pregnancy. *Midwifery.* **26**(1): 13–17.

Pratt RJ, Curran ET (2006) Personal respiratory protection and tuberculosis: national evidence-based guidelines in England and Wales. *Br J Infect Cont.* **7**(3): 15–17.

Pratt R J, Grange JM, Williams VG (2005) *Tuberculosis: a foundation for nursing and healthcare practice.* London: Hodder Arnold.

Public Health England (PHE) (2013a) *Seasonal Influenza Vaccine Uptake amongst Frontline Healthcare Workers (HCWs) in England: Winter season 2012/13* [online]. Available at: www.gov.uk/government/uploads/system/uploads/attachment_data/file/245605/Seasonal_Influenza_Vaccine_Uptake_HCWs_2012_13.pdf (accessed 23 November 2013).

Public Health England (PHE) (2013b) *Tuberculosis in the UK: 2013 report* [online]. Available at: www.hpa.org.uk/webc/HPAwebFile/HPAweb_C/1317139689583 (accessed 25 March 2014).

Ramussen SA, Kissin DM, Yeung LF, *et al.* (2011) Preparing for influenza after 2009 H1N1: special considerations for pregnant women and newborns. *Am J Obstet Gynecol.* **204**(6): S13–20.

Ross S, Furrows S (2014) *Rapid Infection Control Nursing.* Oxford: Wiley, Blackwell.

Royal College of Obstetricians and Gynaecologists (RCOG), Royal College of Midwives (RCM) (2009) *Guidance on Swine Flu (H1N1v) for Pregnant Mothers: a joint statement from the Royal College of Obstetricians and Gynaecologists and the Royal College of Midwives* [online]. Available at: www.rcm.org.uk/college/policy-practice/position-statement/swine-influenza-h1n1/#sthash.BrvGjAsm.dpufhttp://www.rcm.org.uk/college/policy-practice/position-statement/swine-influenza-h1n1/ (accessed 1 April 2014).

Rubinstein F, Micone P, Bonotti A, *et al.* (2013) Influenza A/H1N1 MF59 adjuvanted vaccine in pregnant women and adverse perinatal outcomes: multicentre study. *BMJ.* **346**: f393.

Smith KC (2002) Congenital tuberculosis: a rare manifestation of a common infection. *Curr Opin Infect Dis.* **15**(3): 269–74.

Steelfisher GK, Blendon RJ, Bekheit MM, *et al.* (2011) Novel pandemic A (H1N1) influenza vaccination among pregnant women: motivators and barriers. *Am J Obstet Gynecol.* **204**(6): S116–23.

Steinhoff MC, MacDonald N, Pfeifer D, *et al.* (2014) Influenza vaccine in pregnancy: policy and research strategies. *Lancet.* **383**(9929): 1611–12.

Stokes S, Ismail KM (2011) Uptake of the H1N1 vaccine by maternity staff at a university hospital in the UK. *Int J Gynaecol Obstet.* **112**(3): 247.

Stone S, Nelson-Piercy C (2012) Respiratory disease in pregnancy. *Obstet Gynecol Reprod Med.* **22**(10): 290–8.

Tamma P, Ault K, del Rio C, *et al.* (2009) Safety of influenza vaccination during pregnancy. *Am J Obstet Gynecol.* **201**(6): 547–52.

Tanaka T, Nakajima K, Murashima A, *et al.* (2009) Safety of neuraminidase inhibitors against novel influenza A (H1N1) in pregnant and breastfeeding women. *CMAJ.* **181**(1–2): 55–8.

Thompson MG, Li DK, Shifflett P, *et al.* Pregnancy and Influenza Project Workgroup (2014) Effectiveness of seasonal trivalent influenza vaccine for preventing influenza virus illness among pregnant women: a population-based case-control study during the 2010–2011 and 2011–2012 influenza seasons. *Clin Infect Dis.* **58**(4): 449–57.

Uyeki TM (2009) Human infection with highly pathogenic avian influenza A (H5N1) virus: review of clinical issues. *Clin Infect Dis.* **49**(2): 279–90.

Varner MW, Rice MM, Anderson B, *et al.* (2011) Influenza-like illness in hospitalized pregnant and postpartum women during the 2009–2010 H1N1 pandemic. *Obstet Gynecol.* **118**(3): 593–600.

World Health Organization (WHO) (2010) *Treatment of Tuberculosis Guidelines.* Geneva: WHO [online]. Available at: www.who.int/tb/publications/2010/9789241547833/en/ (accessed 4 March 2014).

World Health Organization (WHO) (2011) *Guidelines for Intensified Tuberculosis Case-Finding and Isoniazid Preventative Therapy for People Living with HIV in Resource-Constrained Settings.* Geneva: WHO.

World Health Organization (WHO) (2013) *Global Tuberculosis Report 2013* [online]. Available at: www.who.int/tb/publications/global_report/en/ (accessed 4 March 2014).

Zenner D, Kruijshaar ME, Andrews N, *et al.* (2012) Risk of tuberculosis in pregnancy: a national, primary care-based cohort and self-controlled case series study. *Am J Respir Crit Care Med.* **185**(7): 779–84.

APPENDIX 1

ARTERIAL BLOOD GAS MONITORING: AN EXPLANATION OF THE PHYSIOLOGY THAT UNDERPINS INTERPRETATION

The body is continually producing acid as a by-product of metabolism. However, the pH of blood needs to be maintained within a narrow range to allow normal enzyme activity essential for healthy cellular activity. Acidosis occurs when the pH is <7.35; alkalosis occurs when the pH is >7.45. Small changes to pH outside the normal ranges create significant problems in the body. Controls of acid–base homeostasis involve chemical buffers, respiration and adjustments by the kidneys.

- Buffers respond quickly and act like sponges, soaking up the excess hydrogen or wringing themselves out to release hydrogen. Buffers include phosphate and plasma proteins such as albumin, although the most significant is the carbonic acid–bicarbonate system.
- Chemoreceptors in the body detect any build-up of acid and quickly send a message to the respiratory centre in the brain to increase the rate and depth of breathing. This is why the assessment of the respiratory rate is such an important basic observation in detection of developing ill health.
- The renal control of acid–base balance works more slowly but is effective. The kidney tubules influence pH by selectively reabsorbing and eliminating chemicals including bicarbonate, phosphate, hydrogen and chloride (Coggins 2008b).

When looking at the ABG result, the midwife should first note whether the pH is within the normal range or not. Then she should look at the $PaCO_2$ and then the level of HCO_3. Table 9.3 summarises the possible findings when there is an acid–base imbalance indicating whether it is a respiratory cause or a metabolic cause.

TABLE 9.3 Causes of acid–base imbalance

	Acidosis	Alkalosis
Respiratory	CO_2 ↑ (inadequate respiration, including pneumonia)	CO_2 ↓ (hyperventilation)
Metabolic	Bicarbonate/base excess ↓ (chronic renal failure – not enough bicarbonate) or Metabolic acid ↑ (ketoacidosis)	Bicarbonate/base excess ↑ (vomiting – loss of acids)

(Margereson & Withey 2012)

CHAPTER 10

Whooping cough (pertussis)

INTRODUCTION

Pertussis, commonly known as whooping cough, is a prolonged, distressing, contagious disease caused by a small Gram-negative coccobacillus bacterium known as *Bordetella pertussis* (Bannister *et al.* 2006). Pertussis is a notifiable disease, and when a substantial outbreak was noted in 2012 a temporary programme of vaccination for pregnant women at 28–38 weeks' gestation was introduced (HPA 2012a, JCVI 2012). The majority of pertussis-related deaths and severe complications occur in infants aged less than 3 months and the aim was to protect newborn and young babies via passive immunity acquired from the mother. Midwives were required to implement the vaccination programme at short notice. The most challenging aspect of this was for midwives to understand the rationale, provide information to parents, be knowledgeable about pertussis and, most important, answer questions regarding the validity and safety of the vaccination programme. Midwives may come into contact with women and their family members who have an upper respiratory tract infection. They will need to be able to recognise the need for referral and take appropriate action should whooping cough be suspected.

CLINICAL FEATURES

Three stages in the course of pertussis are recognised: (1) the catarrhal stage, with symptoms similar to a common cold; (2) a spasmodic stage lasting about 2 weeks and involving distressing frequent coughing that may cause cyanosis; and (3) a recovery phase, which can be prolonged, lasting up to several months. Typical symptoms of a 'whoop' or vomiting can be absent in older children or adults (HPA 2012b). *See* Box 10.1 for a detailed description of the clinical features of pertussis.

BOX 10.1 CLINICAL FEATURES OF PERTUSSIS – THE THREE STAGES

1. *Catarrhal* (lasts 2 weeks): non-specific symptoms including runny nose, sore throat, conjunctivitis. A cough develops after 4–5 days.
2. *Spasmodic* (lasts 2 weeks): intense bouts of coughing (sometimes referred to as 'paroxysms'), with no inspiration between them. They are very distressing and can lead to cyanosis. These episodes can occur spontaneously or they can be precipitated by external factors such as cold and noise. The paroxysm ends with a characteristic gasp for air that causes an inspiratory cry (a 'whoop'), which is sometimes accompanied by a vomit, although the features may also occur separately. Infants may appear to 'gag' or 'gasp' and may temporarily stop breathing.
3. *Convalescent* (lasts from 2 weeks to several months): coughing gradually subsides.

(Bannister *et al.* 2006, DH 2013, Goering *et al.* 2013, HPA 2012b)

Complications in young infants include apnoea, hypoxia, bronchopneumonia and repeated vomiting leading to weight loss (Wood & McIntyre 2008). Lengthy hospitalisation and oxygen supplementation is often required (Cortese *et al.* 2008, Castagnini & Munoz 2010). Venous pressure raised during coughing can cause nosebleeds, conjunctival haemorrhage and facial petechiae. Bruised ribs can result from the intense coughing (HPA 2012b). Intracranial haemorrhage and encephalitis can occur in infants, leading to lifelong complications (Bannister *et al.* 2006). A number of babies died during the 2012 outbreak (HPA 2012b).

TRANSMISSION

Pertussis is highly contagious. Coughing by an infected person generates airborne aerosol droplets that can infect a vulnerable host. A person is considered infectious from 2–4 days before he or she starts to cough to around 21 days after the coughing starts (HPA 2012b). Incubation is around 7–10 days (HPA 2012a). Many infants acquire *B. pertussis* from household contacts, including their parents and older siblings, although for up to a third the source of infection is not identified (Wiley *et al.* 2013). Healthcare and children's workers have also been identified as a potential source for spreading pertussis infection (Bechini *et al.* 2012, Wood & McIntyre 2008).

EPIDEMIOLOGY

Before the era of pertussis vaccination in the late 1950s, pertussis was an endemic disease, affecting an average of 120 000 people in the UK each year, with peaks occurring approximately every 3 years (DH 2013).

It is now estimated that more than 80% of infants worldwide routinely receive pertussis vaccination as part of the diphtheria, tetanus and pertussis combination. However, protection from pertussis following immunisation or natural infection is not lifelong. Immunity following infant immunisation lasts only 4–12 years, and 4–20 years following natural infection (Bechini *et al.* 2012). This waning immunity has created a reservoir of infection among older children, adolescents and adults that provides a potential source for transmission to susceptible infants prior to vaccination (Bechini *et al.* 2012, Woods & McIntyre 2008).

In 2012 a significant increase in cases of pertussis was reported. The outbreak was mainly among teenagers and young adults but the highest rate of the most serious consequences was seen in babies under 3 months old (HPA 2012a, JCVI 2012). Similar peaks were seen in the United States and in Australia, New Zealand and Canada (HPA 2012b). The dramatic increase in numbers and the impact on young infants prompted the Joint Committee on Vaccination and Immunisation to review current prevention strategies for the control of pertussis (JCVI 2012).

STRATEGIES TO CONTROL WHOOPING COUGH INFECTION

The main strategy for controlling the impact of pertussis infection is the current childhood vaccination programme (*see* Box 10.2). Uptake rates in the UK for the primary course of three doses is high, at around 95%, by the age of 12 months (HPA 2012b).

BOX 10.2 THE CHILDHOOD VACCINATION PROGRAMME IN THE UK

- The five-in-one multivalent vaccine Pediacel is used, which combines diphtheria, tetanus, acellular pertussis, inactivated polio and *Haemophilus influenzae* type b (DTaP/IPV/Hib) (HPA 2012a)
- It is an accelerated programme offered to infants at 2, 3 and 4 months of age.
- A booster dose of pertussis-containing vaccine is given to children from about 3 years and 4 months of age.

(HPA 2012b)

A further variety of strategies for prevention of pertussis in young infants before the age of full vaccination have been proposed. These may be implemented as a general extension of the childhood vaccination programme or be cascaded during times of outbreak or in relation to specific case notification.

These strategies include the following:

- vaccinating adolescents and adults with a low-dose adult formula of diphtheria, tetanus and acellular pertussis vaccine (DTPa) to boost waning immunity in this population – vaccination interval has been reduced from 10 years down to 5 years

- vaccinating pregnant women between 28 and 32 weeks' gestation and up to 38 weeks' gestation (*see* later section 'Vaccination of pregnant women')
- cocoon strategy – this targets vaccination to those most closely associated with the newborn, including postpartum mothers, fathers and close household contacts
- vaccination of healthcare and childcare workers, particularly those working with infants and pregnant women
- early administration of a prophylactic course of recommended antibiotics in addition to vaccination for those in contact with someone with whooping cough – this may include pregnant women following individual assessment based on gestational age and suitability of antibiotics.

(Woods & McIntyre 2008, Bechini *et al.* 2012, Murphy *et al.* 2008, Gall *et al.* 2011, HPA 2012a, PHE 2013)

TYPES OF VACCINE

The first pertussis vaccines developed in the late 1950s were whole-cell vaccines. These vaccines were associated with a higher incidence of side effects, which included fever, malaise and pain at the injection site. Febrile convulsions thought to be associated with the vaccine occurred in about 0.5% of those vaccinated. Rare but serious side effects (estimated rate of 1 in 100 000 vaccinations (<0.001%)) included encephalopathy with permanent neurological damage. Understandably, professionals and parents were concerned and vaccination rates fell to around 30%, triggering a resurgence of pertussis in the 1980s (Goering *et al.* 2013, DH 2013).

Acellular pertussis vaccines have now replaced the whole-cell pertussis vaccine in many countries including the UK. These new types of vaccines contain up to five key specific purified or recombinant *B. pertussis* antigens (Bechini *et al.* 2012, Wood & McIntyre 2008). They were developed in Japan in the late 1970s and have been used there since 1981. These newer vaccines provide the same or better protection but cause fewer side effects (Goering *et al.* 2013).

There are different acellular pertussis-containing vaccines available, the main difference between them being the number of pertussis antigen components they contain and what other vaccines they are combined with. The preparation currently advised for pregnant women is Repevax, which contains low-dose diphtheria, tetanus, five-component acellular pertussis and inactivated polio antigens (DTaP/IPV) (JCVI 2012). No monovalent pertussis preparation is available (DH 2013).

VACCINATION OF PREGNANT WOMEN

During pertussis outbreaks, immunisation of pregnant women during the third trimester is recommended (Murphy *et al.* 2008). This is thought to be the most effective way to protect newborn infants at a time when whooping cough is circulating in the population. This policy of temporary immunisation was implemented in the UK in September 2012 (HPA 2012a, JCVI 2012). The aim was to vaccinate pregnant women between 28 and 38 weeks' gestation (ideally between 28 and 32 weeks) (JCVI 2012). The timing of vaccination was aimed at boosting antibody levels at an optimum time for antibodies to pass from mother to baby and thus provide temporary passive immunity for the newborn until the age of vaccination (Gall *et al.* 2011). After vaccination it takes about 2 weeks for high levels of antibodies to be produced by the mother, and the maximum time for transfer of these antibodies to the fetus occurs after 34 weeks' gestation (HPA 2012b). Vaccination during pregnancy also protects the mother from acquiring pertussis and being a potential source of transmission (HPA 2012a, b).

The *Green Book: Immunisation against infectious disease* (DH 2013:285) (which provides the most up-to-date advice on all immunisation schedules) states:

> Pertussis-containing vaccines may be given to pregnant women when protection is required without delay. There is no evidence of risk from vaccinating pregnant women or those who are breast-feeding with inactivated viral or bacterial vaccines or toxoids.

Monitoring of pertussis-containing vaccination in pregnant women has not noted any elevated frequency of adverse events (CDC 2013, Rasmussen *et al.* 2013), although this remains an area of ongoing research.

The patient information leaflet provided for Repevax (the current vaccine preparation advised for pregnant women) states that the vaccine is not recommended in pregnancy (Sanofi Pasteur MSD 2012). The Health Protection Agency (2012b) and the Joint Committee on Vaccination and Immunisation (2012) explain that this is because there have been no clinical trials with pregnant women, and not because there are any specific concerns or evidence of harm in pregnancy. The Health Protection Agency (2012b) recommends that guidance from the Joint Committee on Vaccination and Immunisation should be followed. It is advised that those administering the vaccine should be familiar with the *Green Book* (DH 2013) advice regarding administration, special considerations and adverse side effects. They should also read the vaccine packet before administration. Box 10.3 provides general information on some of the practical aspects of pertussis vaccination. A study of midwives in Australia showed that midwives' confidence in their skill and knowledge in delivery of vaccinations was an important determinant in their motivation to support a vaccination programme (Robbins *et al.* 2011). Education programmes and skills workshops for midwives will be needed when new policies of vaccination are implemented. In an era of potential 'information overload' for women, improved ways of providing information to women needs to be considered, although the personal communication by the midwife will remain key in supporting women in decision-making.

BOX 10.3 PRACTICAL POINTS REGARDING ADMINISTRATION OF PERTUSSIS-CONTAINING VACCINE TO PREGNANT AND POSTPARTUM WOMEN*

- Informed consent must be obtained.
- The midwife should advise women on possible adverse reactions, including pain, redness and swelling at the site of injection; a small painless nodule may form at the injection site and they may develop a slightly raised temperature accompanied by shivering, headache and muscle or joint pain.
- The vaccine is inactivated and therefore cannot cause the diseases from which it protects.
- The pre-filled syringe needs to be shaken to form a cloudy white suspension before use.
- The vaccine should be given as an intramuscular injection into the deltoid muscle.
- It can be given at the same time as other vaccines such as influenza (use different arm).
- It can be given at the same time as anti-D.
- Avoid giving the vaccine at a time of acute illness.
- Check to ensure the woman has not already had the vaccination recently.
- Check that the woman has not had a previous anaphylactic reaction to any component in the vaccine.
- Record the vaccination in the general practitioner and maternity notes.
- Breastfeeding is not contraindicated.
- The vaccine is latex and thiomersal free.
- Egg allergy is not a contraindication to the Repevax vaccine.

* Information relates to use of Repevax; readers should access specific local guidelines and up-to-date recommended online resources.

(HPA 2012b, DH 2013)

Midwives should remind women of the importance of starting their babies' schedule of vaccinations at 8 weeks in order to achieve longer-term protection (HPA 2012b). They should also ensure older siblings are up to date with their immunisations.

MIDWIVES AND CONTACT WITH CASES OF WHOOPING COUGH

Midwives may be alerted to suspected cases of whooping cough in community settings. They should advise potentially affected individuals to stay at home and to separate themselves from young infants and pregnant women. Midwives will need to ensure urgent referral to a doctor for diagnosis, treatment, management of contacts, follow-up and notification. Detailed documentation including demographic details, clinical features, gestation, immunisation record and close contacts should be recorded for all suspected cases of pertussis.

Diagnosis can be made by culture of *B. pertussis* on a swab taken from the posterior nasopharynx using an ultrafine flexible nylon swab. Accurate details regarding onset of symptoms should be provided on the laboratory request form and the specimen processed promptly. For older children aged 5–16 years who have not had a pertussis vaccine in the last year, oral fluid testing using a specially designed kit is recommended. For infants under 12 months who are acutely ill, polymerase chain reaction analysis can be performed on pernasal samples and provide a more rapid diagnosis than waiting for results of culture (PHE 2013). Serological testing is used for diagnosis of cases in adults. Onset of symptoms and vaccination history are required to aid interpretation of this test.

If a pregnant woman contracts whooping cough, her symptoms may be more intense because of the enhanced respiratory demand of pregnancy, but it is not thought she is more at risk of complications than non-pregnant adults and no adverse fetal outcomes have been reported (HPA 2012a). However, if she contracts pertussis late in pregnancy, there is a risk of transmitting the illness to her newborn (HPA 2012a).

Antibiotics have been shown to be effective at eliminating *B. pertussis* and may be useful in reducing transmission of pertussis, but they seem to have little effect on reducing the symptoms or shortening the length of illness (Altunaiji *et al.* 2013, PHE 2013). Age-specific guidance for antibiotic treatment and post-exposure prophylaxis, including recommendations for pregnancy, are provided by Public Health England (PHE 2013).

Contacts of cases of whooping cough considered a priority for identification and treatment include those that are vulnerable to complications (newborn and infants who have not yet received their three vaccinations) and those at risk of transmitting pertussis to this vulnerable group. This includes pregnant women over 32 weeks' gestation, midwives and other healthcare workers working with pregnant women, infants and household contacts (HPA 2012a). The management of contacts may include chemoprophylaxis with recommended antibiotics and immunisation (HPA 2012a, c).

The Health Protection Agency has produced guidance for the management of pertussis incidents in healthcare settings that deal with notification and prevention of transmission (HPA 2012c). Box 10.4 summarises key actions advised in these guidelines although reference to the full guidelines is recommended.

BOX 10.4 SUMMARY OF HEALTH PROTECTION AGENCY GUIDELINES FOR THE MANAGEMENT OF PERTUSSIS INCIDENTS IN HEALTHCARE SETTINGS

- Cases of pertussis should be notified to Public Health England (formerly the Health Protection Agency). Infection and prevention control teams in local units should be alerted and where staff illness is suspected, occupational health should also be advised.
- Hospitalised patients should be cared for in respiratory isolation.
- Pregnant women, infants under 1 year who have not completed a vaccination programme and healthcare workers working with infants and pregnant women are priority groups for contract tracing and prophylaxis.
- Chemoprophylaxis with antibiotics and vaccination should be offered to priority contacts as appropriate.

(HPA 2012c)

ROLE OF THE MIDWIFE

- Keep up to date with current recommendations regarding whooping cough vaccination in pregnancy.
- Provide women with accessible information regarding whooping cough vaccination that includes the rationale for current recommendations.
- Ensure prompt referral of any cases of suspected whooping cough in women or their families along with advice to avoid contact with other people.
- Remind women that it is important for all family members to keep up to date with vaccinations, as this will be the best way to protect the newborn baby.
- Midwives should ensure they keep up to date with their own vaccinations.

USEFUL RESOURCES

- Health Protection Agency (2012) *Vaccination against Pertussis (Whooping Cough) for Pregnant Women: An update for healthcare professionals.* [online] Available at www.hpa.org.uk/webc/ HPAwebFile/HPAweb_C/1317136495835
- Health Protection Agency (2012) *Public Health Management of Pertussis: HPA guidelines for the public health management of pertussis incidents in healthcare settings.* [online] available at www.hpa.org.uk/webc/HPAwebFile/HPAweb_C/1317136713302
- National Health Service (2012) *Pertussis (Whooping Cough) Immunisation for Pregnant Women: Factsheet October 2012* [online]. Available at: www.gov.uk/government/uploads/system/

uploads/attachment_data/file/138194/DoH_8153_-whoopingCough_factsheet_12pp_07.pdf (accessed 31 March 2014).

REFERENCES

Altunaiji S, Kukuruzovic R, Curtis N, *et al.* (2013, reprint) Antibiotics for whooping cough (pertussis) (Review). *Cochrane Database Syst Rev.* (3): CD004404.

Bannister B. Gillespie S, Jones J (2006) *Microbiology and Management.* 3rd ed. Oxford: Blackwell Publishing.

Bechini A, Tiscione E, Boccalini S, *et al.* (2012) Acellular pertussis vaccine in risk groups (adolescents, pregnant women, newborns and health care workers): a review of evidence and recommendations. *Vaccine.* **30**(35): 5179–90.

Castagnini LA, Munoz FM (2010) Clinical characteristics and outcomes of neonatal pertussis: a comparative study. *J Pediatr.* **156**(3): 498–500.

Centers for Disease Control and Prevention (CDC) (2013) Updated recommendations for use of tetanus toxoid, reduced diptheria toxoid, and acellular pertussis vaccine (Tdap) in pregnant women – Advisory Committee on Immunization Practices (ACIP), 2012. *MMWR Morb Mortal Wkly Rep.* **62**(7): 131–5 [online]. Available at: www.cdc.gov/mmwr/preview/mmwrhtml/mm6207a4.htm (accessed 31 March 2014).

Cortese MM, Baughman AL, Zhang R, *et al.* (2008) Pertussis hospitalizations among infants in the United States, 1993 to 2004. *Pediatrics.* **121**(3): 484–92.

Department of Health (DH) (2013) Pertussis. In: *The Green Book: Immunisation against infectious disease* [online]. Available at: www.gov.uk/government/publications/pertussis-the-green-book-chapter-24 (accessed 24 March 2014). pp. 277–94.

Gall SA, Myers J, Pichichero M (2011) Maternal immunization with tetanus-diphtheria-pertussis vaccine: effect on maternal and neonatal serum antibody levels. *Am J Obstet Gynecol.* **204**(334): e1–5.

Goering RV, Dockrell HM, Zuckerman M, *et al.* (2013) *Mims' Medical Microbiology.* 5th ed. Oxford: Elsevier, Saunders.

Health Protection Agency (HPA) (2012a) *HPA Guidelines for the Public Health Management of Pertussis* [online]. Available at: www.hpa.org.uk/webc/HPAwebFile/HPAweb_C/1287142671506 (accessed 24 March 2014).

Health Protection Agency (HPA) (2012b) *Vaccination against Pertussis (Whooping Cough) for Pregnant Women: an update for healthcare professionals* [online]. Available at: www.hpa.org.uk/webc/HPAwebFile/HPAweb_C/1317136495835 (accessed 24 March 2014).

Health Protection Agency (HPA) (2012c) *Public Health Management of Pertussis: HPA guidelines for the public health management of pertussis incidents in healthcare settings* [online]. Available at: www.hpa.org.uk/webc/HPAwebFile/HPAweb_C/1317136713302 accessed 24 March 2014.

Joint Committee on Vaccination and Immunisation (JCVI) (2012) *Minute of teleconference on Thursday Wednesday 30 August 2012 10.00am–12.00am and post-teleconference discussion* [online]. Available at: www.gov.uk/government/uploads/system/uploads/attachment_data/file/223497/JCVI_minutes_Aug_2012_Pertussis_-_final.pdf (accessed 24 March 2014).

Murphy TV, Slade BA, Broder KR, *et al.* Advisory Committee on Immunization Practices (ACIP); Centers for Disease Control and Prevention (CDC) (2008) Prevention of pertussis, tetanus, and diphtheria among pregnant and postpartum women and their infants recommendations of the Advisory Committee on Immunization Practices (ACIP). *MMWR Recomm Rep.* **57**(RR-4): 1–51.

Public Health England (PHE) (2013) *Pertussis Factsheet for Healthcare Professionals* [online]. Available at: www.hpa.org.uk/webc/HPAwebFile/HPAweb_C/1317139762805 (accessed 23 March 2014).

Rasmussen SA, Watson AK, Kennedy ED, *et al.* (2013) Vaccines and pregnancy: past, present, and future. *Semin Fetal Neonatal Med.* **19**(3): 161–9.

Robbins SC, Leask J, Hayles EH, *et al.* (2011) Midwife attitudes: an important determinant of postpartum pertussis booster vaccination. *Vaccine.* **29**(34): 5591–4.

Sanofi Pasteur MSD (2012) *Patient Information Leaflet for the User: Repevax* [online]. Available at: www.medicines.org.uk/EMC/history/17377/PIL/REPEVAX (accessed 31 March 2014).

Wiley KE, Zuo Y, Macartney KK, *et al.* (2013) Sources of pertussis infection in young infants: a review of key evidence informing targeting of the cocoon strategy. *Vaccine.* **31**(4): 618–25.

Wood N, McIntyre P (2008) Pertussis: review of epidemiology, diagnosis, management and prevention. *Paediatr Respir Rev.* **9**(3): 201–12.

CHAPTER 11

Viral rash illnesses in pregnancy that may affect the fetus

→ Overview
→ Rubella
→ Parvovirus B19
→ Measles
→ Chickenpox (varicella)
→ Cytomegalovirus

OVERVIEW

Pregnant women may come into contact with a range of viral illnesses that commonly affect children. The midwife requires good knowledge of the presentation and implications of these illnesses to facilitate effective health education, make an accurate assessment, document relevant details and refer women exposed to viral rash illnesses. It is particularly important to identify those illnesses that pose a risk to the mother, fetus or neonate and for which timely intervention can improve the outcome (MacMahon 2012). The mother most often contracts the infections from her own children. Pregnant childcare workers and teachers are also at risk. This chapter will first look at how to prevent rash illness in pregnancy, principles of assessment, documentation and referral. Public Health England, formerly the Health Protection Agency, provides detailed guidance for health professionals on the management of rash illness in pregnancy – details for accessing this are provided at the end of this chapter (HPA 2011a).

Sections on each of the five conditions – (1) rubella, (2) parvovirus, (3) measles, (4) varicella and (5) cytomegalovirus (CMV) – will elaborate on the specific assessment, features and complications of these individual infections for mother and baby.

It is important to note that CMV infection does not cause a rash and women are

TABLE 11.1 Summary of the features of common viral rash illness and their impact on pregnancy

	Varicella zoster (chickenpox)	Rubella (German measles)	Parvovirus B19 (slapped cheek syndrome)	Rubeola (measles)	Cytomegalovirus (CMV)
Estimates of % young female adults without immunity*	Varies with country of origin 1%–14% in temperate climates Up to 50% in tropical climates	3%–4%	40%–50%	<5%	50%
Infectivity: risk of transmission from close contact	High (70%–90%)	High (90%)	Medium (50%)	Very high (99%)	
Incubation period	10–21 days	14–21 days	4–14 days	10–14 days	
When is it infectious for contacts?	48 hours before onset of rash until lesions have all crusted over	From 7 days before rash until 4 days after onset of rash	From 10 days before onset of rash, ending when rash appears	From 4 days before rash until 4 days after onset of rash	Viral shedding of CMV continues in body fluids for months to over 1 year
Type of rash	Vesicular	Maculopapular	Maculopapular	Maculopapular	None
Satisfactory evidence of immunity following rash exposure in pregnancy	History of chickenpox (less reliable in tropical countries) Two doses of varicella vaccine	Two doses of rubella-containing vaccine	History unreliable No vaccine available	Two doses of measles-containing vaccine	Immunity does not preclude reactivation nor reinfection

	Varicella zoster (chickenpox)	Rubella (German measles)	Parvovirus B19 (slapped cheek syndrome)	Rubeola (measles)	Cytomegalovirus (CMV)
Risks to susceptible mother	Serious pneumonitis	Minimal Possible acute joint pain	Minimal Possible acute joint pain, anaemia	Serious pneumonitis	Minimal May have glandular fever-type illness
Risk to fetus or neonate	Congenital varicella syndrome: <20 weeks, 1%–2% Childhood zoster: 25–36 weeks Neonatal varicella: 4 days before to 2 days after delivery, 20%	<11 weeks: 90%: congenital rubella syndrome 11–16 weeks: 20%: congenital rubella syndrome 16–20 weeks: small risk of deafness	<20 weeks: 9% excess fetal loss 3% develop fetal hydrops, with 50% fatality	0–40 weeks, increased fetal loss, preterm delivery and low birthweight perinatal; severe measles, encephalitis	Majority of infants are asymptomatic Around 10%–15% present with CMV manifestations at birth, of which about half will develop serious outcomes including cerebral palsy and hearing loss; however, 10%–15% of those appearing normal at birth will later go on to develop a problem – usually hearing loss

* Percentages are estimates only, as they will vary according to maternal age (affected by coverage of vaccination programmes), ethnicity and source of data collection (sources: MacMahon 2012, HPA 2011a).

unlikely to be aware of this infection. However, as it may cause significant fetal damage it is discussed in this chapter. Table 11.1 gives an overview of the key features and implications for pregnancy of the conditions.

REDUCING THE RISK OF RASH ILLNESS IN PREGNANCY

Vaccination provides the most effective intervention for reducing the burden of disease from a viral rash illness during pregnancy. MMR (measles, mumps, rubella) vaccination is offered to children at around the time of their first birthday, with a second dose given just prior to starting school. However, the vaccine can be given at any age and is also offered to older children, teenagers, healthcare workers and adults, including non-immune women of childbearing age. Women found to be non-immune during antenatal screening are offered MMR vaccination in the immediate postnatal period. The immunisation programme has been effective in reducing morbidity related to rubella and measles in pregnancy (DH 2013a), although negative publicity in the late 1990s affected parent confidence and rates of vaccination were affected at that time. (*See* further details under 'MMR vaccination' headings in both the 'Rubella' and the 'Measles' sections in this chapter.) Vaccination for chickenpox is available in countries outside the UK including the United States and Japan but is not a part of the UK childhood vaccination schedule, although chickenpox vaccination is offered to non-immune healthcare workers (DH 2012) and may be recommended to non-immune women prior to pregnancy. There is no reliable vaccine for parvovirus and a vaccine for CMV is under development (Townsend 2011).

Antenatal booking assessment provides further opportunities for prevention of the consequences of common childhood viral infections. The midwife should enquire about any rash illness or contact with rash illness. This questioning not only uncovers a recent exposure to infection but also raises awareness and enables the midwife to provide further verbal and written information. Antenatal screening tests include assessment of immunity to rubella, and the midwife should also ask the woman if she has had chickenpox. Women born outside the UK may not have benefited from vaccination programmes, and if recently arrived from areas where these infections are common may have had recent exposure. Midwives need to tailor information and provide access to effective translation to optimise the quality of communication with these women. Midwives should explain what women should do if they come into contact with a rash illness and/or develop a rash themselves. They should also give information on the importance of handwashing when in contact with the urine and secretions of young children. Box 11.1 provides an overview of strategies to reduce the risk of rash illness in pregnancy.

BOX 11.1 REDUCING THE RISK OF RASH ILLNESS IN PREGNANCY

PRIOR TO PREGNANCY
- Check history of chickenpox and shingles
- Check vaccination status of available vaccines such as MMR and postpone pregnancy to enable vaccination to be given. Pregnancy should be avoided for 1 month following MMR vaccination (DH 2013a)

BOOKING
- Enquire if the woman has had a rash illness or contact with someone with rash illness in the current pregnancy
- Advise women to seek assistance of a health professional (by telephone) if they develop a rash illness or have contact with someone with a rash illness during the pregnancy
- Record vaccinations the woman has had and enquire and record if she has had chickenpox or shingles
- Routine screen for rubella IgG on booking bloods
- Storage of booking bloods enables subsequent comparison for serological testing

POST-PARTUM
- Vaccination as indicated for those found not immune

GENERAL ADVICE
- Advise women to avoid contact with rash illness when they are pregnant
- If they do have contact, they should seek advice as soon as possible, preferably by telephone

(MacMahon 2012)

THE PREGNANT WOMAN WHO HAS CONTACT WITH RASH ILLNESS AND/OR DEVELOPS A RASH

All pregnant women should contact their midwife, general practitioner (GP) or obstetrician urgently if they develop a rash in pregnancy or have contact with someone who has a rash, regardless of their immune status. However, they should avoid going to the maternity unit or antenatal clinic. The contact – that is, the person with the rash – is known as the index case. The type of rash should be identified to determine what specific infection the index case may have and details of the diagnosis sought. The nature, timing and duration of exposure need to be determined. Household contact is associated with the highest risk of transmission (HPA 2011a). Exposure to varicella, rubella and parvovirus is defined as face-to-face for 15 minutes in same room, whereas lesser exposure to measles may be relevant (HPA 2011a, MacMahon 2012).

The mother's susceptibility to infection needs to be ascertained. This can be specific where the index case has a definite diagnosis. Immunity to rubella, for example, can be checked from results of booking bloods. Where immune status is uncertain and significant contact confirmed, the woman requires urgent referral to specialist virology, microbiology or infectious diseases consultant for serological testing and counselling (MacMahon 2012).

Where a woman has a rash, a doctor should examine her and a clinical history obtained to aid diagnosis. The appearance of a rash on darker skin may be more difficult to see. Those with non-vesicular rash illness should be investigated for rubella and parvovirus B19 infection (HPA 2011a). A maculopapular rash is a feature of measles, rubella and parvovirus and a vesicular rash is chickenpox.

Laboratory investigation to aid diagnosis and management will be sought. Box 11.2 details the information required for the laboratory when investigating a woman with a rash illness. Box 11.3 details the details required when investigating a woman who has been exposed to a rash illness. The midwife will assist in enhancing the accuracy of the information by keeping detailed records of the information provided by the woman.

BOX 11.2 INFORMATION REQUIRED WHEN REQUESTING LABORATORY INVESTIGATION FOR RASH ILLNESS

- Name, date of birth, hospital number and telephone contact
- State clearly that woman is pregnant; include date of last menstrual period and estimated date of delivery and gestational age
- Clinical features of illness, type and distribution of rash, date of onset of symptoms and rash
- Past history of infection, vaccination and recent antibody testing
- Any known contact with individual with rash illness; date of contact?

(MacMahon 2012, HPA 2011a)

Women should be given written information about the testing and possible outcomes as a backup to verbal discussion They should be largely reassured that the incidence of rubella (the infection with highest morbidity for the fetus), is very low and tests are likely confirm an absence of rubella infection (NICE 2013). Use of competent interpreters and language-appropriate material for women who don't speak English is good practice. The woman will need contact numbers and follow-up details, and all discussions and care plans need to be documented. Treatment with immunoglobulins may be indicated for susceptible women to reduce the impact of illness and are used in the management of exposure to measles and chickenpox. Referral to a specialist in fetal medicine is recommended if the potential for congenital damage is established, for discussions, detailed ultrasound and management that may include offer of termination of pregnancy (HPA 2011a). Continuity of care by the midwife may provide valuable support for the woman during the period of uncertainty while diagnosis and assessment is made.

BOX 11.3 INFORMATION TO COLLECT WHEN A PREGNANT WOMAN IS EXPOSED TO A RASH ILLNESS

- Name, date of birth, hospital number and telephone contact
- Gestational age, last menstrual period and estimated date of delivery, date of booking bloods
- Current date and date of reported exposure
- Rash in index case:
  - is it maculopapular or vesicular?
  - if a diagnosis, where was this made?
  - date of onset of the rash?
  - is there an associated local outbreak?
- Nature of maternal exposure: household? face-to-face? prolonged?
  - dates and duration
  - contact prior to rash?
- Details of the pregnant woman; history of chickenpox or shingles, vaccination status MMR and varicella.

RUBELLA

INTRODUCTION

Rubella, also known as German measles, is a mild disease caused by an RNA virus spread by droplet contact from nasopharyngeal secretions. When a pregnant woman contracts rubella in the first trimester there is a 90% risk of the virus causing damage to the developing fetus. Midwives need to understand the impact of rubella and they have a role in educating the wider public of the dangers of rubella in pregnancy. Antenatal screening for rubella immunity and postnatal immunisation of susceptible women are an established part of midwifery care. Recent public concern over the MMR vaccine has led to suboptimal levels of vaccination in the UK. In addition, women born outside of the UK may not have been vaccinated or exposed to rubella in their country of origin.

FEATURES OF RUBELLA

Rubella is a mild disease and up to 50% of women may be asymptomatic (Gruslin & Faden 2008). The incubation period is 14–21 days, with the rash appearing in most people 14–17 days after exposure (DH 2013a). Symptoms may precede rash by 1–5 days and include slight rise in temperature, mild sore throat, conjunctivitis and tender swollen neck lymph glands. Painful joints (arthralgia), particularly in the hands and feet, are common in adults and may last some weeks. The typical rash lasts 1–3 days and consists of fine red spots that begin on the face, neck and behind the ears and then spreads to the rest of body (Bannister *et al.* 2006). The virus can infect others from 1 week before symptoms up until 4 days after the rash first appears (period of infectivity), (DH 2013a).

TRANSMISSION

Transmission of the virus is by inhalation of aerosol from nasopharynx secretions. The virus replicates in the lymph nodes of the upper respiratory tract and spreads via blood throughout the body and can cross the placenta to cause congenital infection (Gruslin & Faden 2008, Banatvala & Brown 2004).

CONGENITAL RUBELLA SYNDROME

There is a high rate (80%–90%) of congenital defect and/or fetal loss when a woman has rubella in the first trimester, as the virus damages the dividing cells during fetal development. Deafness is the most commonly occurring defect. After 16 weeks' gestation, the frequency and severity of fetal damage decreases dramatically (Banatvala & Brown 2004). Rubella between 16 and 20 weeks carries a minimal risk of deafness only (HPA 2011a). Fetal defects are unlikely when infection occurs prior to conception and after 20 weeks' gestation (Gruslin & Faden 2008, Banatvala & Brown 2004). Features of Congenital rubella syndrome (CRS) may be permanent and evident at birth, others are transient and some may not be evident until adolescence. *See* Figure 11.1 for the possible features of CRS.

ANTENATAL SCREENING

Screening for rubella in pregnancy aims to find the small percentage of women who do not have rubella immunity, with the aim to offer vaccination in the immediate postnatal period. Screening for rubella immunity (presence of rubella-specific IgG) is part of the routine antenatal booking tests. When ordering these tests the midwife should enquire if the woman has had recent exposure or possible infection during the current pregnancy. This information is essential for the laboratory to determine the difference between past exposure and immunity (IgG antibodies) or current infection (IgM antibodies). If found to be non-immune, the midwife should give the woman specific information about rubella and advise her to report immediately

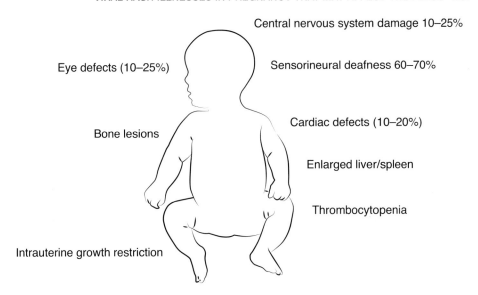

FIGURE 11.1 Possible features of congenital rubella syndrome

any symptoms of rash illness to her midwife, GP or obstetrician. Susceptible women should also report if they have contact with someone who has rash illness. A significant contact is usually defined as face-to-face contact, or being in the same room for over 15 minutes (HPA 2011a). The importance of postnatal immunisation should be discussed.

Rubella reinfection is possible following immunity, although is more likely following immunisation than naturally occurring disease (Banatvala & Brown 2004). Women with reinfection usually don't have any symptoms and it is diagnosed when changes to antibody concentration are detected when they are being investigated for contact with an infected person. The risk to the fetus of subclinical maternal reinfection in the first trimester is thought to be approximately 5%–10%; that is, much lower than primary rubella infection in a non-immune woman (HPA 2011a).

The Joint Committee on Vaccination and Immunisation (JCVI 2012) are considering changing the current screening approach to the recording of a woman's history of MMR vaccination. Problems of recall and non-immunity despite previous vaccination may make this approach less effective (Matthews *et al.* 2013).

EXPOSURE TO RASH ILLNESS AND RUBELLA IN PREGNANCY

All pregnant women should contact their midwife, GP or obstetrician urgently, by telephone, if they develop a rash in pregnancy or have contact with someone who has a rash or symptoms of rubella, regardless of their immune status. Identification of the diagnosis of the index case, the woman's immune status, level of contact and assessment of symptoms are evaluated. (*See* section entitled 'The pregnant women who has contact with rash illness and/or develops a rash' earlier in this chapter for details of the management of this situation).

It is unreliable to diagnose rubella by symptoms only, as a number of illnesses can have a similar rash, including parvovirus B19 infection, measles, herpes viruses and in tropical areas dengue fever and others (Banatvala & Brown 2004). Testing will be referred to the health protection unit and may involve a number of blood tests, depending on individual circumstances. Rubella is now a notifiable disease, which means clinicians are required to provide details of the case to the health protection unit to facilitate monitoring of the spread of the disease.

Laboratory testing for confirmation or not of recent rubella infection can be problematic, particularly when investigation begins 4 weeks or more after the onset of the rash illness (HPA 2011a). Midwives will assist the process of diagnosis by ensuring rapid referral of women accompanied by detailed accurate information. Serological diagnosis is greatly assisted by the archived availability of booking blood samples, which are kept for 2 years (UK NSC 2010). These samples can be used to help identify immunity or the timing of an infection by comparison with the later blood sample (MacMahon 2012).

Accurate diagnosis will be pursued regardless of gestational age for a number of reasons, including risk of CRS and also for management of possible contacts in maternity settings (NICE 2013). Women will be simultaneously investigated for parvovirus B19 (HPA 2011a). Referral to a virologist and fetal medicine specialist is indicated to assess risk of CRS. Termination of pregnancy can be considered where CRS is thought likely. Human normal immunoglobin (HNIG) is thought not to be effective in providing post-exposure protection from rubella and is only considered when termination of pregnancy is considered unacceptable (MacMahon 2012, DH 2013a).

Women with rubella infection are advised to avoid contact with other pregnant women for 6 days after the start of the rash. They should rest, drink plenty of fluids and take paracetamol for relief of symptoms. (NICE 2013).

MMR VACCINATION

The main objective of rubella vaccination is to prevent CRS. The current MMR vaccination programme aims to reduce the risk to pregnant women by both individual immunity and by reducing the general spread of infection by increasing 'herd' immunity, which aims to vaccinate enough people that the spread of infection is diminished. Rubella immunisation was introduced in the UK in 1970 and was made available to teenage schoolgirls and non-immune women of childbearing age. This policy aimed to protect women individually when pregnant. By 1987, 98% of women of childbearing age were immune to rubella and rates of congenital rubella were low but had not been completely eliminated. The combined measles, mumps and rubella vaccine MMR was introduced in 1988 with the aim of halting the spread of rubella among young children and thus protecting the small number of women who remained susceptible, as well as reducing the morbidity associated with mumps and measles. In 1993, there was a large increase in rates of rubella among school-age children who had not been eligible for the vaccination programme introduced only 5 years earlier. A catch-up programme of vaccination for school children aged 5–16 years was run in 1994. These children were immunised with the MR (measles and rubella only) vaccine, as there were insufficient stocks of MMR at that time (DH 2013a). About 5% of the population do not respond to the first dose of rubella vaccine and remain susceptible (Khare & Khare 2007). The two-dose MMR schedule was introduced in 1996.

In 1998, Wakefield *et al.* published controversial research in the *Lancet*, based on a 12-patient case series that proposed a link between MMR, autism and bowel disease. Widespread negative publicity for MMR suggested that single vaccines were safer and this led to a reduction in the uptake of MMR vaccination. (*See* Chapter 1 for discussion on multiple vaccine use under the heading 'Vaccination'.) Following investigations into research misconduct, the *Lancet* fully retracted the 1998 research article in 2010. In May 2010, Wakefield and a colleague, Walker–Smith, were both found guilty of serious professional misconduct and were removed from the medical register (Deer 2011). Unfortunately, after such poor publicity it takes time for public confidence to be restored. The coverage of MMR vaccination of children by their second birthday fell to 79.9% in 2003–04. The rate has now recovered, with 92.3% of children receiving the MMR vaccine by 2 years of age in 2012–13, although figures remain slightly below the World Health Organization's recommended target rate of 95% (HSCIC 2013). Lower rates of MMR vaccination occur in more affluent areas (Elliman & Bedford 2007).

Single-preparation vaccines for MMR are not available from the National Health Service. They are imported into the UK and are only available privately. Public Health England reports that they are less effective and less safe than MMR and have not been tested for potency and toxicity (PHE 2014). Single-preparation injections for these illnesses require six separate injections and it is not known what the optimum spacing of these injections should be. The lapse time between completing the six-injection schedule leaves the children vulnerable to these illnesses for a longer period. Children are also subjected to the six injections with the accompanying discomfort rather than two and the possibility of missed appointments is increased (PHE 2014).

Impact of vaccination on immunity, rates of rubella and congenital rubella syndrome

A recent study in the North Thames region of England used samples from newborn blood spot screening to measure maternally acquired rubella IgG antibody levels. The aim was to determine the extent of maternal immunity to rubella in the population. The study found a rate of 2.7% of mothers from the 18 882 tested were non-immune

(Hardelid *et al.* 2009). A smaller study in South Wales found a higher rate of 6.4%, indicating local differences (Matthews *et al.* 2013). Mothers who were born abroad, particularly those from sub-Saharan Africa and South East Asia, were more likely to be non-immune than mothers born in the UK (Hardelid *et al.* 2009, Tookey *et al.* 2002, Banatvala and Brown 2004). Midwives need to be aware of this higher incidence in non-UK-born women, provide information that is tailored to individual require-ments and ensure opportunity for postnatal vaccination.

Before vaccination, 200–300 babies a year were born with CRS in the UK (Price 2008). However, numbers of congenital rubella have reduced substantially and there have only been 20 cases reported to the national surveillance programme since 1999, and none in 2012. Most cases of CRS infants have been born to women who them-selves were born overseas. For many they acquired the infection overseas in early pregnancy (Tookey *et al.* 2013). The need for continued work in worldwide vaccina-tion programmes is evident.

Postnatal vaccination

Vaccination should be offered to non-immune women in the postnatal period with the aim to achieve a 100% vaccination rate. The Department of Health recommends two doses of MMR given 1 month apart, with advice to avoid pregnancy for 1 month after vaccination (DH 2013a). However, studies reveal that postnatal immunisation cover-age appears to fall well below the 100% standard and this appears to be for a number of reasons. Yung *et al.* (2008) carried out an audit on post-partum immunisation for non-immune women at two maternity units in England. Each unit used a different approach to postnatal vaccination. One unit referred women for vaccination by the GP, while the second unit offered immunisation before discharge. Not surprisingly, uptake of immunisation was greater when offered before going home from hospital, although still only achieving a rate of 60%. Similarly, Matthews *et al.* (2013), who audited postnatal immunisation over a 1-year period, found that a third of women left maternity services without the first dose of MMR. For those who received the first dose there are no data to confirm how many women visit the GP for the second dose. Early discharge policies have been suggested as a cause for reduced rates of immunisa-tion prior to leaving the hospital (Matthews *et al.* 2013). Studies have reported errors in the recording of immune status in the notes from the antenatal period, although this accounts for a very small number of those missed for vaccination (Bloom *et al.* 2006, Matthews *et al.* 2013).

Women who have had anti-D can also receive their vaccination for MMR, as it is thought the response to the vaccination should be adequate. However, if the woman has had a blood transfusion, this may interfere with the antibody response to a vacci-nation (Blackburn 2013). The MMR should be given but the antibody response should be measured 6–8 weeks after vaccination and repeated if required (DH 2013a). Mild egg allergy is not a reason to withhold MMR vaccination. It is recommended that MMR is given intramuscularly into the upper arm or anterolateral thigh (DH 2013a).

MMR vaccination is not recommended in pregnancy, as it is a live vaccine. Inadvertent vaccination with rubella vaccine during pregnancy may occur. In the UK and other countries surveillance of such incidents has provided reassuring data and termination of pregnancy is not recommended. MMR vaccine is safe to be given when breastfeeding (DH 2013a).

PARVOVIRUS B19

INTRODUCTION

Parvovirus B19 (colloquially known as 'slapped cheek syndrome') is a relatively mild viral illness common in childhood. Parvoviruses are the smallest viruses (*parvo* meaning small) known to cause human disease (Collier & Oxford 2006). Parvovirus B19 was discovered in 1975 by chance during routine screening for hepatitis B among blood donors. It is named after the location of the lab sample in which it was found – namely, panel B, number 19 (Cossart *et al.* 1975). The formal title for the condition is *erythema infectious* and it is also sometimes referred to as 'fifth disease', a reference to an old classification of childhood diseases where it was placed fifth in a list of common childhood conditions (Molyneaux 2007, Gruslin & Faden 2008, Lamont *et al.* 2010).

In 20%–30% of infections with parvovirus B19 there are no symptoms. For the remainder, the infection may just cause a mild illness and most people don't remember if they have had the condition (Gruslin & Faden 2008). In children it may present with a distinct 'slapped cheek' rash on the face.

The incubation range is 4–14 days (Tolfvenstam & Broliden 2009). The initial symptoms, when present, are fever, headache and generally feeling unwell. It is at this stage the individual is infectious (Gruslin & Faden 2008). Later the facial rash appears (more common in children) and even later there may be a 'lacy' red rash on the body, legs and arms. Joint pain of hands, wrists, knees and ankles is a more common feature of disease in adult females (Gruslin & Faden 2008, Riley 2011). Parvovirus B19 appears as a very similar condition to rubella and can only be reliably distinguished from rubella through laboratory testing. Parvovirus B19 in pregnancy is usually a mild illness for the mother (Khare & Khare 2007). After recovery, immunity is usually lifelong (Tolfvenstam & Broliden 2009).

However, a complicating feature of parvovirus B19 is that it targets the rapidly dividing precursor cells of red blood cells (RBCs) in order to multiply, and in the process of that replication, damages these cells (Elliot *et al.* 2007). Consequently, about 10 days after the initial infection a temporary anaemia develops (Molyneaux 2007). This is not problematic for healthy people but can be serious for those with underlying hematological diseases such as sickle-cell disease (Collier & Oxford 2006).

Where individuals are immunocompromised such as with human immunodeficiency virus, parvovirus B19 may result in persistent infection and chronic anaemia (Collier & Oxford 2006). For a small number of infants, this destruction of RBCs underlies the development of hydrops fetalis in the fetus (*see* further details under heading 'Implication for the fetus' later in this section).

EPIDEMIOLOGY

Parvovirus infections occur worldwide, with outbreaks occurring in spring and summer, with a 3- to 4-year epidemic cycle. It spreads mostly among school children aged 6–10 years (NICE 2010). During epidemics, 50% of susceptible children and 25% of susceptible teachers acquire parvovirus B19 infection (Lamont *et al.* 2010). By childbearing age, 50% of women are immune (MacMahon 2012). Parvovirus B19 infection probably occurs in 0.25%–1% of pregnancies, with the majority of these infections going unnoticed (Gruslin & Faden 2008).

TRANSMISSION

Parvovirus B19 is spread by respiratory secretions, blood and from mother to fetus via the placenta (Molyneaux 2007, Gruslin & Faden 2008, Collier & Oxford 2006). Mothers, teachers and health workers dealing with young children are at risk of contracting parvovirus B19 during pregnancy (Khare & Khare 2007). In household contacts, the rate of transmission is around 50%, thus women are most likely to become infected from their own children (Crowcroft *et al.* 1999, Ismail & Kilby 2003).

PREVENTION

Routine screening for antibody B19, to determine those women who are not immune, is not justified, as there is no prophylactic treatment or vaccine available. However, Khare and Khare (2007) suggest that screening may be considered for those women in at-risk occupations, such as childcare workers and primary school teachers. They suggest that pregnant women without immunity should stay away from their workplace at times of known outbreaks of the disease. Frequent handwashing and avoiding contact with children suspected of parvovirus infection seems a reasonable approach, although in practical terms this would be difficult, as a child is most contagious before obvious symptoms appear (Elliot *et al.* 2007). For mothers, it would be difficult to avoid their own children. Blanket decisions regarding exclusion from work areas are not advocated (NICE 2010, Ismail & Kilby 2003, Tolfvenstam & Broliden 2009).

MATERNAL TESTING

Pregnant women should be advised to inform their GP, midwife or obstetrician if they develop a rash, have painful joints or are in contact with someone with rash-like illness, although many women with parvovirus B19 will not have symptoms. Diagnosis for parvovirus B19 may also be sought as part of investigations for intrauterine death or when an ultrasound scan reveals hydrops fetalis (Ismail & Kilby 2003).

Following exposure to parvovirus B19, women should have immediate serological testing for both B19 virus-specific IgG and B19 virus-specific IgM. (*See* section entitled 'The pregnant women who has contact with rash illness and /or develops a rash' earlier in this chapter for details of the management of this situation.) Presence of B19 virus-specific IgG and absence of IgM suggests prior exposure and immunity, whereas IgG negative and IgM positive suggests acute infection (Riley 2011). Women can be advised about the low risk of fetal loss in the first trimester and the low risk of hydrops and fetal loss in the second trimester.

IMPLICATION FOR THE FETUS

When a pregnant woman suffers B19 infection, the virus can cross the placenta to the fetus before maternal antibodies have developed and crossed the placenta to protect the fetus (Molyneaux 2007). When maternal infection is confirmed, regular fetal monitoring should be undertaken. Weekly ultrasound scans will look for features of developing hydrops and this fetal surveillance should continue for 12 weeks after infection (Riley 2011).

Infection in the first 20 weeks of pregnancy results in an approximately 9% risk of intrauterine death, with the greatest risk of loss occurring between 13 and 20 weeks (Gruslin & Faden 2008, Riley 2011). The risk of fetal loss after 20 weeks is much lower, at less than 1% (Riley 2011). In the third trimester the fetal immune response is more developed and helps protect the fetus, although the newborn may still be anaemic (Molyneaux 2007).

Hydrops fetalis and fetal death occur mainly as a result of the anaemia caused by the destruction of the immature fetal RBCs by the parvovirus. Fetal anaemia reduces oxygenation of the endothelial cells that line the blood vessels. Damage to these cells, increasing pressure within the vessels, and reduced albumin causes the characteristic leaking of fluid into the tissues (oedema) and body spaces (ascites) indicative of hydrops fetalis. Reduced albumin, infection of the fetal cardiac muscle (myocarditis) and degenerative changes to the placenta are also implicated as a cause of fetal demise (Lamont *et al.* 2010, Tolfvenstam & Broliden 2009). Fetal loss is usually 4–6 weeks after maternal infection.

The most critical time for fetal infection seems to be at around 16 weeks' gestation. At this time, fetal production of RBCs is significantly increased, as the fetus becomes more dependent on its own RBCs (Lamont *et al.* 2010). Hydrops most often occurs 2–5 weeks after maternal infection. The fetus with hydrops due to B19 may spontaneously recover (Riley 2011), although intrauterine transfusion improves survival rates (Molyneaux 2007). When fetal hydrops is diagnosed, the woman should be referred to a fetal medicine specialist promptly. Intrauterine fetal transfusion may be undertaken to correct significant fetal anaemia (Gruslin & Faden 2008). Risks of in utero transfusion include rupture of membranes, bradycardia, immediate delivery, chorioamnionitis and intrauterine death (Smith & Whitehall 2008). It is important to remember that hydrops fetalis is rare and only occurs in 3% of pregnancies where the mother had B19 between 9 and 20 weeks (HPA 2011b).

For those infants who survive fetal infection the long-term outcome is good, as it seems the virus does not produce any teratogenic effect. For this reason, termination of pregnancy is not indicated (Molyneaux 2007, Gruslin & Faden 2008, Riley 2011).

In addition to ultrasound scans, fetal testing in cases of proven maternal parvovirus infection may include polymerase chain reaction testing to detect B19 virus in amniotic fluid and Doppler studies to identify fetal anaemia. The velocity of blood flow during systole in the middle cerebral artery increases as the blood thins in anaemia (Smith & Whitehall 2008, Riley 2011).

MEASLES

INTRODUCTION

Measles infection (also known as rubeola) may cause adverse affects for the mother and fetus during pregnancy. It is a highly infectious illness and although rare in the population, outbreaks have occurred recently. Midwives need to ensure timely referral of women when exposed to measles during pregnancy for assessment of their vulnerability to infection. The administration of MMR vaccination to non-immune women in the postnatal period is part of the midwife's responsibility.

FEATURES OF MEASLES

Measles is a highly infectious viral illness spread by respiratory droplets. Prior to widespread vaccination, measles was a common illness in children (Khare & Khare 2007). The incubation period for measles is 10–14 days (Riley 2011). Symptoms appear around 10 days after infection and last for 14 days. The initial prodromal symptoms include cold-like symptoms, fever and conjunctivitis. After 2–4 days, a characteristic red-brown spotty rash appears, initially behind the ears, and then spreads over the body for the next 4 days, and lasts for a week. A distinguishing feature of measles is greyish-white spots in the mouth and throat, known as Koplik's spots (Khare & Khare 2007). A saliva or blood test can confirm the diagnosis. Measles is a notifiable disease and cases are therefore reported to the local health protection unit (DH 2013b). A person with measles is infectious from the beginning of the prodromal symptoms (2–4 days before the rash appears) and for about 4 days after the rash appears. Diagnosis is based on clinical features including Koplik's spots and can be confirmed by serology (Riley 2011). Where immunisation rates are below 95%, measles may spread through the community (Bannister et al. 2006).

Widespread vaccination for measles has made this an uncommon illness. However, in resource-poor settings, outbreaks of measles can have devastating effects. Secondary bacterial pneumonia is a common complication of measles. Post-measles encephalitis occurs in 1 in 1000 cases and can be life-threatening or lead to permanent neurological damage (Bannister *et al.* 2006). Death due to pneumonia or encephalitis is reported to occur in 1–2 per 1000 cases (Riley 2011). Subacute sclerosing panencephalitis (SSPE) is a serious neurological complication that leads to involuntary spasms, mental deterioration and severe neurological impairment. These complications are more common in the very young, those with reduced immunity and adults (DH 2013b). Box 11.4 lists the range and incidence of complications of measles.

BOX 11.4 COMPLICATIONS OF MEASLES

- Otitis media (7%–9%)
- Pneumonia (1%–6%)
- Diarrhoea (8%)
- Convulsions (0.5%)
- Encephalitis (1 per 1000)
- SSPE (1 in 25 000)
- Death (1 in 5000)

(DH 2013b)

IMPACT ON PREGNANCY

The main problem of contracting measles during pregnancy is that the high fever may stimulate uterine contractions, which may lead to miscarriage or preterm delivery (Khare & Khare 2007, White *et al.* 2012). Medication and tepid sponging to keep the fever down is a priority (Riley 2011). It is not clear whether measles poses any greater threat to the pregnant woman although some studies have reported a higher rate of hospitalisation, pneumonia and death related to measles infection in pregnancy (Riley 2011, Chiba *et al.* 2003, White *et al.* 2012). Pregnant women with measles should be monitored for respiratory complications (Riley 2011) (*see* Chapter 9). A few cases of SSPE have also been reported in pregnant women (Campbell *et al.* 2007).

It is generally thought that the measles virus is not teratogenic. Measles is not associated with any specific congenital syndrome and no consistent pattern of fetal abnormality has been observed following maternal measles infection (Campbell *et al.* 2007). Complications to the fetus or newborn are generally those related to preterm delivery. However, when maternal infection occurs around the time of delivery, the newborn may develop severe measles. The paediatrician should be informed and appropriate isolation and monitoring of the neonate is indicated (Riley 2011). Premature infants who acquire measles are vulnerable to life-threatening pneumonia and SSPE (Campbell *et al.* 2007).

CONTACT WITH MEASLES DURING PREGNANCY

All pregnant women should contact their midwife, GP or obstetrician urgently, by telephone, if they develop a rash in pregnancy or have contact with someone who has a rash or symptoms of measles, regardless of their immune status. Identification of the diagnosis of the index case, the woman's immune status, level of contact and assessment of symptoms are evaluated. (*See* section entitled 'The pregnant women who has contact with rash illness and /or develops a rash' earlier in this chapter for details of the management of this situation.)

Measles is highly infectious and where a woman is at significant risk of becoming infected with measles, the midwife should ensure rapid referral to appropriate medical services where administration of HNIG can be considered. Immunogloblin is a concentrated antibody preparation derived from pooled plasma originating from blood donations and is considered a scarce commodity (DH 2013b). It can be given intramuscularly or intravenously and it provides immediate but short-term protection against infection. There is a narrow window of opportunity (within 6 days of exposure) in which the administration is likely to be effective. The assessment for suitability for HNIG will include determining the woman's immune status based on her age, country of origin, history of previous measles infection, known immunisation record and a blood test for antibodies (if time allows) (HPA 2013a).

MMR VACCINATION

MMR vaccination began in 1988 with the two-dose schedule being introduced in 1996. This has led to a substantial reduction in measles transmission in the UK. Complications following measles such as SSPE and death were almost eliminated. However, an increase in cases of measles since early 2012, particularly among school-age children, has been seen. The age group most affected is 10- to 14-year-olds, and is thought to be linked to the poor coverage of MMR vaccination between 1999 and 2005 following negative publicity. (*See* section on MMR vaccination in the 'Rubella' section earlier in this chapter.) Hospital admissions and complications of measles have risen (PHE 2013).

Women contemplating pregnancy who are not immune should arrange with their GP to have the MMR vaccination before pregnancy. Vaccination can also be given in the immediate postnatal period. Vaccination is safe for breastfeeding mothers. A second dose can be given after 1 month. An advantage of MMR vaccination prior to pregnancy is that maternal antibodies will provide protection in young infants until about 6 months of age (Bannister *et al.* 2006).

However, as MMR is a live vaccine, vaccination in pregnancy is not recommended and reliable contraception should be used to avoid pregnancy up to 1 month after vaccine administration. Should inadvertent vaccination of MMR in pregnancy occur, surveillance data is reassuring with regard to any long-term affects, and for that reason, termination of pregnancy is not advocated (DH 2013b).

CHICKENPOX (VARICELLA)

INTRODUCTION

Varicella zoster virus (VZV) is a member of the herpes virus family and is the virus responsible for chickenpox (varicella) and shingles (herpes zoster) (DH 2012). It is a highly infectious disease that mainly affects children. Primary infection generally provides lifelong immunity (Lamont *et al.* 2011). The incubation period is 10–21 days and it is infectious for 2 days before the rash appears until after all of the ruptured vesicles have crusted over, which takes about 5 days (Khare & Khare 2007, MacMahon 2012).

Symptoms involve:

- fever, malaise and general aching 1–2 days before rash
- vesicular rash, which erupts in crops over the trunk, face, oropharynx and scalp
- the rash is intensely itchy and the vesicles become filled with pus, which then crust over.

(Johannessen & Ogilvie 2012, Khare & Khare 2007)

Complications for children and adults can include bacterial infection of the vesicles, pneumonia and encephalitis (Johannessen & Ogilvie 2012). Chickenpox is estimated to complicate 3 in 1000 pregnancies (RCOG 2007) and can cause congenital varicella syndrome, maternal varicella pneumonia and neonatal varicella. The development of varicella pneumonia is more likely in the third trimester (Lim *et al.* 2001). The effects of maternal varicella infection on the fetus and newborn are related to the timing of infection.

TRANSMISSION

Transmission occurs through direct contact with vesicular fluids, airborne droplets from infected respiratory secretions and contact with infected articles (Khare & Khare 2007, Riley 2011). The virus enters through the upper respiratory tract or conjunctiva and may multiply for a few days in the local lymph tissue before entering the blood, spreading through the body and making its way to skin tissue (Johannessen & Ogilvie 2012). Chickenpox is very contagious and will infect about 90% of those who come into contact with it (Khare & Khare 2007). In temperate countries including the UK, most children contract chickenpox between 4 and 10 years of age and thus develop immunity, with only around 10% of adults remaining at risk (Johannessen & Ogilvie 2012). However, women from tropical and subtropical areas are more likely to be seronegative (as high as 75%) for varicella zoster virus and therefore are more susceptible to chickenpox (RCOG 2007, Lamont *et al.* 2011).

SHINGLES

VZV will normally remain dormant but may surface in times of physiological, hormonal or immunological stress. This second manifestation of VZV after what may be a long time since the primary infection with chickenpox is known as shingles (herpes zoster). The virus travels from the sensory root ganglia to a peripheral site usually in the upper thoracic zone. It is characterised by a patch of painful, itchy, vesicles on a red base distributed along a dermatome (an area of skin supplied by a particular branch of nerve fibres) (Johannessen & Ogilvie 2012). More than one episode is uncommon and the stimulus for reactivation is unknown. Maternal shingles is thought unlikely to cause fetal abnormality (Banatvala 2002, Lamont *et al.* 2011) and does not usually cause neonatal infection, as maternal antibodies normally protect the neonate.

COMPLICATIONS OF CHICKENPOX FOR THE FETUS OR NEWBORN

Varicella can cross the placenta when the mother has chickenpox and infect the fetus. Risks to the fetus and neonate when the mother has chickenpox are related to the time of infection.

In the first 20 weeks of pregnancy

Congenital (or fetal) varicella syndrome is a rare consequence of fetal infection resulting in a number of complications (*see* Box 11.5). The risk of congenital varicella syndrome is approximately 2% when mothers have chickenpox before 20 weeks'

BOX 11.5 CONGENITAL VARICELLA SYNDROME

- Intrauterine growth restriction
- Skin loss or scarring
- Hypoplasia of limbs and muscle, rudimentary digits
- Abnormalities of the central nervous system including microcephaly
- Eye deformities
- Developmental delay

(Price 2008, Riley 2011, Lamont *et al.* 2011)

gestation (Riley 2011, Johannessen & Ogilvie 2012, Price 2008). One case has been reported following maternal infection between 20 and 28 weeks (RCOG 2007).

Women who have chickenpox in early pregnancy may be referred to a fetal medicine specialist for antenatal diagnosis and counselling. Detailed ultrasound may aid the diagnosis of congenital varicella syndrome although the structural changes to the fetus will not be evident until at least 5 weeks after the infection. Findings may include limb deformity, microcephaly, hydrocephalus, calcification of soft tissue and intrauterine growth restriction. DNA detection of VZV in amniotic fluid can be done but results may not be helpful in determining whether the fetus is affected and is therefore not routinely used (RCOG 2007, Lamont et al. 2011).

In the second and third trimesters of pregnancy

Maternal infection at 21–36 weeks is not usually associated with adverse fetal effects, although the newborn may develop herpes zoster (shingles) in early childhood (Banatvala 2002, Khare & Khare 2007). Shingles in the neonate is reactivation of the virus after a first infection of varicella that occurs in utero (RCOG 2007).

A week before to a week after delivery

There is a high risk of varicella in the newborn when the baby is born within 7 days of the first time the mother notices the rash or if the rash appears within 7 days after delivery (RCOG 2007). Neonatal chickenpox may result from transplacental transmission, ascending infection or via the newborn's respiratory tract (Lamont et al. 2011). If maternal rash begins 7 days or more before delivery the antibodies have developed and have transferred across the placenta and thus the baby is protected (Johannessen & Ogilvie 2012). The exception to this is babies born at less than 28 weeks' gestation; they are at risk because they have less protection from maternally acquired antibodies (Lamont et al. 2011).

Siblings are another source of infection for the newborn, but if the mother is immune the newborn is protected by passively acquired antibodies. If the mother has no immunity the newborn baby will be susceptible.

Neonatal varicella is a serious illness characterised by fever, a vesicular rash and spread to organs. The mortality rate is 7%–10% but was 30% before the use of prophylaxis and treatment (Khare & Khare 2007, Riley 2011, Lamont et al. 2011).

MANAGEMENT OF INFANTS EXPOSED TO CHICKENPOX AROUND THE TIME OF BIRTH

Newborn infants whose mothers develop varicella 7 days before to 7 days after delivery may be prescribed varicella zoster immunoglobulin (VZIG). VZIG is considered not to be of any benefit once the newborn shows signs of infection. The baby may also benefit from acyclovir (an antiviral medication) if the onset of maternal varicella was

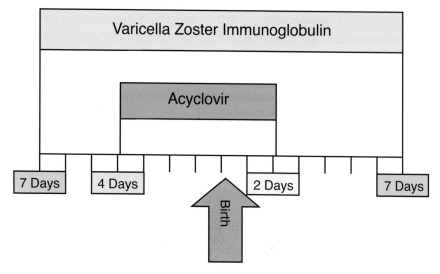

Onset of mother's chickenpox symptoms

FIGURE 11.2 Treatment that may be prescribed for infants exposed to varicella around the time of birth (Riley 2011, RCOG 2007)

between 4 days before birth and up to 2 days after (Riley 2011, RCOG 2007). A neonatologist will direct treatment with VZIG and acyclovir. Consultation with a virologist is advised. The infant should be monitored for signs of infection until 28 days after onset of maternal infection (RCOG 2007) (*see* Figure 11.2).

About half of neonates exposed to maternal varicella will develop chickenpox despite immunoglobulin prophylaxis but severe complications and mortality is significantly reduced with this treatment (RCOG 2007). VZIG may extend the incubation period to up to a month and infants should be followed up over that period for signs of chickenpox (RCOG 2007).

MANAGEMENT OF CHICKENPOX IN PREGNANCY

Antenatal care

The occurrence rate of varicella fetal syndrome when a mother has chickenpox is minimal when compared with the 85% risk of rubella fetal damage. Consequently, in the UK, there is no programme for vaccination, nor is there coordinated screening for immune status (Price 2008). The midwife, as part of the booking interview, should enquire with regard to history of chickenpox or shingles. When women report they have had chickenpox in the past this has been shown to correlate closely with blood tests finding that they have immunity to chickenpox (RCOG 2007). If the woman has not had chickenpox, or if she is not sure, the midwife should advise the woman to avoid contact with chickenpox in pregnancy and to notify the midwife or doctor if she has contact and/or she develops a chickenpox-type rash (HPA 2011a). Those women from tropical and subtropical countries such as the Caribbean, South India and sub-Saharan Africa, where background prevalence is low, are more likely not to have had chickenpox (RCOG 2007, MacMahon 2012). Although not routinely recommended, postnatal vaccination may be considered for those women without immunity to varicella (Lamont *et al.* 2011). Pregnancy should be avoided for 3 months following vaccination (DH 2012).

Care following exposure to chickenpox in pregnancy or development of chickenpox in pregnancy

Management of exposure to chickenpox

The woman who has contact with someone with chickenpox and/or develops symptoms of chickenpox when she is pregnant should seek advice by telephone from her GP, midwife or obstetrician. (*See* section entitled 'The pregnant women who has contact with rash illness and/or develops a rash' earlier in this chapter for details of the management of this situation.)

For those women who have contact with chickenpox but have no symptoms, it will be important to establish the woman's immune status with regard to varicella zoster. It is advised that a non-immune pregnant woman who is exposed to chickenpox or herpes zoster during pregnancy be offered post-exposure prophylaxis with VZIG within 10 days of exposure (DH 2012).

Management of maternal chickenpox

Most children with chickenpox have a relatively uncomplicated recovery. However, for adults chickenpox can be a serious illness. Pregnant women who have chickenpox late in their pregnancy and those who smoke are particularly vulnerable to developing pneumonia with a mortality rate of up to 10%, even with antiviral treatment and intensive care (RCOG 2007, Khare & Khare 2007). Other maternal complications include neurological problems, thrombocytopenia, disseminated intravascular coagulation and bleeding (Khare & Khare 2007, RCOG 2007). Prompt treatment including intravenous acyclovir improves survival (Riley 2011).

If a woman develops chickenpox she should contact her midwife or doctor immediately, noting when she first noticed the lesions. The midwife should refer the pregnant women with symptoms of chickenpox to her GP, although liaison with an obstetrician for advice is also advised. Oral acyclovir may be prescribed to women beyond 20 weeks of pregnancy, if seen by a doctor within 24 hours of the development of the rash. This medication may decrease the duration of the temperature and symptoms (RCOG 2007, Riley 2011). If her condition remains uncomplicated, the woman should stay at home, although daily review may be advised. Women should be advised to avoid contact with other pregnant women and babies at least until all the vesicles have crusted over (Khare & Khare 2007, RCOG 2007).

However, a pregnant woman with varicella who develops respiratory symptoms such as cough, increased respiratory rate, fever or shortness of breath, has other medical problems or is near to term, should be immediately referred for hospital assessment (RCOG 2007). The woman will need to be isolated away from other mothers and babies when in hospital (Khare & Khare 2007) and advice from the hospital infection control team should be sought.

Labour

Delivery during the period of infection should be avoided if possible, as this is the most hazardous time for mother and baby. Delaying delivery (in the absence of spontaneous labour) for at least a week is beneficial, as this will allow the transfer of protective antibodies from mother to fetus. The mother is at risk of bleeding due to coagulation disorders at the time of infection. However, delivery may be required for obstetric reasons or to improve ventilation for the mother if she develops respiratory failure subsequent to pneumonia (RCOG 2007). (For further details see the section on pneumonia in Chapter 9.) Infected pregnant women will require a negative-pressure room, if available, for labour and delivery and isolation procedures followed (Riley 2011).

The anaesthetist will need to decide the best option for anaesthesia if required for delivery. General anaesthetic may exacerbate varicella pneumonia. There is a theoretical risk that the varicella virus in vesicles on the skin surface could be introduced into the central nervous system during spinal anaesthesia and therefore epidural anaesthesia, which avoids puncture of the dura, may be preferable. The site for needle insertion should avoid any vesicles (RCOG 2007).

Postnatal

Following delivery, the mother may remain unwell. If she is still in the infectious period she will need to be cared for in isolation. Frequent assessment for maternal well-being will be required. The baby will require assessment by the neonatologist and preventive treatment given as indicated (see earlier section, 'Management of infants exposed to chickenpox around the time of birth'). The midwife will need to monitor the baby for signs of varicella infection. It is advised that breastfeeding be avoided until the mother has passed the infectious period (Khare & Khare 2007). Separation of mother and baby and the use of expressed breast milk has been advocated where mothers have infectious varicella at the time of delivery (AAP 2012). Others have suggested that separation of mother and baby is not helpful (Sendelbach & Sanchez 2012) although prevention of postnatal transmission from mother to newborn will be difficult. Midwives should seek advice from the neonatologist and hospital infection control team for guidance in individual circumstances. Where separation is advocated, full discussion and ongoing liaison with the mother, taking into account her preferences, will be required, to minimise the impact of this.

PRECAUTIONS FOR HEALTHCARE WORKERS

Occupational health screening should establish immune status of healthcare workers and non-immune staff should be offered varicella vaccination (RCOG 2007). Vaccinated healthcare workers, and those with a definite history of having had chickenpox, can be considered protected if they are exposed to varicella in the course of their work. However, if they feel unwell or develop a fever or a rash they should attend occupational health before having any contact with mothers or babies (DH 2012). Midwives with herpes zoster should also seek advice from occupational health before having contact with mothers and babies (RCP 2010).

CYTOMEGALOVIRUS

INTRODUCTION

CMV is the most common cause of congenital infection in the UK, although mothers are usually unaware of the infection when pregnant. The virus can cause infection in the fetus and yet not all cases of fetal infection cause any long-term damage. However, in up to 20% of infants with sensorineural hearing loss and other adverse outcomes including cerebral palsy, congenital CMV infection may be the cause (Townsend 2011). Despite a prevalence of around 3 per 1000 births, congenital CMV is a relatively unknown condition among parents. Due to problems of detection, poor ability to identify those infants at risk of serious outcomes, a lack of an effective vaccine and limited treatment, screening for CMV is not advocated. Currently the only method of preventing CMV infection in pregnancy is for midwives to advise women about the risk of acquiring CMV, mainly through contact with the urine and respiratory secretions of young infants. Midwives need to be knowledgeable about CMV to support women through the lengthy and uncertain process of diagnosis and management should CMV infection be suspected.

FEATURES OF CYTOMEGALOVIRUS

CMV is common throughout the world, with most people acquiring primary infection when they are children. As a result, approximately 50% of women of reproductive age have antibodies to CMV (CMV seropositive) (Roos & Baker 2011). The name cytomegalovirus means 'large cell virus', which describes the swollen cells that characterise infections caused by the virus (Collier & Oxford 2006). CMV is a member of the herpes family of viruses, which includes herpes simplex, Epstein–Barr virus and varicella zoster. A characteristic of this family of viruses is the ability of the virus to lay dormant (or latent) in the body after a primary infection. Reactivation of latent CMV can occur during pregnancy and is usually asymptomatic (Roos & Baker 2011, Gilbert 2002). CMV is a relatively mild disease in healthy people and maternal infection may go unnoticed. However, infection when acquired as a fetus can cause significant morbidity (Gillespie & Bamford 2012). Congenital infection can occur after maternal primary infection, reactivation or possibly reinfection with a different strain of CMV and it is not known which type of infection is more likely to be associated with congenital damage (Townsend 2011). A vaccine for CMV that may reduce the risk of contracting CMV when pregnant and may boost the immune responses of seropositive women is under development (Sabbaj *et al.* 2011). However, further research is needed to determine if such a vaccine would be beneficial in reducing the rates of congenital CMV disease (Townsend 2011).

COMPLICATIONS OF CYTOMEGALOVIRUS IN PREGNANCY

CMV has a gestational age-related profile whereby the impact of disease is different according to when it is first contracted. Figure 11.3 shows possible manifestations of CMV. The impact of congenital infection can range from there being no effect on the fetus or newborn to it causing long-term serious health complications including deafness and neurological impairment (*see* the heading 'Diagnosis of maternal or fetal infection and morbidity for the fetus' later in this section for further details). CMV infection, including reactivation of CMV, poses a threat to the health of those women who are immunocompromised, such as those with the human immunodeficiency virus (Collier & Oxford 2006, Gillespie & Bamford 2012).

TRANSMISSION

It is generally thought that CMV is not very contagious. Transmission requires close contact with a person secreting CMV in body fluids (Gruslin & Faden 2008). CMV virus can be shed in urine, saliva, blood, genital secretions and breast milk (Peckham *et al.* 2002, Gilbert 2002). CMV is thought to be commonly spread between children attending childcare nurseries, and children will shed CMV virus in saliva and urine for up to 18 months after the initial infection (Nigro & Adler 2011). Most women therefore acquire CMV after contact with young children, usually their own (Adler *et al.* 2004). Seronegative childcare workers are also at significant risk (Nigro & Adler 2011). Studies have shown benefit in preventing primary CMV infection in mothers and carers through education with regard to hygiene when dealing with young children. This includes basic measures such as handwashing after nappy changing (Vauloup-Fellous *et al.* 2009, Adler *et al.* 2004). Heating, soap, detergent and disinfectant destroy the virus (Malm & Engman 2007).

Sexual transmission of CMV and, rarely, transmission via blood transfusion and organ transplant can occur (Gruslin & Faden 2008, Collier & Oxford 2006).

Mother-to-child transmission

Transmission from the mother to the fetus or newborn can occur via the placenta and from vaginal secretions and blood during delivery and postnatally via breast

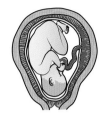

(**a**) fetal infection is associated with morbidity and mortality; intrauterine transmission is more likely when maternal infection occurs later in pregnancy, although late transmission is associated with lower risk of damage to the fetus (Townsend 2011);

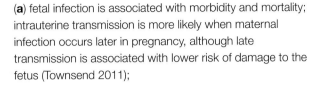

(**b**) CMV infection during delivery or in the postnatal period from breastfeeding does not cause long-term problems for healthy term infants (Gillespie & Bamford 2012, Gruslin & Faden 2008, Malm & Engman 2007); however, in very premature infants (less than 32 weeks' gestation) complications may occur (Malm & Engman 2007);

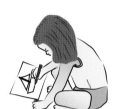

(**c**) children may readily become infected at daycare centres, as the virus sheds through saliva and urine;

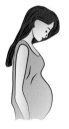

(**d**) CMV can spread by kissing and sexual intercourse; usually no clinical symptoms, but in 5% of cases CMV causes an infectious mononucleosis syndrome like that caused by the Epstein–Barr virus; this is a febrile illness with enlarged spleen, impaired liver function and the appearance of abnormal lymphocytes (Collier & Oxford 2006, Malm & Engman 2007);

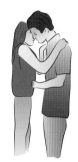

(**e**) adults usually have no symptoms, although some (less than 25%) will have flu-like syndrome with persistent sore throat, fatigue and muscle aching.

FIGURE 11.3 Manifestations of CMV according to age when infection occurs

milk (Malm & Engman 2007). Risk of fetal infection is greatest in the third trimester (Nigro & Adler 2011), although the likelihood of major complications from CMV congenital infection is widely thought to be greatest when the mother has a primary infection in early pregnancy (Gruslin & Faden 2008, Gilbert 2002, Azam *et al.* 2001, Goering *et al.* 2013). The risk of primary infection in pregnancy is about 2% (in non-immune women) (Malm & Engman 2007) resulting in fetal infection in about 40% of cases (Townsend 2011). Congenital CMV infection can also occur following maternal reactivation and possibly reinfection by CMV, although the risk to the infant is unclear (Townsend 2011).

Where CMV is transmitted via genital secretions at birth or via breast milk, it is not thought to cause any significant clinical illness in the newborn unless the infant is very premature. There are no recommendations against breastfeeding by mothers known to be shedding the virus and the potential benefits of breast milk versus the risk of CMV transmission need to be considered when contemplating breastfeeding in very premature infants (AAP 2012). When assessing the impact of CMV on the fetus it is important to distinguish between the fetus being infected and the fetus suffering damage as a result of that infection (Langford & Banatvala 2000). Even when fetal infection is confirmed, most fetuses will not be affected (Price 2008), although the uncertainty will cause significant anxiety for parents.

DIAGNOSIS OF MATERNAL OR FETAL INFECTION AND MORBIDITY FOR THE FETUS

Most CMV infections in pregnancy will go unnoticed. Investigation will only be undertaken if the woman presents with a flu-like illness similar to infectious mononucleosis (glandular fever), has significant contact with someone with CMV, or following detection of ultrasound scan findings suggestive of congenital CMV infection (Yinon *et al.* 2010, Khare & Khare 2007). Referral to the medical team, including virologist and fetal medicine specialist, is essential for appropriate and detailed investigation and counselling with regard to fetal CMV infection.

Maternal blood tests will help the diagnosis, although interpretation of results is complex and it can be difficult to determine the timing of infection. The use of paired samples from booking bloods and a good clinical history is required. The tests will look at changes in antibody titres and the presence of CMV IgM, although this is unreliable, as it can persist for many months following infection (Kriebs 2008, Gilbert 2002).

When maternal CMV infection is thought likely, examination of the amniotic fluid can be done to determine fetal infection. This may need to be undertaken after 21 weeks' gestation when there is adequate fetal renal function, and at least 7 weeks after the presumed time of maternal infection. The interval is important, as it takes up to 6 weeks for sufficient replication of the virus in the fetal urine to enable detection in the amniotic fluid (Gilbert 2002, Yinon *et al.* 2010). The identification of the virus in the amniotic fluid is a reliable indicator of fetal infection but this does not confirm if the fetus has been affected or not by the virus (Azam *et al.* 2001). Absence of fetal infection will make serious abnormality unlikely and provide reassurance to parents (Gilbert 2002). When fetal infection is confirmed the gestation of the pregnancy, the viral load in the amniotic fluid and ultrasound evidence will inform decision-making with regard to possible termination of pregnancy (Gilbert 2002, Yinon *et al.* 2010, Bhide & Papageorghiou 2008, Nigro & Adler 2011). Serial ultrasound is suggested to look for features suggestive of CMV damage such as intrauterine growth restriction, intracranial calcification, ventriculomegaly or microcephaly (Nigro & Adler 2011).

MANAGEMENT OF INFANT WITH CMV INFECTION

Of those infants who are infected with CMV in utero, only 10% will have features of congenital CMV syndrome at birth, with 90% appearing normal. However, 5%–15%

of those appearing normal at birth will later go on to develop a problem (Townsend *et al.* 2011).

Blood, urine and throat swabs are used to make the diagnosis of CMV in the neonate. Congenital infection is confirmed when tests are positive in the first 3 weeks of life. Postnatal infection may cause positive test results after 3 weeks (Bannister *et al.* 2006).

Permanent defects occur in about half of those infants who display symptoms at birth (Bannister *et al.* 2006). Microcephaly and sensorineural hearing loss are the commonest problems. Prognosis is understandably worse for those with neurological deficit at birth (Bannister *et al.* 2006). Box 11.6 lists characteristic manifestations of congenital CMV.

The involvement of a specialist paediatrician to direct treatment will be required. Intravenous or oral antiviral medication may be prescribed for those infants with neurological manifestations. It is used with the aim of improving outcome although requires long hospital stays for administration and there are concerns regarding toxic side effects (Townsend 2011).

BOX 11.6 CHARACTERISTIC MANIFESTATIONS OF CONGENITAL CYTOMEGALOVIRUS

- Prematurity and/or growth restriction
- Neurological involvement including microcephaly, seizures and abnormal muscle tone
- Chorioretinitis
- Petechiae
- Sensorineural hearing loss
- Enlarged liver and spleen
- Prolonged jaundice
- Anaemia
- Thrombocytopenia

(Gruslin & Faden 2008, Azam *et al.* 2001, Bannister *et al.* 2006, Malm & Engman 2007)

Infants who have congenital CMV infection but have no symptoms at birth still have a 5%–15% risk of developing neurological problems and hearing loss in the first 6 years of childhood (DeVries 2007, Malm & Engman 2007, Townsend 2011). The midwife should ensure appropriate communication regarding requirements for follow-up with specialist paediatric services, the GP and the health visitor.

SCREENING AND PREVENTION OF CYTOMEGALOVIRUS

Antenatal screening to prevent poor outcomes from CMV is not feasible for a number of reasons. Blood tests for CMV lack the sensitivity required to be useful for screening in pregnancy. There is currently no vaccine for CMV, although this is under development. Prediction of infants at long-term risk is difficult, and there are limits to the availability of effective treatments (Townsend 2011). Identification of asymptomatic newborns through the newborn blood spot screening or from saliva tests may be possible in the future. If newborns affected by CMV are identified early, regular monitoring of hearing may enable early detection of hearing loss. Timely interventions may improve speech and language outcomes for those infants with hearing loss (Townsend 2011).

The best way to prevent CMV transmission is frequent handwashing. Midwives can advise pregnant women to wash their hands after changing nappies or when handling respiratory secretions in young children (Vauloup-Fellous *et al.* 2009). This is particularly important for the 50% of the population who are CMV negative, although not exclusively, as there remains the possibility of reinfection of CMV. The absence of screening, however, means most women do not know their immune status and therefore it is difficult to target those who would most benefit from education regarding this risk (DeVries 2007). Pregnant childcare workers are at significant risk of primary CMV infection during pregnancy if they are not immune, and this is a group that would benefit from educational intervention (Nigro & Adler 2011).

ROLE OF THE MIDWIFE

- Recognise characteristics of viral rash illness or CMV in women or their close contacts.
- Make arrangements for the referral of women with contact or symptoms of a viral infection to the obstetrician, microbiologist, fetal medicine specialist, neonatologists and GP as indicated.
- The woman who has contact with, or symptoms of, a rash illness will need to be cared for away from other pregnant women. The midwife will need to make arrangements to continue routine antenatal care as well as provide support for the woman through the processes of investigation regarding maternal and fetal well-being.
- Offer advice regarding handwashing, care with respiratory secretions and/or separation from young children at times of outbreak.
- Contribute to health education and involvement in vaccination programmes as indicated.

USEFUL RESOURCES

- CMV Action website (http://cmvaction.org.uk).
- Health Protection Agency (HPA) (2011) *Guidance on Viral Rash in Pregnancy* [online]. Available at: www.hpa.org.uk/webc/HPAwebFile/HPAweb_C/1294740918985 (check for updates of this guidance from Public Health England website www.gov.uk/government/organisations/public-health-england).
- Royal College of Obstetrics and Gynaecology (RCOG) 2007 Green-top guideline No. 13. *Chickenpox in Pregnancy.* London: RCOG.

REFERENCES

Adler SP, Finney JW, Manganese AM, *et al.* (2004) Prevention of child-to-mother transmission of cytomegalovirus among pregnant women. *J Pediatrics.* **145**(4): 485–91.

American Academy of Pediatrics (AAP) (2012) Breastfeeding and the use of human milk. *Pediatrics.* **129**(3): e827–41.

Azam AZ, Vial Y, Fawer CL, *et al.* (2001) prenatal diagnosis of congenital cytomegalovirus infection. *Obstet Gynecol.* **97**(3): 443–48.

Banatvala JE (2002) Viral infections in pregnancy. In: de Swiet M (editor). *Medical Disorders in Obstetric Practice.* Oxford: Blackwell Science. pp. 513–31.

Banatvala JE, Brown DW (2004) Rubella. *Lancet.* **363**(9415): 1127–37.

Bannister B, Gillespie S, Jones J (2006) *Infection: microbiology and management.* Oxford: Blackwell.

Bhide A, Papageorghiou AT (2008) Managing primary CMV infection in pregnancy. *BJOG.* **115**(7): 805–7.

Blackburn ST (2013) *Maternal, Fetal and Neonatal Physiology: a clinical perspective.* 4th ed. Maryland Heights: Elsevier.

Bloom SA, Trepka MJ, Nobles RE, *et al.* (2006) Low postpartum rubella vaccination rates in high-risk women, Miami, Florida 2001. *Am J Prev Med.* **30**(2): 119–24.

Campbell H, Andrews N, Brown KE, *et al.* (2007) Review of the effect of measles vaccination on the epidemiology of SSPE. *Int J Epidemiol.* **36**(6): 1334–48.

Chiba ME, Saito M, Suzuki N, *et al.* (2003) Measles infection in pregnancy. *J Infect.* **47**(1): 40–4.

Collier L, Oxford J (2006) *Human Virology.* 3rd ed. Oxford: Oxford University Press.

Cossart YEAM, Field B, Widdows C, *et al.* (1975) Parvovirus-like particles in human sera. *Lancet.* **1**(7898): 72–3.

Crowcroft NS, Roth CE, Cohen BJ, *et al.* (1999) Guidance for control of parvovirus B19 infection in healthcare settings and the community. *J Public Health Med.* **21**(4): 439–46.

Deer B (2011) Secrets of the MMR scare: how the vaccine crisis was meant to make money. *BMJ.* **342**: c5258.

Department of Health (DH) (2012) Varicella. In: *Immunisation against Infectious Disease (the Green Book)* [online]. Available at: www.gov.uk/government/organisations/public-health-england/series/immunisation-against-infectious-disease-the-green-book (accessed 30 April 2014).

Department of Health (DH) (2013a) Rubella. In: *Immunisation against Infectious Disease (the Green Book)* [online]. Available at: www.gov.uk/government/organisations/public-health-england/series/immunisation-against-infectious-disease-the-green-book (accessed 30 April 2014).

Department of Health (DH) (2013b) Measles. In: *Immunisation against Infectious Disease (the Green Book)* [online]. Available at: www.gov.uk/government/organisations/public-health-england/series/immunisation-against-infectious-disease-the-green-book (accessed 30 April 2014).

DeVries J (2007) The ABCs of CMV. *Adv Neonatal Care.* **7**(5): 248–55.

Elliman D, Bedford H (2007) MMR: where are we now? *Arch Dis Child.* **92**(12): 1055–7.

Elliot T, Worthington T, Oman H, *et al.* (2007) *Medical Microbiology and Infection.* 4th ed. Oxford: Blackwell Publishing.

Gilbert GL (2002) Infections in pregnant women. *Med J Aust.* **176**(5): 229–36.

Gillespie SH, Bamford K (2012) *Medical Microbiology and Infection at a Glance.* 4th ed. Oxford: Wiley-Blackwell.

Goering RV, Dockrell HM, Zuckerman M, *et al.* (2013) *Mims' Medical Microbiology.* 5th ed. Oxford: Elsevier, Saunders.

Gruslin A, Faden Y (2008) Toxoplasmosis, cytomegalovirus, herpes simplex virus, rubella, parvovirus and listeria infections. In: Rosene-Montella K, Keely E, Barbour LA, *et al.* (editors). *Medical Care of the Pregnant Patient.* 2nd ed. Philadelphia: ACP Press. pp. 687–708.

Hardelid P, Cortina-Borja M, Williams D (2009) Rubella seroprevalence in pregnant women in North Thames: estimates based on newborn screening samples. *J Med Screen.* **16**(1): 1–6.

Health Protection Agency (HPA) (2011a) *Guidance on Viral Rash in Pregnancy* [online]. Available at: www.hpa.org.uk/webc/HPAwebFile/HPAweb_C/1294740918985 (accessed 18 September 2014).

Health Protection Agency (HPA) (2011b) *General Information on Parvovirus* [online]. Available at: www.hpa.org.uk/Topics/InfectiousDiseases/InfectionsAZ/ParvovirusB19/General Information/ (accessed 18 September 2014).

Health and Social Care information Centre (HSCIC) (2013) *NHS Immunisation Statistics, England – 2012–13 [NS]* [online]. Available at: www.hscic.gov.uk/catalogue/PUB11665 (accessed 30 April 2014).

Ismail KMK, Kilby MB (2003) Human parvovirus B19 infection and pregnancy. *Obstet Gynaecol.* **5**(1): 4–9.

Johannessen I, Ogilvie MM (2012) Herpesviruses. In: Greenwoood D, Baner M, Slack RC, *et al.* (editors). *Medical Microbiology.* 18th ed. Edinburgh: Churchill Livingston Elsevier. pp. 419–45.

Joint Committee on Vaccination and Immunisation (JCVI) (2012) *Minute of the Meeting held on Wednesday 1 February 2012* [online]. Available at: http://webarchive.nationalarchives.gov.uk/20120907090205/https://www.wp.dh.gov.uk/transparency/files/2012/04/JCVI-meeting-1-February-2012_draft-minutes.pdf (accessed 30 April 2014).

Khare MM, Khare MD (2007) Infections in pregnancy. In: Greer IA, Nelson-Piercy C, Walters BJN (editors). *Maternal Medicine: medical problems in pregnancy.* Edinburgh: Churchill Livingstone. pp. 217–35.

Kriebs JM (2008) Breaking the cycle of infection: TORCH and other infections in women's health. *J Midwifery Womens Health.* **53**(3): 173–4.

Lamont RF, Sobel JD, Carrington D, *et al.* (2011) Varicella-zoster virus (chickenpox) infection in pregnancy. *BJOG.* **118**(10): 1155–62.

Lamont RF, Sobel JD, Vaisbuch E, *et al.* (2010) Parvovirus B19 infection in human pregnancy. *BJOG.* **118**(2): 175–86.

Langford KS, Banatvala JE (2000) Infections that affect the fetus. *Curr Obstet Gynecol.* **10**(4): 178–82.

Lim WS, Macfarlane JT, Colthorpe CL (2001) Pneumonia and pregnancy. *Thorax.* **56**(5): 398–405.

MacMahon E (2012) Investigating the pregnant woman exposed to a child with a rash. *BMJ.* **344**: e1790.

Malm G, Engman ML (2007) Congenital cytomegalovirus infections. *Semin Fetal Neonatal Med.* **12**(3): 154–9.

Matthews l, Gray S, Gray D, *et al.* (2013) Post-partum MMR vaccination rates in rubella-susceptible antenatal women. *Br J Midwifery.* **21**(1): 16–22.

Molyneaux PJ (2007) Parvoviruses B19 infection: erythema infectious. In: Greenwood D, Slack R, Peutherer J, *et al.* (editors). *Medical Microbiology.* 17th ed. Edinburgh: Churchill Livingstone, Elsevier. pp. 467–75.

National Institute for Health and Care Excellence (NICE) (2010) Clinical Knowledge Summary (CKS): Parvovirus B19 infection [online]. Available at: http://cks.nice.org.uk/parvovirus-b19-infection (accessed 18 September 2014).

National Institute for Health and Care Excellence (NICE) (2013) Clinical Knowledge Summary (CKS): *Rubella* [online]. Available at: http://cks.nice.org.uk/rubella (accessed 18 September 2014).

Nigro G, Adler SP (2011) Cytomegalovirus infections during pregnancy. *Curr Opin Obstet Gynecol.* **23**(2): 123–8.

Peckham C, Tookey P, Giaquinto C (2002) Cytomegalovirus: to screen or not to screen. In: Donders G, Stray-Pedersen B (editors). *Viral Infection in Pregnancy.* Paris: Elsevier. pp. 83–96.

Price LC (2008) Infectious disease in pregnancy. *Obstet Gynaecol Reprod Med.* **18**(7): 173–9.

Public Health England (PHE) (2013) Measles cases in England: update to end April 2013. *Health Protection Report.* **7**(23) [online]. Available at: www.hpa.org.uk/hpr/archives/2013/hpr2313.pdf (accessed 18 September 2014).

Public Health England (PHE) (2014) Measles, mumps, rubella(MMR): Use of combined vaccine instead of single vaccines [online]. Available at: www.gov.uk/government/publications/mmr-vaccine-dispelling-myths/measles-mumps-rubella-mmr-maintaining-uptake-of-vaccine (accessed 18 September 2014).

Riley LE (2011) Rubella, measles, mumps, varicella and parvovirus. In: James D, Steer PJ, Weiner CP, *et al.* (editors). *High Risk Pregnancy: management options.* 4th ed. New York: Elsevier Saunders pp. 493–502.

Roos T, Baker DA (2011) Cytomegalovirus, herpes simplex virus, adenovirus, Coxsackievirus and human papillomavirus. In: James D, Steer PJ, Weiner CP, *et al.* (editors). *High Risk Pregnancy: management options.* 4th ed. New York: Elsevier Saunders. pp. 503–20.

Royal College of Obstetrics and Gynaecology (RCOG) (2007) *Chickenpox in Pregnancy.* Green-top Guideline 13. London: RCOG.

Royal College of Physicians (RCP) (2010) *Varicella Zoster Virus: occupational aspects of management; a national guideline* [online]. Available at: www.nhshealthatwork.co.uk/images/library/files/Clinical%20excellence/Varicella_zoster_guidelines_web_navigable.pdf (accessed 5 March 2013).

Sabbaj S, Pass RF, Goepfert PA, *et al.* (2011) Glycoprotein B vaccine is capable of boosting both antibody and CD4 T-cell responses to cytomegalovirus in chronically infected women. *J Infect Dis.* **203**(11): 1534–41.

Sendelbach DM, Sanchez PJ (2012) Varicella, influenza: not necessary to separate mother and infant. *Pediatrics.* **30**(2): e464.

Smith J, Whitehall J (2008) Human parvovirus B19: a literature review and case study. *Infant.* **4**(3): 101–4.

Tolfvenstam T, Broliden K (2009) Parvovirus B19 infection. *Semin Fetal Neonatal Med.* **14**(4): 218–21.

Tookey PA, Cortina–Borja, Peckham CS (2002) Rubella susceptibility among pregnant women in North London, 1996–1999. *J Public Health Med.* **24**(3): 211–16.

Tookey PA, Bedford H, Peckham CS (2013) Congenital rubella: act now to prevent re-emergence of congenital rubella [letter]. *BMJ.* **347**: f4498.

Townsend C (2011) *Review of Screening for Cytomegalovirus in the Antenatal and/or the Neonatal Periods* [online]. Available at: www.screening.nhs.uk/policydb_download.php?doc=198 (accessed 30 April 2014).

Townsend C, Peckham CS, Tookey PA (2011) Surveillance of congenital cytomegalovirus in the UK and Ireland. *Arch Dis Child Fetal Neonatal Ed.* **96**(6): F398–403.

UK National Screening Committee (UK NSC) (2010) *Infectious Diseases in Pregnancy Screening Programme: programme standards* [online]. Available at: http://infectiousdiseases.screening. nhs.uk/publications (accessed 22 August 2013).

Vauloup-Fellous C, Picone O, Cordier AG, *et al.* (2009) Does hygiene counseling have an impact on the rate of CMV primary infection during pregnancy? Results of a 3-year prospective study in a French hospital. *J Clin Virol.* **46**(Suppl. 4): S49–53.

Wakefield A, Murch SH, Anthony A, *et al.* (1998) Illeal-lymphoid-nodular hyperplasia, non-specific colitis, and pervasive developmental disorder in children. *Lancet.* **351**(9103): 637–41 [retracted].

White SJ, Boldt KL, Holditch SJ, *et al.* (2012) Measles, mumps, rubella. *Clin Obstet Gynaecol.* **55**(2): 550–9.

Yinon Y, Farine D, Yudin MH (2010) Screening, diagnosis, and management of cytomegalovirus infection in pregnancy. *Obstet Gynecol Surv.* **65**(11): 736–43.

Yung C, Skidmore S, Lord S (2008) Postpartum MR immunisation uptake in non-immune women. *Br J Midwifery.* **16**(5): 288–91.

CHAPTER 12

Food-borne infections in pregnancy

> → Listeria
> → Salmonella
> → Toxoplasmosis

INTRODUCTION

Food safety is a concern for all people but it is even more important for pregnant women, as they appear to be more susceptible to some food-related infections and these infections may cause harm to the fetus or newborn. It is interesting to note some authors have suggested that the nausea and vomiting of early pregnancy is benefi-cial in protecting the fetus from food-borne pathogens, as the mother becomes more sensitive in what she chooses to eat (Sherman & Flaxman 2002). However, illness affecting the mother with vertical transmission to the fetus or newborn remains a concern, in particular for cases of listeria, salmonella and toxoplasmosis. A number of food safety recommendations, including lists of foods to avoid in pregnancy, add to an information-saturated environment that the pregnant woman is required to navigate. It is important to note that the transmission of toxoplasmosis goes beyond food safety and includes transmission via cats. In addition, working with farm ani-mals, particularly during lambing, is another source of contact with these infections. Midwives will need to recognise ill health and ensure prompt referral for women with food-borne illness and will have a significant role in providing health education advice to women that aims to prevent these illnesses.

LISTERIA

Listeria monocytogenes is a small Gram-positive rod-shaped bacterium that is widespread in the environment and can be found in soil, fruit and vegetables, and sewerage (Goering *et al.* 2013, Yudin 2011). *Listeria* can also be found in the digestive tract of animals, without causing illness, but it may subsequently contaminate meat and dairy products (Delgado 2008). Listeriosis is a relatively uncommon infection but more likely to cause problems for those with some degree of immunosuppression including pregnant women and newborn infants.

Laboratories are instructed to notify local health protection units of listeriosis cases to ensure effective public health follow-up – there are around 30 cases a year affecting pregnant women in England and Wales (HPA 2011a). Investigation of previous outbreaks of listeriosis has led to improved food standards, and where food is correctly prepared, handled and stored the risk of being infected with *Listeria* is low (Tam *et al.* 2010), although pregnant women are still advised to avoid consumption of certain foods. Box 12.1 lists some of the variety of foods that can become contaminated with *Listeria*. Contaminated food smells, looks and tastes normal (Yudin 2011). Unlike most bacteria, *Listeria* can survive and multiply in food stored in a domestic fridge, but it is killed with pasteurisation and/or proper cooking (Yudin 2011, Ridgeway 2002). Advice for pregnant women should include aspects of food preparation and storage alongside a list of foods to avoid.

BOX 12.1 FOODS THAT MAY BECOME CONTAMINATED WITH *LISTERIA*

- Uncooked meat
- Uncooked, unwashed vegetables
- Unpasteurised milk
- Unpasteurised milk-containing products including cheese
- Soft ripened cheese*
- Refrigerated ready-to-eat delicatessen-type meats and salads*
- Seafood*

* Risk considered low when purchased from reputable shops (Tam *et al.* 2010)

Women who become infected with *Listeria* by eating contaminated food can pass that infection on to the fetus or newborn. This vertical transmission from mother to child may occur in utero (via blood and placenta), causing congenital listeriosis. Where a mother is infected with *Listeria* in the gastrointestinal tract or vaginal secretions (as a result of contamination from the gastrointestinal tract), she may also pass on the infection during birth or from direct contact following delivery (Gillespie & Bamford

2012, Posfay-Barbe & Wald 2009, Elliot *et al.* 2007, Bannister *et al.* 2006). Studies have identified that *Listeria* can transiently colonise the gastrointestinal tract of women without causing illness (Lamont *et al.* 2011).

The incidence of listeriosis in pregnant women is approximately 12 per 100 000, which is 17 times the rate in the general population (0.7 per 100 000) (Mylonakis *et al.* 2002, Lamont *et al.* 2011). The relative suppression of cell-mediated immunity in pregnancy and the placenta's susceptibility to this microorganism are possible explanations as to why listeriosis is more common among pregnant women (Posfay-Barbe & Wald 2009, Yudin 2011). Apart from immune vulnerability, other factors that influence the extent of illness include the virulence of a particular strain of *Listeria* and the amount of bacteria ingested. The duration of the incubation period is unknown but is thought to be around 3 weeks (Lamont *et al.* 2011).

Pregnant women with listeriosis most commonly suffer flu-like symptoms with a high temperature ($\geq$38.2°C), back or abdominal pain, headache, aching joints and generally feeling unwell. A small number of women may experience vomiting and diarrhoea. Occasionally listeriosis causes meningitis and sepsis in women; however, up to a third of women have no symptoms (Lamont *et al.* 2011, Mylonakis *et al.* 2002). The symptoms (when present) are similar to many infectious conditions, including sepsis, and the midwife should immediately refer any woman who is unwell to a medical practitioner for review.

Identifying the bacteria from blood culture will normally confirm the diagnosis, although samples for testing can be taken from a number of locations from both mother and newborn. These will include, in addition to blood culture, samples taken from cervical and vaginal secretions, placental tissue, amniotic fluid, lochia, gastric aspirate and cerebrospinal fluid (Gillespie & Bamford 2012, Yudin 2011).

Listeriosis in early pregnancy often leads to miscarriage or premature delivery (Bannister *et al.* 2006). A review of 222 cases of listeriosis in pregnancy over a 10-year period examined the features of maternal listeriosis, diagnosis, and outcomes for the babies of pregnancies complicated by listeriosis. This study found that 20% of pregnancies ended in miscarriage or stillbirth. Of those babies who were live-born, many of whom were born prematurely, approximately 60% recovered, 25% were neonatal deaths, and 12% had neurological or other long-term disability. For the remainder the outcome was unknown (Mylonakis *et al.* 2002).

As symptoms of maternal listeriosis may go unnoticed, the first indication of *Listeria* infection may be when the newborn baby becomes unwell. The symptoms of neonatal listeriosis are similar to group B streptococcus (*see* Box 12.2). There is an early presentation (within 1–2 days of birth) or a late presentation (1–3 weeks after birth). In late presentations the newborn is more likely to develop sepsis and meningitis (Bannister *et al.* 2006, Delgado 2008, Posfay-Barbe & Wald 2009).

BOX 12.2 SYMPTOMS OF NEONATAL LISTERIOSIS

- Severe respiratory distress
- Enlarged liver or spleen
- Fever
- Neurological symptoms including irritability
- Skin rash (raised pale patches with bright erythematous (red) base)
- Rarely the newborn will present with granulomatosis infantisepticum, where the infant has granuloma abscesses in the lung, skin, liver and other locations; this condition has a high mortality rate

(Yudin 2011, Gruslin & Faden 2008)

Listeriosis will respond to treatment by antibiotics and treatment of the mother may improve the outcome for the unborn baby (Gruslin & Faden 2008). Serial ultrasound scans to assess fetal growth are recommended, and consultation with the neonatal team prior to delivery is essential to plan for adequate and timely treatment of the neonate (Gruslin & Faden 2008, Delgado 2008). After delivery the placenta should be sent to histology for examination. Characteristic abscesses and inflammation of the villi may be found (Gruslin & Faden 2008). Antibiotics may improve the outcome for the neonate when diagnosis is made early (Lamont *et al.* 2011). Mothers and babies with listeria will require isolation, particularly when diarrhoea is present (Bannister *et al.* 2006, Gillespie & Bamford 2012).

PREVENTION OF LISTERIOSIS AND OTHER FOOD-BORNE PATHOGENS

Prevention of listeriosis aims to reduce ingestion of contaminated food, although for many infections the source is not determined (Gruslin & Faden 2008, Goering *et al.* 2013). Food items implicated in outbreaks of listeriosis have included ready-to-eat meats, meat pâté, hot dogs, unpasteurised milk and milk products, and soft cheese (Ross *et al.* 2006). These are the main foods targeted to avoid. Box 12.3 summarises the guidance on how to avoid listeriosis in pregnancy.

Midwives are in a key position to inform women about food safety in pregnancy, but it is challenging to provide effective health education when there are so many competing demands on both the time the midwife has with the woman and the priorities of health messages. Studies have shown that pregnant women are not aware of the increased risk of food-borne illness in pregnancy. Many have not heard of listeriosis and said they had not been given information by their caregivers (Kirkham & Berkowitz 2010, Cates *et al.* 2004, Bondarianzadeh *et al.* 2007, Ogunmodede *et al.* 2005). Pregnant women may not understand, or they may find it confusing or difficult,

---

BOX 12.3 GUIDANCE ON HOW TO AVOID LISTERIOSIS IN PREGNANCY

- Do not eat unpasteurised dairy products* including milk, soft ripened cheeses that have a rind such as Brie and Camembert, and soft blue veined cheeses such as Gorgonzola.
- Pre-prepared meals and ready-to-eat poultry need to be stored below 5°C, eaten by the due date and reheated thoroughly according to the manufacturer's guidelines.
- Cook all meat and chicken thoroughly.
- When reheating food, make sure it is steaming hot all the way through.
- Do not eat meat spreads and pâté, including vegetable pâté.
- Avoid ready-to-eat food from salad bars, sandwich bars, delicatessens and smorgasbords where food is left out for long periods.
- Wash fruit and vegetables.
- The risk of *Listeria* infection is low in cold meats and smoked fish, but pregnant women may choose to avoid these products as well.
- Keep your fridge clean and ensure it is maintaining a temperature below 5°C.

* Unpasteurised milk can be a source of a range of virulent pathogens, not just *Listeria monocytogenes* but also *Campylobacter jejuni*, *Salmonella* spp, *Brucella* spp, *Toxoplasmosis gondii* and *Escherichia coli*.

(NHS 2014, Food Standards Agency n.d., Committee on Infectious Diseases *et al.* 2014)

---

to adhere to the guidance. Many of those that did know which foods to avoid admitted to eating high-risk foods (Wong *et al.* 2013). Those preparing food for them, both in the home and commercially, also need to be aware of the recommendations (Delgado 2008). Women from deprived backgrounds and those from ethnic minority groups are at greater risk of contracting listeriosis (HPA 2011a, Gillespie *et al.* 2010) indicating perhaps that health messages are not as effective for some of the most vulnerable groups of women. Busy clinics, language barriers, reduced provision for parent education, reliance on written materials and the relative rareness of listeriosis will hamper the effectiveness of health education in this area. Messages need to promote positive behaviours and include what women can eat (not just what they cannot) and how to reduce risk by cooking and heating. This may help reduce the negative burden of the advice, which may be overwhelming for some women. Use of high-quality Internet-based information that includes video clips and mobile phone apps may provide innovative ways to improve communication.

ROLE OF THE MIDWIFE IN RELATION TO LISTERIOSIS

- Midwives need to seek innovative ways to advise women regarding food hygiene and information on what foods to avoid in pregnancy. Presenting what foods women can eat is just as important as listing what they can't eat.
- Midwives should refer all cases of febrile illness for medical assessment.
- The midwife should observe the neonate for signs of early or late *Listeria* infection, which will include signs of sepsis, respiratory distress or neurological impairment.
- Isolation of mothers and babies with listeriosis may be required.
- Where a pregnant woman is found to have listeriosis, referral to the neonatal team fetal medicine specialist is required.
- The midwife should ensure good communication regarding listeriosis after discharge to the community team in view of the possibility of late-onset neonatal disease. For this reason the community midwife may need to visit for longer.

SALMONELLA

Salmonella spp are bacteria that most commonly cause food poisoning. More than 2500 different strains of *Salmonella* have been identified. Outbreaks of salmonella food poisoning occur sporadically and have been associated with travel and attendance at large social gatherings. Beef, poultry, unpasteurised milk and eggs are implicated as sources of salmonella; however, all food including vegetables can become contaminated. Contamination of kitchen surfaces, poor handwashing and failure to reach adequate cooking temperatures are all recognised as factors contributing to transmission of the bacteria (HPA 2011b, Ross & Furrows 2014).

Symptoms of illness include fever, diarrhoea and abdominal cramps and usually appear 12–72 hours after eating the contaminated food (Coughlin *et al.* 2003).

Pregnant women are not thought to be at more risk than others of contracting salmonella (Tam *et al.* 2010), but they are generally more susceptible to complications of food poisoning, so midwives should ensure prompt referral for assessment. There have been case reports of intrauterine death, premature delivery and neonatal infection associated with salmonella, making early diagnosis and treatment a priority (Schloesser *et al.* 2004). The associated fever should be treated, as any febrile illness in pregnancy is associated with miscarriage and premature labour. Fluid replacement may be required to avoid any complications of dehydration. Obtaining a stool sample for microbiology may aid diagnosis.

Laboratories will require relevant clinical information to be written on the request form. This should include the stage of pregnancy, symptoms, travel history and any particular suspected pathogen. Enquiries should be made about possible source of the infection and any others who display similar symptoms (NICE 2009).

Salmonella infection is usually self-limiting and does not normally require antibiotic treatment, as routine use of antibiotics contributes to the emergence of antibiotic-resistant strains. However, antibiotics may be indicated in cases of systemic disease and in pregnancy (Coughlin *et al.* 2003).

The illness usually lasts around 4–7 days and maternal prognosis is good. However, occasionally the fetus may be affected. Spread via the blood, through the placenta to the fetus, is thought to occur in a small number of cases. Evidence of fetal illness may appear 1–2 weeks after initial gastrointestinal symptoms in the mother (Coughlin *et al.* 2003).

PREVENTION OF SALMONELLA

Box 12.4 summarises some of the key recommendations for prevention of salmonella.

BOX 12.4 KEY RECOMMENDATIONS FOR PREVENTION OF SALMONELLA

- Good hand hygiene
- Rigorous kitchen hygiene
- Avoid raw or partially cooked eggs and be aware that raw eggs may be an ingredient in fresh mayonnaise or chocolate mousse
- Adequate cooking of meat, poultry
- Care with regard to eating when on holidays
- Care with regard to the storage, freezing, unfreezing and cooking of food
- Vegetables eaten raw should be washed thoroughly
- Keep raw and cooked food separate (including utensils)
- Do not reheat food more than once

ROLE OF MIDWIFE IN RELATION TO SALMONELLA

- Prompt referral for medical assessment if a pregnant woman appears to have symptoms of food poisoning
- Aim to reduce maternal temperature and encourage hydration
- Provide information to pregnant women with regard to food hygiene

TOXOPLASMOSIS

T. gondii is a protozoan parasite. It can infect almost all warm-blooded animals, including humans, and up to a third of the world's population has been infected (Pappas *et al.* 2009). The parasite has a complex life cycle and cats are hosts for the infective stage of the parasite (Bannister *et al.* 2006, Montoya & Liesenfeld 2004). Women may acquire toxoplasmosis through contact with cat litter, eating under-cooked meat or unpasteurised milk products and from inadvertent ingestion of contaminated soil particles in water and on vegetables. The main threat posed by toxoplasmosis is when pregnant women contract it for the first time in or just before pregnancy, where it can pass via the placenta and infect the fetus, leading to mis-carriage or stillbirth. The newborn exposed to toxoplasmosis in utero may develop congenital toxoplasmosis, a condition featuring major eye and neurological damage (Petersen 2007, Bannister *et al.* 2006).

Midwives need to understand the transmission of toxoplasmosis as the basis for giving accurate information to women to help them prevent contracting this infec-tion when pregnant. They also have a role in timely referral and support of parents who encounter this infection.

LIFE CYCLE OF *TOXOPLASMA GONDII*

T. gondii has a complicated life cycle, taking different forms starting with oocysts (*see* Figure 12.1). The reproduction of the parasite takes place in the cat's intestine, resulting in the production of millions of oocysts. These oocysts are passed on in cat faeces, and under favourable conditions (warm, moist soil) can remain viable in the soil for up to a year (Franco & Ernest 2011, Wilson 2006). Animals and humans can ingest the oocysts via contaminated soil or water. For example, humans may ingest them on unwashed vegetables. Animals grazing on grass contaminated by cat faeces may ingest the oocysts (Wilson 2006).

After ingestion the parasite reproduces. Tachyzoites, as the name implies (*tachy* = fast), are the rapidly multiplying stage of the parasite. At this stage they cir-culate throughout the body, establishing cysts in tissues such as the brain, muscle, the eye and placenta. In immune-competent adults and children, the immune sys-tem deals effectively with this invasion by tachyzoites and under pressure from the host's immune system, tachyzoites are brought under control and transformed into bradyzoites, the slow-multiplying, dormant quiescent stage (*brady* = slow). Tissue cysts are formed with the bradyzoites contained within them (Wilson 2006, Bannister *et al.* 2006, Montoya & Liesenfeld 2004).

EPIDEMIOLOGY

Although occurring worldwide, the prevalence of *T. gondii* infection varies according to climate, cultural habits and socio-economic status (Pappas *et al.* 2009). There is a

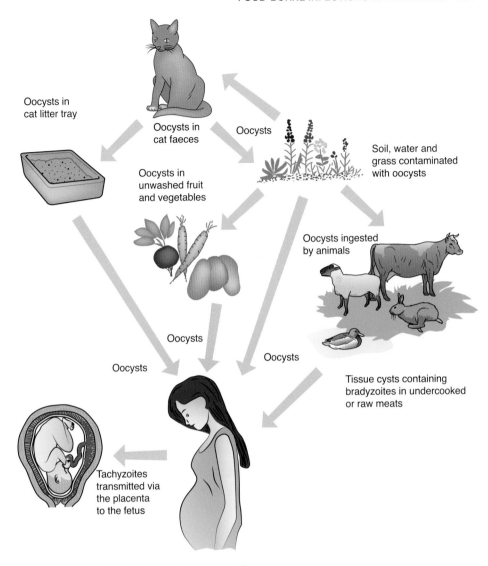

Oocysts in
cat litter tray

Oocysts in
cat faeces

Oocysts

Soil, water and
grass contaminated
with oocysts

Oocysts in
unwashed fruit
and vegetables

Oocysts ingested
by animals

Oocysts

Oocysts

Oocysts

Tissue cysts containing
bradyzoites in undercooked
or raw meats

Tachyzoites
transmitted via
the placenta
to the fetus

FIGURE 12.1 Life cycle of *Toxoplasma gondii*

higher prevalence in warm countries, where oocysts will survive well, and therefore countries with a higher incidence of toxoplasmosis include southern Europe, South America and Africa (Petersen 2007, Gruslin & Faden 2008). Habits in food preparation and consumption also influence seroprevalence rates (Pappas *et al.* 2009).

About 9%–17% of women in the UK have been previously exposed to toxoplasmosis infection at the time of booking, and women born outside the UK or living in rural areas are more likely to test positive for toxoplasmosis (Pappas *et al.* 2009, Flatt & Shetty 2013). In the UK, toxoplasmosis infection is rare in pregnancy (Khare & Khare 2007). In 2013, there were 36 cases of toxoplasmosis among pregnant women in England and Wales, with two confirmed cases of congenital toxoplasmosis (PHE 2014). It is more common in France and other southern European countries, where up to 6% of pregnancies may be affected (Bannister *et al.* 2006).

CLINICAL FEATURES

Toxoplasmosis is controlled effectively by cell-mediated immunity, so for immune-competent individuals, the infection poses little risk. Most individuals (including pregnant women) who acquire infection with *T. gondii* do not have any obvious symptoms. If symptoms do occur (only in around 10%), they may involve some enlargement of lymph nodes accompanied by fever, malaise and headache, which may persist for some weeks (Gruslin & Faden 2008, Bannister *et al.* 2006, Montoya & Liesenfeld 2004). However, in immune-suppressed individuals, including those with the human immunodeficiency virus, complications of toxoplasmosis can be severe and include myocarditis, encephalitis and pneumonitis (Bannister *et al.* 2006, Gruslin & Faden 2008).

TRANSMISSION

Of importance to midwives, vertical transmission of toxoplasmosis can occur from mother to fetus. In settings such as the UK, where seroprevalence to the infection is low, a woman is unlikely to be infected, as the habits and environment where she lives makes her low risk. However, if she does become infected, it is more likely to be a primary infection, which carries the greatest risk of harm to the fetus (Pappas *et al.* 2009). Transmission to adults and children of *T. gondii* is predominantly by the oral route and thus individuals can acquire toxoplasmosis by:

- ingestion or handling of raw or undercooked meat that contain tissue cysts
- handling cat faeces
- consuming water or food that has been in contact with soil that has been contaminated by the faeces of infected cats (e.g. from eating unwashed vegetables or salad, drinking contaminated unfiltered water)
- contact with contaminated soil via hands (e.g. gardening)
- consuming unpasteurised milk or dairy products.

(Petersen 2007, Cook *et al.* 2000, Wilson 2006, Franco & Ernest 2011, Boyer *et al.* 2005)

Studies that have looked specifically at risk factors for contracting toxoplasmosis in pregnancy have, unsurprisingly, found similar risks to that in the general population as already listed (Flatt & Shetty 2012, Cook *et al.* 2000). Cleaning the cat litter box is a known risk factor for toxoplasmosis, but, interestingly, cat ownership was not a risk factor for contracting toxoplasmosis in pregnancy (Cook *et al.* 2000, Flatt

& Shetty 2012, Pappas *et al.* 2009). Authors suggest that health messages about the risk of toxoplasmosis in pregnancy from contact with cat litter have been effective in preventing transmission via this route but that women are less aware of the risk associated with eating undercooked meat. However, in a study of 131 mothers of infants with congenital toxoplasmosis in the United States, less than half the mothers could recall any risk exposure or features of illness during pregnancy (Boyer *et al.* 2005). The authors of this study argued that antenatal screening was needed to improve detection of toxoplasmosis in pregnancy. The unreliability of recall and small sample sizes will hamper studies of risk, but information on these factors is useful for preventive health education.

Mother-to-child transmission

When the mother acquires toxoplasmosis for the first time during pregnancy the parasite may enter the fetal circulation via the placenta. Maternal infection acquired before pregnancy poses little or no risk to the fetus except when infection occurs within a few weeks (3 at most) before conception (Montoya & Liesenfeld 2004, McClure & Goldenberg 2009).

Transplacental infection of toxoplasmosis will occur in about a third of infected pregnancies, although the risk of the fetus being infected increases with gestation. If maternal infection occurs in early pregnancy the risk of congenital toxoplasmosis is low (15%–25%), whereas the rate of transmission is greater than 60% in the last trimester. However, if the fetus is infected in the first and second trimester, more serious complications of congenital toxoplasmosis occur. In summary, the risk of congenital infection increases throughout pregnancy but the severity of impact on the fetus decreases (Gruslin & Faden 2008, Franco & Ernest 2011, Bannister *et al.* 2006).

CONGENITAL TOXOPLASMOSIS

A fetus severely affected with congenital toxoplasmosis may be stillborn or die soon after birth. Significant abnormalities may be evident on ultrasound. Box 12.5 lists some of the manifestations of congenital toxoplasmosis before and after birth. These symptoms are not unique to toxoplasmosis and can result from other infections including cytomegalovirus, herpes simplex virus, rubella and syphilis.

There is often no evident abnormality present at birth in a fetus affected in the last trimester. However, chorioretinitis with consequent visual impairment and neurological complications can develop up to 15 years after birth (Boyer *et al.* 2005, Bannister *et al.* 2006). Treatment of infected infants in the first year of life and good follow-up improves outcomes (Boyer *et al.* 2005, Berrébi *et al.* 2010).

BOX 12.5 POSSIBLE MANIFESTATIONS OF CONGENITAL TOXOPLASMOSIS BEFORE AND AFTER BIRTH

FETUS: ULTRASOUND FINDINGS

- Intracranial calcification
- Ventricular dilation
- Liver enlargement
- Ascites
- Increased thickness of the placenta

INFANT SIGNS

- Intracranial calcification
- Hydrocephalus
- Microcephaly
- Early or late chorioretinitis
- Psychomotor or neurological developmental delay
- Epilepsy

(Montoya & Liesenfeld 2004, Gruslin & Faden 2008)

SCREENING AND DIAGNOSIS OF TOXOPLASMOSIS IN PREGNANCY

Strategies for control and prevention of congenital toxoplasmosis vary between countries. National antenatal screening is performed in France, Austria and Slovenia. The first booking blood sample is tested for specific IgM and IgG antibodies. France offers the most vigilant testing, with seronegative women (i.e. those most vulnerable to primary toxoplasmosis infection in pregnancy) being further tested monthly during pregnancy (Petersen 2007).

Most European countries, including the UK, do not recommend screening. The rationale for this includes that screening is not cost-effective, with the cost of screening not returning sufficient benefit, particularly where the incidence of congenital toxoplasmosis is low. The diagnostic test for acute *T. gondii* infection is not straightforward because the specific IgM antibodies can be long-lasting and so their presence in a sample does not necessarily indicate recent infection (Bannister *et al.* 2006). The treatment available is not entirely satisfactory, with studies examining the outcomes for children following treatment not proving conclusive benefit (Petersen 2007). However, some authors disagree, offering evidence regarding the benefits of screening that includes reduced morbidity from congenital toxoplasmosis when treatment is started promptly and options of termination of pregnancy where the fetus is severely affected (Boyer *et al.* 2005, Berrébi *et al.* 2010).

In countries, including the UK, where routine screening is not done, tests are available on demand or based on an individual risk assessment (Petersen 2007). Serology tests on maternal blood can detect antibodies to the organism. These will reflect whether the woman has ever been infected. A *negative* result will mean the woman has never had toxoplasmosis. However, this does indicate she is not immune and therefore should take precautions to avoid infection before and during pregnancy. A *positive* result means the woman has had toxoplasmosis at some point in her life. The blood will then be sent to the national Toxoplasma Reference Laboratory, where further testing is required to determine whether or not this is a recent (acute) infection (Petersen 2007, Tommy's 2013). When an acute infection is diagnosed in the mother during or just before pregnancy, further assessment is required to assess the risk of the infection affecting the fetus. Ultrasound findings (*see* Box 12.5) and amniocentesis are used to aid diagnosis of toxoplasmosis infection of the fetus (Gruslin & Faden 2008). Box 12.6 lists tests used for diagnosis.

BOX 12.6 DIAGNOSTIC TESTS FOR TOXOPLASMOSIS

- In **pregnant women**, serological tests for specific antibodies are used where infection is suspected; serial samples may be needed.
- In the **fetus**, PCR test or culture of amniotic fluid samples are required to reliably diagnose fetal infection.
- In the **neonate**, IgM specific antibody in blood or PCR test or culture of blood, cerebrospinal fluid, placenta or products of conception.

(Bannister *et al.* 2006, Khare & Khare 2007, Petersen 2007)

MANAGEMENT

Medical practitioners, including an obstetrician, fetal medicine specialist and a paediatrician, should direct treatment discussing the relative benefits and possible disadvantages of management options. This will be an anxious time for women, and support by the midwife that includes sensitivity to their needs in decision-making and access to specialist counselling and information will be essential.

Specific antibiotics may be prescribed as soon as maternal infection is confirmed. This will aim to reduce the transmission and severity of fetal infection, although it is thought the parasite will cross the placenta at an early stage of the infection (Montoya

& Liesenfeld 2004, Petersen 2007). In addition to antibiotics, treatment with an antiparasitic medication is commenced if fetal infection is confirmed following amniocentesis (Franco & Ernest 2011, Khare & Khare 2007). Antiparasitic medication may inhibit folate synthesis and is therefore best avoided in the first trimester. Supplements of folic acid are required when this medication is prescribed (Bannister *et al.* 2006, Franco & Ernest 2011). Infected infants may be treated with the same medication, for 6–12 months (Bannister *et al.* 2006).

Prospective cohort studies have demonstrated there may be improved outcomes for infants where treatment is started early and continued into the neonatal period (SYROCOT study group 2007, Gras *et al.* 2005, Berrébi *et al.* 2010). The paediatric team should be informed with regard to congenital toxoplasmosis so appropriate neonatal care and follow-up can be organised.

Termination of pregnancy may be considered following confirmation of fetal infection. Referral to fetal medicine specialists for investigations and assessment will provide parents with accurate information. Factors affecting decision-making will include individual fetal assessment, maternal preferences and gestational age (Gruslin & Faden 2008).

Toxoplasmosis is not directly transmitted from person to person and therefore no special infection control measures are required (Ross & Furrows 2014). Neither the mother nor the infant pose any risk of transmission to healthcare professionals or others and the midwife should ensure mother and baby are cared for in the normal way (Franco & Ernest 2011).

PREVENTION

The most effective way to prevent congenital toxoplasmosis is for midwives to give women clear, accurate and timely information on how to avoid contracting toxoplasmosis when they are pregnant or are planning pregnancy. Box 12.7 summarises the key aspects of that advice. Some of this advice concerns food preparation, which can be included in general advice about eating in pregnancy and linked to how to avoid other food-borne infections. Further specific information regarding contact with cat faeces is specific to toxoplasmosis. In common with listeriosis, general public awareness of toxoplasmosis is probably low. Pregnant women can feel overwhelmed by the amount of information given in early pregnancy, and the challenge for midwives is to provide some verbal information backed up with written information in an accessible form.

BOX 12.7 ADVICE FOR PREGNANT WOMEN AND THOSE PLANNING PREGNANCY ON HOW TO AVOID TOXOPLASMOSIS

- Avoid eating raw or undercooked meat or poultry
- Avoid eating cured meats such as prosciutto and salami
- Wash your hands and all utensils, chopping boards, plates and surfaces that have been in contact with raw meat
- Wash fruit, vegetables and salad before eating
- Don't drink unpasteurised milk or eat any dairy products made from it
- Wear gloves when gardening or handling soil or sand, and wash your hands well afterwards
- Ask someone else to clean out the cat litter box; this should be done daily – if you can't avoid this job, wear gloves and wash your hands well afterwards
- Cover your child's play sandpit to avoid cats using it as a litter box
- Do not handle lambing ewes
- If you visit a farm, wash your hands thoroughly after contact with sheep and avoid handling newborn lambs

(Jones *et al.* 2003, Tommy's 2013, BMJ Group 2009)

ROLE OF THE MIDWIFE IN RELATION TO TOXOPLASMOSIS

- Provision of timely, concise, accurate and clear health education information regarding how to avoid toxoplasmosis infection just before and during pregnancy.
- Prompt referral of women who think they may have infection or contact with toxoplasmosis when they are pregnant.
- Support for women undergoing testing and treatment for themselves and their fetus or newborn with regard toxoplasmosis.
- Information for women on support groups and further information on toxoplasmosis. A list of some useful resources for women is provided at the end of this chapter.
- Ensure women with toxoplasmosis are not subject to any strict isolation procedures beyond normal policies and that they are treated normally.

USEFUL RESOURCES

- BMJ Group (2009) *Patient Leaflets from the BMJ Group: toxoplasmosis in pregnancy* [online] Available at http://bestpractice.bmj.com/best-practice/pdf/patient-summaries/congenital-toxoplasmosis-standard.pdf
- NHS Choices (n.d.) *Foods to Avoid in Pregnancy* [online]. Available at: www.nhs.uk/conditions/pregnancy-and-baby/pages/foods-to-avoid-pregnant.aspx#close Provides specific information on how to avoid listeria, with useful lists of which cheeses can be eaten, along with other advice about food safety.
- Food Standards Australia New Zealand (n.d.) *Advice for People at Risk: listeria and food* [online]. Available at: www.health.gov.au/internet/main/publishing.nsf/Content/01922F453 4D07BFCCA257BF0001CAC00/$File/Listeria.pdf (accessed 15 March 2014). Useful lists of food to avoid but also alternative safe foods.
- Tommy's (2013) *Toxoplasmosis and Pregnancy.* [online] available at www.tommys.org/page. aspx?pid=193

REFERENCES

Bannister B, Gillespie S, Jones J (2006) *Infection: microbiology and management.* 3rd ed. Oxford: Blackwell Publishing.

Berrébi A, Assouline C, Bessières, *et al.* (2010) Long-term outcomes of children with congenital toxoplasmosis. *Am J Obstet Gynecol.* **203**(552): e1–6.

BMJ Group (2009) *Patient Leaflets from the BMJ Group: toxoplasmosis in pregnancy* [online]. Available at: http://bestpractice.bmj.com/best-practice/pdf/patient-summaries/congenital-toxoplasmosis-standard.pdf (accessed 24 March 2014).

Bondarianzadeh D, Yeatman H, Condon-Paoloni D (2007) Listeria education in pregnancy: lost opportunity for health professionals. *Aust N Z J Public Health.* **31**(5): 468–74.

Boyer KM, Holfels E, Roizen M, *et al.* (2005) Risk factors for *Toxoplasma gondii* infection in mothers with congenital toxoplasmosis: implications for prenatal management and screening. *Am J Obstet Gynecol.* **192**(2): 564–71.

Cates SC, Carter-Young HL, Conley S, *et al.* (2004) Pregnant women and listeriosis: preferred educational messages and delivery mechanisms. *J Nutr Educ Behav.* **36**(3): 121–7.

Committee on Infectious Diseases; Committee on Nutrition; American Academy of Pediatrics (2014) *Policy Statement: consumption of raw or unpasteurized milk and milk products by pregnant women and children. Pediatrics.* **133**(1): 175–9.

Cook AJ, Gilbert RE, Buffolano W, *et al.* (2000) Sources of toxoplasma infection in pregnant women: European multicentre case-controlled study. European Research Network on Congenital Toxoplasmosis. *BMJ.* **321**(7254): 142–7.

Coughlin LB, McGuigan J, Haddad NG, *et al.* (2003) Salmonella sepsis and miscarriage. *Clin Microbiol Infect.* **9**(8): 866–8.

Delgado AR (2008) Listeriosis in pregnancy. *J Midwifery Womens Health.* **53**(3): 255–9.

Elliot T, Worthington T, Oman H, *et al.* (2007) *Medical Microbiology and Infection.* 4th ed. Oxford: Blackwell Publishing.

Flatt A, Shetty N (2013) Seroprevalence and risk factors for toxoplasmosis among antenatal women in London: a re-examination of risk in an ethnically diverse population. *Eur J Public Health.* **23**(4): 648–52.

Food Standards Agency (n.d.) *Listeria: keeping food safe* [online]. Available at: http://multimedia. food.gov.uk/multimedia/pdfs/publication/listeriafactsheet0708.pdf (accessed 14 March 2014).

Franco A, Ernest JM (2011) Parasitic infections. In: James D, Steer P, Weiner CP, *et al.* (editors). *High Risk Pregnancy: management options.* 4th ed. New York: Elsevier Saunders. pp. 543–62.

Gillespie IA, Mook P, Little CL, *et al.* (2010) Human listeriosis in England, 2001–2007: association with neighbourhood deprivation. *Euro Surveill.* **15**(27): 7–16.

Gillespie SH, Bamford K (2012) *Medical Microbiology and Infection at a Glance.* 4th ed. Oxford: Wiley-Blackwell.

Goering RV, Dockrell HM, Zuckerman M, *et al.* (2013) *Mims' Medical Microbiology.* 5th ed. Oxford: Elsevier, Saunders.

Gras L, Wallon M, Pollak A, *et al.* European Multicenter Study on Congenital Toxoplasmosis (2005) Association between prenatal treatment and clinical manifestations of congenital toxoplasmosis in infancy: a cohort study in 13 European centres. *Acta Paediatr.* **94**(12): 1721–31.

Gruslin A, Faden Y (2008) Toxoplasmosis, herpes simplex virus, rubella, parvovirus and listeria infections. In: Roseanne-Montella K, Keely E, Barbour RVL (editors). *Medical Care of the Pregnant Patient.* 2nd ed. Philadelphia: ACP. pp. 687–708.

Health Protection Agency (HPA) (2011a) Decrease in listeriosis incidence in England and Wales in 2010 [online]. *Health Protection Report.* **5**(13): 11 April. Available at: www.hpa.org.uk/hpr/archives/2011/news1311.htm#list#wnv (accessed 13 March 2014).

Health Protection Agency (HPA) (2011b) *Salmonella: clinical information* [online]. Available at: www.hpa.org.uk/Topics/InfectiousDiseases/InfectionsAZ/Salmonella/GeneralInformation/salmClinicalinformation/ (accessed 14 March 204).

Jones J, Lopez A, Wilson M (2003) Congenital toxoplasmosis. *Am Fam Physician.* **67**(10): 2131–8.

Khare MM, Khare MD (2007) Infections in pregnancy. In: Greer IA, Nelson–Piercy C, Walters BNJ (editors). *Maternal Medicine: medical problems in pregnancy.* Edinburgh: Churchill Livingstone, Elsevier. pp. 217–35.

Kirkham C, Berkowitz J (2010) Listeriosis in pregnancy: survey of British Columbia practitioners' knowledge of risk factors, counseling practices, and learning needs. *Can Fam Physician.* **56**(4): 158–66.

Lamont RF, Sobel J, Mazaki-Tovi S, *et al.* (2011) Listeriosis in human pregnancy: a systematic review. *J Perinat Med.* **39**(3): 227–36.

McClure EM, Goldenberg RL (2009) Infection and stillbirth. *Semin Fetal Neonatal Med.* **14**(4): 182–9.

Montoya JG, Liesenfeld O (2004) Toxoplasmosis. *Lancet.* **363**(9425): 1965–76.

Mylonakis E, Paliou M, Hohmann EL, *et al.* (2002) Listeriosis during pregnancy: a case series and review of 222 cases. *Medicine (Baltimore).* **81**(4): 260–9.

National Health Service (NHS) (2014) *NHS Choices: listeriosis* [online]. Available at: www.nhs. uk/conditions/listeriosis/Pages/Introduction.aspx (accessed 2 October 2014).

National Institute for Health and Care Excellence (NICE) (2009) *Clinical Knowledge Summary: gastroenteritis* [online]. Available at: http://cks.nice.org.uk/gastroenteritis (accessed 2 October 2014).

Ogunmodede F, Jones JL, Scheftel J, *et al.* (2005) Listeriosis prevention and knowledge among pregnant women in the USA. *Infect Dis Obstet Gynecol.* **13**(1): 11–15.

Pappas G, Roussos N, Falagas ME (2009) Toxoplasmosis snapshots: global status of *Toxoplasma gondii* seroprevalence and implications for pregnancy and congenital toxoplasmosis. *Int J Parasitol.* **39**(12): 1385–94.

Petersen E (2007) Toxoplasmosis. *Semin Fetal Neonatal Med.* **12**(3): 214–23.

Posfay-Barbe KM, Wald ER (2009) Listeriosis. *Semin Fetal Neonatal Med.* **14**(4): 228–33.

Public Health England (PHE) (2014) *Health Protection Report: common animal associated infections quarterly report (England and Wales)* [online]. Available at: www.hpa.org.uk/hpr/archives/2014/hpr05-0614.pdf (accessed 15 March 2014).

Ridgeway GL (2002) Fever and non-viral infectious diseases. In: de Swiet M (editor). *Medical Disorders in Obstetric Practice.* 4th ed. Oxford: Blackwell Science. pp. 501–12.

Ross DS, Jones JL, Lynch MF (2006) Toxoplasmosis, cytomegalovirus, listeriosis and preconception care. *Matern Child Health J.* **10**(5 Suppl.): S187–91.

Ross S, Furrows S (2014) *Rapid Infection Control Nursing.* Oxford: Wiley-Blackwell.

Schloesser RL, Schaefer V, Groll AH (2004) Fatal transplacental infection with non-typhoidal Salmonella. *Scand J Infect Dis.* **36**(10): 773–4.

Sherman PW, Flaxman SM (2002) Nausea and vomiting of pregnancy in an evolutionary perspective. *Am J Obstet Gynecol.* **186**(5): S190–7.

SYROCOT (Systematic Review on Congenital Toxoplasmosis) study group; Thiébaut R, Leproust S, Chêne G, *et al.* (2007) Individual patient data meta-analysis of prenatal treatment effect for congenital toxoplasmosis. *Lancet.* **369**(9556): 115–21.

Tam C, Erebara A, Einarson A (2010) Food-borne illnesses during pregnancy: prevention and treatment. *Can Fam Physician.* **56**(4): 341–3.

Tommy's (2013) *Toxoplasmosis and Pregnancy* [online]. Available at: www.tommys.org/page.aspx?pid=193 (accessed 24 March 2014).

Wilson J (2006) *Infection Control in Clinical Practice.* 3rd ed. Edinburgh: Baillière Tindall.

Wong LF, Ismail K, Fahy U (2013) Listeria awareness among recently delivered mothers. *J Obstet Gynaecol.* **33**(8): 814–16.

Yudin MH (2011) Other infectious conditions. In: James (editor). *High Risk Pregnancy Management Options.* 4th ed. Elsevier. pp. 521–42.

CHAPTER 13

Vector-transmitted diseases

→ Malaria
→ Dengue fever
→ Lyme disease
→ Chagas' disease

Vector-transmitted diseases are those that involve the infectious agent having another living organism (vector: for example, an insect) as part of its life cycle, and which will transmit the condition to humans. Although many of these are largely found in tropical areas, UK midwives are seeing vector-transmitted conditions more frequently with the contribution of global temperature changes, as well as travel and immigration becoming increasingly common. All the conditions have potential to affect both the mother and the fetus or newborn, and therefore early suspicion by the midwife may lead to rapid referral and treatment, which may restrict any possible damage. As the midwife is often the first health professional the woman may see, it is vital she has the knowledge to be able to give advice and to assess when referral is necessary.

MALARIA

INTRODUCTION

Malaria is the tropical disease most commonly imported into the UK (RCOG 2010a). While some progress toward eradication has been made in endemic areas – for example, in increasing the number of bed nets and access to drugs – there is also an increase in drug resistance, with no new drugs at present available. A vaccine is vitally needed and much work is being undertaken toward development, although this is proving challenging (Daily 2012, NHS Choices 2013). At present there are no specific actions that a pregnant or breastfeeding woman can take to guarantee she will not become infected with malaria if she travels to an area where it is common, but there is, however, much information that may be effective in keeping her (and her baby) safe.

Pregnancy increases all risks related to malaria: pregnant women appear to be twice as likely to be bitten by mosquitoes of the genus *Anopheles* (Ansell *et al.* 2002, Lindsay *et al.* 2000), to suffer a severe form of the disease (RCOG 2010a, Franco & Ernest 2011) and to die from malaria (Steketee *et al.* 2001) than those women who are not pregnant. Primiparity appears to increase the risk still further (Franco & Ernest 2011).

With increasing drug resistance, ease of travel, the rise in new immigrants and refugees from malaria-endemic regions, and global climate change, malaria in pregnancy in the UK will be increasingly seen. However, at present most malaria seen in the UK appears to be in those who have visited friends and relations in their former country (HPA 2008), and it seems these people are not using chemoprophylaxis (antimalarial drugs) (Smith *et al.* 2008). The midwife, in her public health role, could ensure all women know the risks (this area is explored more fully later in this chapter).

The **ABCD** of malaria prevention underpins advice and care for travellers in malaria endemic areas.

- **A**wareness of risk
- **B**ite prevention
- **C**hemoprophylaxis
- **D**iagnosis and treatment (which must be prompt)

TRANSMISSION

There are four species of *Plasmodium* parasites that cause human malaria: (1) *Plasmodium falciparum*, (2) *Plasmodium vivax*, (3) *Plasmodium malariae* and (4) *Plasmodium ovale*. In addition, a new and rare type has recently been identified in South East Asia: *Plasmodium knowlesi*. *P. falciparum* is the most common and dangerous species and is the cause of the majority of deaths worldwide, probably up to 90%. *P. vivax* and *P. ovale* may take a dormant form in the liver and can cause relapsing malaria years later (Franco & Ernest 2011), and *P. malariae* may also cause a late reoccurrence in future years. Special treatment is necessary to enable the liver to clear the parasite.

The bite of an infected female mosquito of the genus *Anopheles* will transmit *Plasmodium* parasites and the species will determine the severity of the disease. Following the initial bite, sporozoites (the infected form of the *Plasmodium* parasite) are released from the mosquito's salivary glands and enter the blood. Sporozoites infiltrate the woman's liver cells within 30 minutes. In the liver they multiply as merozoites and enter red blood cells (erythrocytes) – thus the circulation. At this time they develop into gametocytes (the reproductive form). Symptoms occur when the parasite enters the erythrocytes.

When circulating in the erythrocytes, gametocytes produce a special protein to protect themselves, which causes adherence to blood vessel walls – this can cause

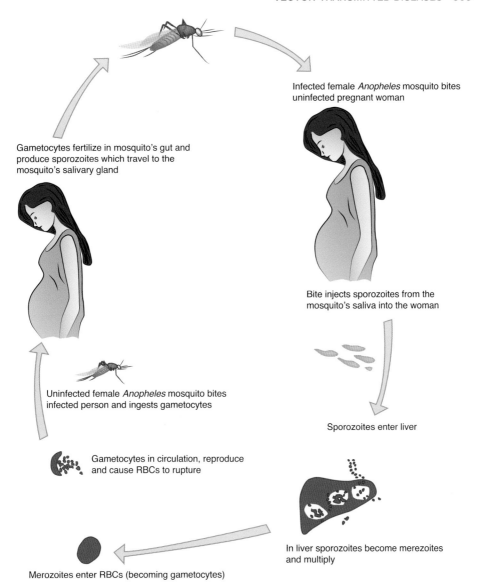

FIGURE 13.1 Life cycle of *Plasmodium* parasites

complications including end-organ damage. However, the main aim of this protection is to prevent the erythrocytes entering the spleen, where they may be destroyed. As the infected erythrocytes containing reproducing gametocytes circulate, the gametocytes destroy the haemoglobin and the red blood cell finally ruptures – and these ruptures occur in a cycle. The body's defence is a pyrexia to try to destroy the parasite and this explains the periodic fever spikes caused by the infection.

An uninfected female anopheline mosquito – which needs blood to produce her eggs – bites the infected person, ingesting gametocytes. These fertilise in her gut and within 1–7 weeks new sporozoites develop, travel to the mosquito's salivary gland and the cycle continues.

Mosquitoes of the genus *Anopheles* breed in shallow fresh water. In many areas, transmission is most common during and just following the rainy season. Some immunity can be developed over years of exposure, although this is never total (Dorman & Shulman 2000) and therefore in areas of greater transmission (good conditions for mosquitoes) young children are most at risk of dying, whereas in areas of less transmission, all age groups are vulnerable.

Transmission can be from mother to fetus or infant, via the placenta or during birth, respectively, or through contaminated blood products (Mali *et al.* 2012) but the vast amount of transmission worldwide is via the bite of an infected female anopheline mosquito.

EPIDEMIOLOGY

Malaria is endemic in more than 100 countries worldwide. Malaria-carrying mosquitoes mainly live in hot countries, with most of the malaria seen in the UK originating in Africa (especially Nigeria and Ghana), Asia (especially India), South and Central America, Hispaniola, Oceania and the Middle East. However, recently there have been reports of malaria diagnosed in non-travellers resident in Greece, albeit at present in very small numbers (CDC 2012a).

Half of the world population is considered at risk of malaria (WHO 2010) and recent estimates have suggested an annual mortality of 0.5–3 million (Franco & Ernest 2011, WHO 2010). One billion people worldwide are estimated to carry the parasite at any one time, and approximately 50 million of these are pregnant women (Franco & Ernest 2011). In some countries, spending on malaria can account for a large proportion (can be up to 40%) of the public health expenditure (WHO 2010) and therefore restricts the potential for the use of resources on other health needs.

One study in Ghana over 2 years (Clerk *et al.* 2009) identified an overall prevalence of malaria parasitaemia in their antenatal clinics of 47%. Associated with reduced risk were older age, multiparity and pregnancy during the dry season (Clerk *et al.* 2009). There is known to be an increased risk for those women who are human immunodeficiency virus (HIV) positive (Van Eijk *et al.* 2003).

Most deaths are related to *P. falciparum* and predominately involve children under 5 years and pregnant women (Franco & Ernest 2011). It is suggested that one child dies of malaria every 45 seconds in Africa, and 10 000–200 000 newborns die annually as a result of infection in pregnancy (Franco & Ernest 2011). Congenital malaria incidence in newborns is estimated at 0.3%–4% (Lee 2008), and placental malaria has also been implicated in impaired development of infants and children, perhaps having lifelong effect (Umbers *et al.* 2011). Malaria is the major cause of intrauterine growth restriction (IUGR) throughout the world (Woensdregt *et al.* 2008).

The number of pregnant women treated for malaria in the UK is not clear, but prevalence studies in the United States demonstrated that 7% of female malaria cases were pregnant women and that the number of pregnant malaria sufferers have almost tripled from 2008 to 2010 (Mali *et al.* 2012).

CLINICAL FEATURES

BOX 13.1 SIGNS AND SYMPTOMS OF MALARIA, FROM MILD (USUALLY NON-SPECIFIC) TO SEVERE (LIFE-THREATENING)

- Pyrexia and/or excessive fatigue (often alternate in a cycle)
- Headache
- Nausea and vomiting
- Myalgia
- IUGR
- Hypertension
- Jaundice may occur, resulting from the haemolysis
- Folate deficiency may develop secondary to haemolysis
- Hepatomegaly
- Splenomegaly
- Anaemia
- Tachypnoea or dyspnoea may lead to pulmonary oedema
- Hypoglycaemia
- Convulsions

Early signs and symptoms of malarial infection are often non-specific (*see* Box 13.1), and may include flu-like symptoms, malaise and headache, with perhaps anaemia, jaundice and/or hepatomegaly (Lagerberg 2008), although pyrexia is often the primary symptom. From 7 to 30 days following infection there will be the distinctive fever cycle – typically, cold with chills, then hot (39°C–40°C) with rigors for up to 6 hours, then sweating, followed by a break, albeit with excessive fatigue – if not treated this may be repeated for several weeks (Lagerberg 2008, Franco & Ernest 2011). Because signs and symptoms may be so vague, it would be advisable to consider malaria as a cause of any high temperature in a woman who has a history of travelling to a high-risk area (Mathew *et al.* 2011).

As malaria can be a multi-organ disease, it may present with renal failure, hypoglycaemia, lactic acidosis, nausea and vomiting, thrombocytopenia, cerebral malaria and/or severe anaemia (Lagerberg 2008). Hyperparasitaemia may lead to intensive care admission and exchange transfusion in extreme cases (Dorman & Shulman 2000).

Sequestration (infiltration) of the placenta by *P. falciparum* often results in the placenta containing a much higher parasitaemia than the woman's blood (Franco & Ernest 2011). Therefore, placental malaria, which is *Plasmodium*-infected erythrocytes pooling in the placenta, can occur without maternal symptoms (Lagerberg 2008), or with non-specific symptoms (Tagbor *et al.* 2008).

Much malaria may be mild and uncomplicated, and those with acquired partial immunity may have fewer and/or less severe symptoms (Lagerberg 2008). However, non-immune pregnant women may have a high rate of miscarriage (up to 60%) and maternal death rates are suggested to be around 10%–50% (WHO 2010). Pregnant women who have some degree of immunity, in areas of high transmission, may also suffer miscarriage or give birth to low-birthweight infants, especially during first and second pregnancies (WHO 2010).

HIV and malaria

It is well known that HIV-positive pregnant women, as well as those who are new mothers, are at greater risk of malaria, probably due to the change in immune status in pregnancy and around the time of delivery (Ladner *et al.* 2003). Women who are HIV-positive are also at increased risk of progression to severe malaria (WHO Expert Committee on Malaria 2000).

Even in stable transmission areas, where women would be expected to be semi-immune to malaria, HIV-positive women are at an increased risk of malaria during pregnancy. WHO (2010) suggests that when co-infected with malaria, there is an increased risk of the baby becoming HIV positive, but there is some controversy regarding this (Msamanga *et al.* 2009). There is also a suggestion that the combination of HIV and malaria may increase complications during pregnancy.

DIAGNOSIS AND TREATMENT

If the midwife learns a woman had travelled to a malaria endemic area in the previous year, she needs to ensure that the woman seeks medical attention for any flu-like illness or fever, which may be malaria. To diagnose malaria, symptoms such as fever and myalgia plus a history of travel (*P. falciparum* can present up to 12 months later) should cause suspicion. Early diagnosis and treatment decreases disease severity; however, definitive diagnosis before treatment is advised, as early symptoms may be vague and unnecessary treatment can lead to drug resistance, which is a growing problem (WHO 2010). In cases of non-specific symptoms with no clear cause and a history of travel, a blood film will usually enable malaria to be quickly diagnosed (RCOG 2010a). *See* Box 13.2 for tests. Misdiagnosis and delay of treatment are commonly cited as contributing to death from malaria in Europe and the United States (RCOG 2010a).

BOX 13.2 TESTING FOR MALARIA

- The current accepted test is microscopic examination of blood films for parasites: two to three drops of blood on a slide are necessary, and this investigation can be done with maternal blood, cord blood and blood from the maternal side of the placenta.
- Rapid diagnostic tests to detect specific parasite antigen or enzyme may be used, usually on a fingertip blood sample, but these are less sensitive than the blood film, and blood films should always be carried out, even if not analysed immediately.
- Polymerase chain reaction (PCR) to detect parasite DNA is highly sensitive, but it is an expensive test and is often not available.
- Results can be compromised – for example, if a woman is taking prophylaxis or parasites may be hidden in the placenta.

In the UK there are expert resources that can be accessed for help in analysing malaria tests (RCOG 2010a).

MANAGEMENT ISSUES

During pregnancy, even those diagnosed with uncomplicated malaria need hospital admission, and those with suspected severe malaria will probably be admitted to intensive care (RCOG 2010a). There is scope for the midwife to be involved in care, whether on the antenatal ward, an infectious diseases ward or intensive care, and she may be best placed to monitor the pregnancy issues and detect any variations from normal in her day-to-day contact with the woman. The multidisciplinary team will direct care, but involvement of the midwife may include psychosocial support as well as monitoring fetal and maternal well-being.

Antenatal examination may show clear signs of fetal compromise, such as oligohydramnious, and maternal tests may show reduced platelets, increased serum urates and signs of proteinuria, and with severe malaria, she may suffer convulsions (suggesting pre-eclampsia or eclampsia); however, antimalarial treatment may cause all these signs to resolve, thus avoiding early delivery. However, regular assessment is necessary, as pre-eclampsia is more common with malaria and IUGR fetuses may become compromised (Adam *et al.* 2011).

Treatment may be oral or intravenous antimalarial drugs. Drug therapy for acute malaria in pregnancy needs expert guidance – an infectious diseases consultant and microbiologists should be part of the multidisciplinary team, and advice sought from specialist centres as necessary, such as the Hospital for Tropical Diseases in London, where 24-hour helplines are available (RCOG 2010a).

During drug therapy the midwife will need to observe for vomiting, which is a symptom of malaria and a side effect of many drugs used, as this may compromise oral medication and is associated with treatment failure (White 1998). Co-infection of malaria and HIV needs a variety of medication with the potential for drug interactions, and there is a need for studies to evaluate this (Uneke & Ogbonna 2009).

During drug treatment, blood films will be used to monitor the women's condition and assess the effects of the drugs, and these are usually done every 24 hours but more frequently if clinical deterioration is seen (RCOG 2010a). Electrolytes, renal and liver functions, and haematology should also be closely monitored (Franco & Ernest 2011). As thrombocytopenia is common in malaria, coagulopathy must be considered (Tan *et al.* 2008, Dorman & Shulman 2000) because of the potential for antepartum haemorrhage, post-partum haemorrhage and disseminated intravascular coagulation. Blood and urine are usually cultured to ensure no other infection is present (Dorman & Shulman 2000). Regular electrocardiograms may be undertaken (Lee 2008).

Blood sugars should be assessed at least on admission, and then regularly, especially if quinine is commenced (Nelson-Piercy 2006). Hypoglycaemia can be asymptomatic, but it may become recurrent or intractable or not occur until the woman seems to be recovering (RCOG 2010a).

In more severe cases there is a risk of pulmonary oedema; therefore, fluid challenges, or overload of intravenous fluid, should be avoided. Lactic acidosis from poor tissue perfusion and oxygenation (Dorman & Shulman 2000) is possible and this must be assessed. Respiration rate and oxygen saturation monitoring should be undertaken frequently, and arterial blood gas assessment may be necessary.

During fetal assessment, fetal heart rate abnormality may be noted, and this may be caused by maternal hypoglycaemia or pyrexia; therefore, treatment of the mother's symptoms and commencement of antimalarials may normalise the fetal heart rate, thus avoiding premature delivery. However, after therapy, it is recommended that vigilance and surveillance for IUGR and preterm labour are maintained (Franco & Ernest 2011).

If labour starts spontaneously while being treated, careful fetal monitoring is necessary, as the baby may be IUGR and compromised (Dorman *et al.* 2000). Cord bloods are usually taken following delivery, and the placenta should be sent for histology. There may be significant parasitaemia in the placenta and cord blood even if the mother has been treated and her levels are negligible (Procop *et al.* 2001). Babies born to 'immune' mothers may have cord parasitaemia but usually they do not demonstrate any symptoms, presumably because they have acquired some immunity from their mothers. Babies with cord parasitaemia born to non-immune women who have not been effectively treated, however, may be very ill and mortality is high (Dorman *et al.* 2000). Even if maternal treatment has been undertaken, there is some evidence that the baby can be infected, and follow-up of the infant is necessary (RCOG 2010a).

Breastfeeding is not contraindicated while being treated with most drugs (Franco & Ernest 2011), but the midwife should ensure that the woman informs her caregivers that she is feeding her baby to confirm this is safe.

POTENTIAL OUTCOMES AND COMPLICATIONS

Factors influencing how well women recover and avoid complications include the level of immunity, gravid status, trimester of pregnancy and co-morbidity (Lagerberg 2008). *See* Box 13.3 for a list of potential complications and it must be noted that the risk of severe and complicated malaria is significantly increased in pregnancy.

BOX 13.3 POTENTIAL COMPLICATIONS OF MALARIA FOR THE MOTHER AND NEWBORN

- Miscarriage, stillbirth, congenital abnormality
- Anaemia
- Pre-eclampsia
- Hypoglycaemia
- Premature labour
- Haemorrhage
- Cerebral malaria
- Puerperal sepsis
- End-organ failure
- Low birthweight – either from prematurity or from IUGR
- Congenital malaria in the newborn
- Neonatal mortality

In a recent study (Bader *et al.* 2010), women with a history of malaria during pregnancy had three times the risk of stillbirth. It is considered that placental damage associated with malaria is the probable cause. There is a higher risk in primiparous women (Shulman *et al.* 2001). Prematurity may be associated with chronic or old malarial infection of the placenta, confirmed by histology in one study (Dorman *et al.* 2000).

The most common complication of malaria is anaemia (Franco & Ernest 2011). Anaemia is caused by:

- haemolysis of erythrocytes containing parasites
- suppression of red blood cell production
- infected erythrocytes concealed in the placenta.

Anaemia contributes to many deaths from haemorrhage (Dorman & Shulman 2000) in resource-poor areas. In the UK, anaemia should be able to be addressed pre-labour, and a haemorrhage, if it occurs, dealt with effectively.

Severe malaria (for which pregnancy increases the risk) and anaemia can result in renal failure (if gross haemoglobinuria, it is sometimes called 'blackwater fever'), pulmonary oedema, jaundice, convulsions and coma (Franco & Ernest 2011). Cerebral malaria is the most common cause of death.

The fetus and newborn

IUGR is common in pregnancies complicated with malaria, and arises from the:
- effect of maternal anaemia
- effect of placental malaria
- association with pre-eclampsia.

The risk of low birthweight is increased with the number of malaria episodes in pregnancy, and it may also be increased if infection is in the second trimester (Kalilani *et al.* 2010). There is also clear evidence that adverse effects can result if the infection is earlier in pregnancy (Rijken *et al.* 2012).

Congenital malaria is defined as the presence of malaria parasites in the erythrocytes of newborns younger than 7 days, and it can result from maternal–fetal transmission (Nelson-Piercy 2006). Although once thought to be uncommon, a recent study has estimated the prevalence at around 10% (Sotimehin *et al.* 2008). The risk factors were found to be primigravidae, a maternal history of pyrexia within 3 months of delivery and maternal peripheral parasitaemia at delivery. The authors suggest that routine screening for babies of these groups in high-risk areas is necessary. In a semi-immune woman, the placenta may be heavily infected, although the woman's peripheral blood film is negative (Dorman & Shulman 2000).

If a breastfeeding baby travels with its mother, her drugs, although present in breast milk, will not protect the baby and the infant will need its own prophylaxis (PHE 2014).

PREVENTION

For those living in countries where malaria is endemic, the degree to which those bitten by mosquitoes of the genus *Anopheles* contract malaria, and the severity of their symptoms, is dependent on the degree of naturally acquired host immunity (Desai *et al.* 2007). However, this immunity depends on repeated exposure to infectious anopheline bites, so women from these countries now living in the UK will have much reduced, or no, immunity (RCOG 2010b). This fact is often unknown by those living in the UK (Morgan & Figueroa-Munoz 2005), which, together with a common belief that malaria is trivial (Morgan & Figueroa-Munoz 2005), probably explains why so few women take precautions when travelling to their former home.

Alongside discussion with a health professional, written literature is also important to ensure the woman has all the information she needs – the Department of Health produces a leaflet (*Think Malaria*) in 11 different languages (*see* Useful Resources section for further information) which may be a very useful resource for both the woman and the midwife.

Personal protection

It is recommended that pregnant women consider the risks of travelling to an area where malaria is endemic and think about postponing their trip unless it is unavoidable (RCOG 2010b).

If travel is necessary, the woman should be advised to explore her specific risk of contracting malaria – for example, travelling in the rainy season would normally increase her risk, as would staying in most rural areas, as opposed to visiting many urban areas and staying in air-conditioned accommodation. The presence of drug-resistant strains of *P. falciparum* or *P. vivax*, and how long she plans to stay are also important considerations. If the woman has a clear idea of where and when she is planning to travel, up-to-date information on her risk can be obtained from centres with expertise on malaria risks (*see* Useful Resources section for websites).

Delaying travel until a less risky time (e.g. the dry season) or modifying travel plans to avoid staying in particularly high-risk environments (e.g. villages with nearby stagnant water) may be an acceptable compromise for women who must travel when pregnant.

Bite prevention

In most of the world, anopheline mosquitoes bite mainly between dusk and dawn. However, other mosquitoes – which may be carrying other diseases such as dengue fever – bite during the day, so applying skin repellents 24 hours a day is advisable (RCOG 2010b). Skin repellents are advised, and DEET is commonly recommended as the most effective and safe – it has not been identified as causing adverse effects in mothers or babies, although DEET has been detected in cord blood (McGready *et al.* 2001). Different strengths are mentioned in the literature, from 20% upwards; however, the RCOG advises 50% DEET (RCOG 2010b). It is worth noting that if others nearby are wearing repellent, an individual not wearing it is at higher risk of being bitten (Moore *et al.* 2007).

Insecticide-treated mosquito nets (ITNs), especially long-lasting ones, are advised (WHO 2010). A Cochrane systematic review (Gamble *et al.* 2006) concluded that ITNs were beneficial for pregnant women at risk of malaria. ITNs have been advised as a reliable and effective practice for many years, but it has been noted that in many areas they are not well used. A study in Nigeria was undertaken to assess use and noted that ITNs were not used because of the cost and also because of the beliefs that it is dangerous in pregnancy, young girls don't get malaria and/or the husband's lack of interest in malaria prevention (Chukwuocha *et al.* 2010). Poor usage has also been demonstrated in other African countries (van Eijk *et al.* 2011).

The use of room sprays containing pryrethroid or permethrin may be appropriate (Yap *et al.* 2001, Srinivasan & Kalyanasundaram 2006). Indoor residual spraying can be effective for up to 12 months, depending on the insecticide used (WHO 2010), and it has been recommended as beneficial. However, there are also studies that demonstrate levels of insecticide residue in breast milk following indoor residual spraying when mothers have been exposed (Bouwman & Kylin 2009). There is a need for research to follow up infants who have been exposed in this way.

A closed air-conditioned room away from water sources that may harbour mosquitoes, together with wearing long sleeves and trousers if it is necessary to go out after dark, in addition to the other specific actions mentioned, and chemoprophylaxis, are the basic recommendations to avoid bites.

Chemoprophylaxis

Basic to prevention and treatment of malaria is the appropriate drug regimen, and since drug resistance is a growing problem, and differs in various areas, it is impossible to give up-to-date information. The use of drugs, both as prophylaxis for travel and in treatment of malaria, should be advised and guided by a professional knowledgeable in this subject. Drug-resistant regions, the potential of fetal toxicity and estimation of the severity of risk are all areas that change rapidly. The online resources listed under Useful Resources at the end of this section should give this information as and when needed, and expert advice should always be sought.

Chemoprophylaxis is normally obtained from the general practitioner or doctors working in specific 'travel clinics', but it would be the responsibility of the midwife to ensure the woman understands the importance of accessing, and taking, the appropriate drugs. Most drug regimens involve starting medication prior to travel and continuing for some time after return – the midwife can support the woman in ensuring she complies with the drug's instructions.

If the woman is breastfeeding when travelling to malaria risk areas she will probably be prescribed the same medicine regimen as in pregnancy (Franco & Ernest 2011), but it would be good practice to ensure the woman has notified the prescribing doctor that she is breastfeeding.

Intermittent preventive treatment in pregnancy (IPTp) is used in some areas of the world in the resident population, because the woman may be asymptomatic with placental malaria (Lagerberg 2008). Various regimens may be used and if HIV positive (or in an area with high HIV prevalence) medication should be given more frequently (Lagerberg 2008). Uptake of IPTp is generally found to be low – one study (Akinleye *et al.* 2009) found this was because about half the women hadn't heard of it, and of those who had, about half were concerned about an adverse effect on their pregnancy. In some countries where IPTp is recommended during pregnancy, adverse reactions to drugs have also been seen to reduce compliance in some regimens (Briand *et al.* 2009).

ROLE OF THE MIDWIFE

Midwives may be the first line of contact for women planning to travel to, or having recently returned from, a malarial area. The midwife may also consider enquiring about plans for travel at booking – midwives now have reduced antenatal contact so need to take all opportunities to ensure they fulfil their public health role. Midwives need to:

- Maintain a knowledge of the signs and symptoms of malaria.
- Provide advice, and referral as necessary, if a woman becomes ill (even mildly) in the year following a visit to a malarial endemic area, or also consider if IUGR is diagnosed (as placental malaria does not always produce symptoms in the mother).
- Ensure a woman from a malarial endemic area understands she may have lost any immunity she had when resident there, and the specific, and increased, risks she may be vulnerable to if she travels when pregnant.
- Provide specific advice if a woman plans to travel to a malarial endemic area, either when pregnant or in the puerperium, and refer for specialist care as necessary.
- Ensure the woman accesses knowledgeable advice when considering chemoprophylaxis.
- As malaria has a high recurrence rate (RCOG 2010a), the midwife should ensure that women who have been treated for malaria attend any scheduled follow-up and are aware of the signs and symptoms and the need to access medical care.

USEFUL RESOURCES

- Arguin P, Steele S (2010) *The Pre-travel Consultation: malaria*. Centers for Disease Control and Prevention Yellow Book: Travellers' Health.
- Department of Health produces a leaflet (*Think Malaria*) in 11 different languages (Available at: www.orderline.dh.gov.uk), which may be a very useful information resource for both the woman and the midwife.
- The Health Protection Agency (now part of Public Health England) maintains a site that is a valuable resource for figures and updated general information. Available at: www.gov.uk/government/publications/malaria

- World Health Organization (2011) *Guidelines for the Treatment of Malaria.* 2nd ed. Available at: www.who.int/malaria/publications

DENGUE FEVER

INTRODUCTION

Dengue fever, a virus transmitted by mosquitoes, is associated with an increased risk of pregnancy complications – in particular, haemorrhage in pregnancy or during labour and the puerperium.

Although at present dengue fever is not diagnosed frequently in the UK, its incidence is increasing worldwide and it is considered endemic in more than 110 countries, including much of Africa (CDC 2013). The rise in numbers is thought to be due to an increase in international travel, urbanisation, population growth and global warming (Whitehorn & Farrar 2010). It has been identified as increasing in numbers in travellers returning to the UK from endemic countries, and Public Health England reported a threefold increase in 2013, compared with 2012 (HPA 2013). However, dengue fever often presents as a self-limiting viral illness; therefore, diagnosis is probably not made in many sufferers, and these numbers may be an underestimation.

In the UK, the majority of cases of imported dengue fever are currently from India, Thailand, Barbados, Sri Lanka and Brazil, although Jamaica and Madeira were implicated in 2012 (NaTHNaC 2013). Dengue fever is usually diagnosed in UK travellers in September and the winter months, probably because these are popular times for travel to areas where dengue fever is present.

There are four different types of the virus, and infection with one can give lifelong immunity to that strain, although it will only provide short-term immunity to the other three (WHO 2009). Subsequent infections with different types can increase the risk of severe complications, although it is not clear why this is the case (Martina *et al.* 2009).

TRANSMISSION

Dengue fever is transmitted via mosquitoes from the genus *Aedes*. Unlike mosquitoes transmitting malaria, these mosquitoes bite during the day – in particular, early morning and evening. Humans and primates are the primary host of the virus, and the disease is transmitted from an infected host, via the mosquito, to an uninfected person. Once infected, the mosquito will remain infected and can continue to spread the virus with every bite. Dengue fever can also be transmitted through infected blood products or organ donation (Stramer *et al.* 2009). Vertical transmission has also been reported (Wiwanitkit 2010).

CLINICAL FEATURES

The incubation period for dengue fever can be from 3 to 14 days (Gubler 2010), and therefore symptoms may first manifest after travellers return home.

Common signs and symptoms of dengue fever include:

- pyrexia – usually sudden onset
- severe headache
- severe myalgia (dengue is often described as 'breakbone fever')
- generalised maculopapular rash (similar to measles)
- mild bleeding, easy bruising
- non-specific flu-like symptoms.

The majority of those infected are asymptomatic or have mild non-specific symptoms (WHO 2009), although they of course still play their part in spreading the disease if bitten by an unaffected mosquito. It is estimated that about 5% will have a severe illness and for some of these it may be life-threatening (Whitehorn & Farrar 2010).

Dengue fever can be particularly dangerous for those with asthma, diabetes or some genetic conditions such as glucose-6-phosphate dehydrogenase (G6PD) deficiency (Guzman *et al.* 2010, Martina *et al.* 2009).

The disease progression is divided into three stages: febrile, critical and recovery (WHO 2009).

1. *Febrile* involves a severe pyrexia (may be >40°C), together with overall aching, perhaps vomiting and a severe headache. Frequently a rash appears around day 4, resembling measles (Knoop *et al.* 2010). The fever may follow various patterns, including resolving and reappearing (Gould & Solomon 2008).
2. The *critical* phase may occur as the fever abates and may only be brief; however, it may involve fluid accumulation in the chest and abdominal cavity, reducing circulating blood supply to the organs. This may result in organ dysfunction and shock (dengue shock syndrome) and/or haemorrhage (dengue haemorrhagic fever), although this only occurs in <5% of those affected (Ranjit & Kissoon 2011).
3. The *recovery* phase usually lasts at least 2 or 3 days and may involve severe itching, a slow heartbeat and a further rash, sometimes associated with peeling of the skin (WHO 2009). Fluid overload is a danger at this time, and following this period the woman may feel overwhelming tiredness for many weeks.

Diagnosis

Although it can be difficult, especially in the initial stages, to differentiate dengue fever from other viral illnesses, diagnosis is generally made based on pyrexia plus other signs listed earlier, and evidence of low white blood cell count, high haematocrit with low platelets or moderately elevated aspartate transaminase (AST) and alanine transaminase (ALT) levels. This can be confirmed by PCR, viral antigen or specific antibodies detection. Expert advice from a specialist in tropical diseases should be sought as soon as suspicion arises.

Impact on pregnancy

If infection occurs in early pregnancy, the loss of the pregnancy or acute fetal abnormality is possible, probably related to the bleeding tendency and/or high fever with which this condition is associated. Chitra and Panicker (2011) examined the impact of dengue fever in pregnancy and identified that those affected mid-trimester, receiving conservative treatment only, appeared to have no complications. However, in late pregnancy the tendency to bleed resulted in severe thrombocytopenia and many needed large amounts of blood products.

Pre-eclampsia, preterm labour and intrauterine growth restriction may be associated with dengue fever (Pouliot *et al.* 2010, Basurko *et al.* 2009), although the potential for bleeding at any time in pregnancy, labour or postnatally must be considered the biggest risk.

Dengue infection in the neonate has been reported, but how commonly this occurs is not certain, as studies are unclear (Chitra & Panicker 2011, Pouliot *et al.* 2010, Chye *et al.* 1997, Maroun *et al.* 2008).

MANAGEMENT AND POTENTIAL OUTCOMES

As already mentioned, most dengue fever infections will be self-limiting, and treatment will be supportive only. However, in approximately 10% of cases, dengue haemorrhagic fever (bleeding, low platelets) or dengue shock syndrome (low blood pressure) may develop, both of which have the potential to be fatal.

It is likely that in the UK any pregnant woman would be admitted to hospital for observation, but unless her condition became complicated, her care would include attention to fluid balance and treatment of symptoms, such as pain and nausea. Non-steroidal anti-inflammatory drugs and aspirin would not be used, as they could increase the potential of bleeding (WHO 2009). Routine care including ongoing screening for pre-eclampsia and fetal assessment, as well as general maternal well-being, would be undertaken.

Outcomes from severe dengue fever will very much depend on the resources available to support the woman if she suffers from complications such as disseminated intravascular coagulation or pregnancy-induced hypertension. Although some studies have reported a maternal mortality of 2.6% (Ismail *et al.* 2006), others suggest this can be greatly reduced with appropriate intensive care (Chitra & Panicker 2011).

PREVENTION

There is no vaccine against dengue fever. Prevention measures described previously under 'malaria' will also protect against bites from mosquitoes transmitting dengue fever; however, these mosquitoes are described as being most active during the day, so precautions against bites need to be taken at all times.

The use of air-conditioning and door and window screens is recommended (CDC 2012b). Since the *Aedes* mosquito larvae are commonly found in 'domestic' water, such as water containers, there have been many initiatives to treat and control conditions in standing water; however, at present this has only been successful in some specific local campaigns.

ROLE OF THE MIDWIFE

- Since the symptoms may only occur after a woman's return from holiday, the midwife must ensure she considers such conditions as dengue fever, enquiring about the woman's recent travel and exposure to mosquitoes, and refer if there is any suspicion.
- If caring for a woman in hospital with dengue fever, undertake comprehensive observations for pre-eclampsia, IUGR, premature labour and, especially, any tendency to bleed.
- Ensure an effective multidisciplinary approach, with advice from the appropriate experts, for any woman with suspected dengue fever.

USEFUL RESOURCES

- Centers for Disease Control and Prevention (CDC) (2012) Dengue fever. Available at WHO (2009) *Dengue: guidelines for diagnosis, treatment, prevention and control.* Available at: http://whqlibdoc.who.int/publications/2009/9789241547871_eng.pdf

LYME DISEASE

INTRODUCTION

Lyme disease (or Lyme borreliosis) is a bacterial infection spread by ticks and may cause a variety of symptoms over several years. Midwives need to ensure they have the knowledge to both advise women about avoiding tick bites and suspect when Lyme disease may be present in order to achieve a timely referral.

Lyme disease is the most common tick-borne infectious disease in Europe and North America. Since national surveillance began in 1982 in the United States, it is estimated that the incidence has increased about 25-fold (Woensdregt *et al.* 2008), and a dramatic increase has also been noted in the past 10 years in the UK (HPA 2012), although this rise is likely to be at least partly due to increased knowledge and awareness.

It is a multi-system disorder and can primarily affect the skin, heart or nervous system. Historically Lyme disease was thought to adversely affect the outcome of pregnancy, with complications such as stillbirth and congenital heart abnormalities (Lakos & Solymosi 2010), but this area is not clear (Bhate & Schwartz 2011a).

TRANSMISSION

Lyme disease is a bacterial infection caused by a group of spirochaetes, *Borrelia burgdorferi*, which have several genospecies varying in geographical distribution. The genospecies is relevant, as they may present with different symptoms or severity. These spirochaetes are transmitted by specific *Ixodes* ticks – the main vector in Europe is *Ixodes ricinus*, with others more common in Asia and North America (Stanek *et al.* 2012).

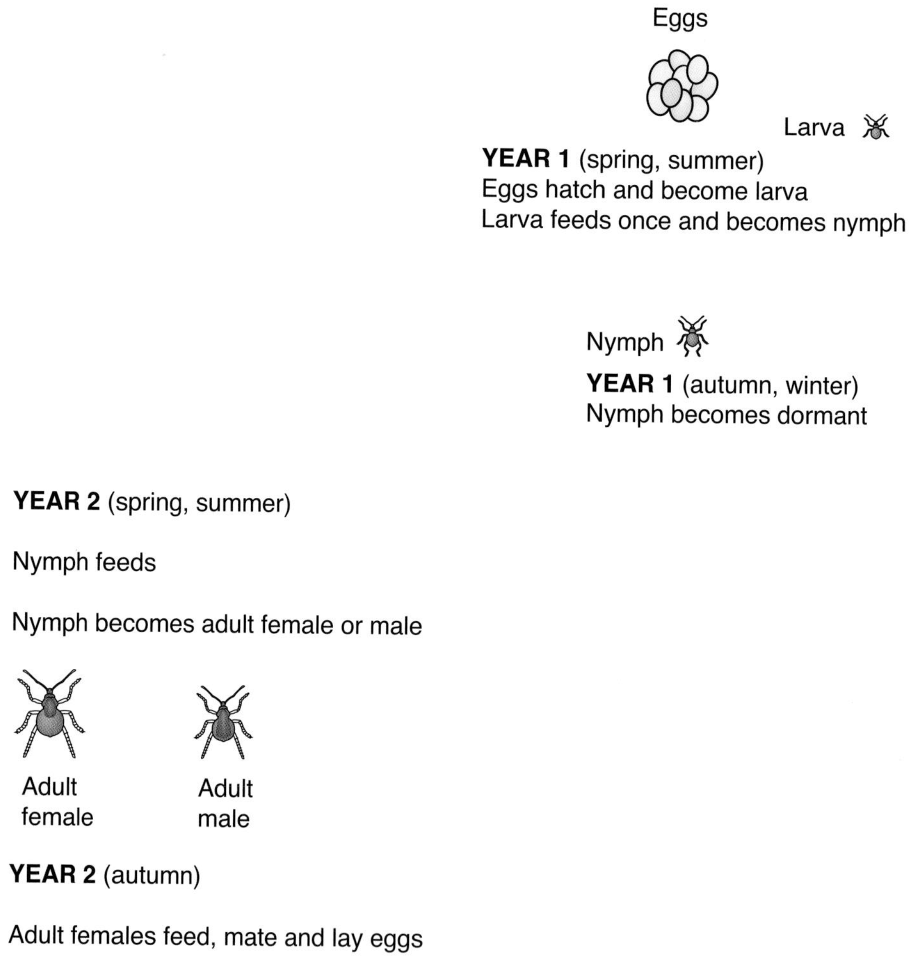

Eggs

Larva

YEAR 1 (spring, summer)
Eggs hatch and become larva
Larva feeds once and becomes nymph

Nymph

YEAR 1 (autumn, winter)
Nymph becomes dormant

YEAR 2 (spring, summer)

Nymph feeds

Nymph becomes adult female or male

Adult
female

Adult
male

YEAR 2 (autumn)

Adult females feed, mate and lay eggs

FIGURE 13.2 Lifecycle of *Ixodes ricinus* tick

I. ricinus ticks go through four stages in their 2-year life cycle: (1) egg, (2) larva, (3) nymph and (4) adult. In the latter three stages they feed once, then drop off to live on the ground, needing 80% humidity for survival and development to their next stage. For this reason they thrive in areas where there is mixed woodland with much underbrush and decaying vegetation. This habitat will also support their main hosts, which are small mammals and some birds, as well as deer, sheep or cattle. In the UK these ticks are reported most commonly in the south of England (South West, South East and London), the Lake District and the Scottish Highlands – popular areas for outdoor recreational activities (HPA 2012).

The most likely time for transmission to humans is during the tick's nymph stage, when their small size (about the size of a poppy seed) makes them difficult to notice (Woensdregt *et al.* 2008). When feeding, the infected tick leaves spirochaetes in the skin (Stanek *et al.* 2012). The tick usually needs to stay in situ for approximately 36–48 hours for successful transmission (Franco & Ernest 2011). The spirochaetes spread from the site of the bite by blood-borne, lymphatic and cutaneous routes, and, in addition to blood, they have been found in spinal, synovial and amniotic fluid (Woensdregt *et al.* 2008).

CLINICAL FEATURES AND DIAGNOSIS

Lyme disease can be asymptomatic (BIA 2011), and when symptoms are present, these may be variable. However, presentation is usually divided into three stages.

1. The *early localised (first) stage* commonly involving a distinctive rash. An erythema migrans or erythema chronicum migrans rash is usually erythematous and well defined around the bite, spreading to cover perhaps quite a large area and commonly described as a 'bullseye'. This is typically found within 1–3 weeks of infection but can appear as late as 16 weeks after the bite, and it may last for many weeks. However, only about 50% of adults and 90% of children have this classic sign (Bhate & Schwartz 2011a). This may be accompanied by non-specific flu-like symptoms.

2. The *early disseminated (second) stage* overlaps the early localised stage, can continue for over a year after the initial infection and may involve less-specific signs such as facial palsy. Other symptoms may be myalgia, arthralgia, mild pyrexia and regional lymphadenopathy (Franco & Ernest 2011), although rarely there may be cardiac symptoms (HPA 2012).

3. The *late (third) stage* is not common and may occur years later (BIA 2011). Late manifestations can include chronic encephalomyelitis, acrodermatitis chronica atrophicans or Lyme arthritis.

Infection of the fetus and placenta are possible during pregnancy, but it is not clear which women are at risk, and when the most common time for this transmission occurs

(Woensdregt *et al.* 2008). Stillbirth, preterm delivery and damage to the fetus and/or the neonate have been reported, but the risk appears low (Woensdregt *et al.* 2008).

Diagnosis can often be difficult. It is usually based on a history of a tick bite in an endemic area, together with the clinical findings. Enzyme-linked immunosorbent assay (ELISA) is the most common laboratory test used to screen for *B. burgdorferi* antibodies, but false positives and false negatives are common (Franco & Ernest 2011). Western blot or PCR tests may also be used for confirmation (Lee 2008). It is suggested that laboratory confirmation is not necessary for a confident clinical diagnosis of erythema migrans but should be used for all later complications of Lyme disease, as symptoms are not specific (BIA 2011).

MANAGEMENT

Treatment (antibiotic, either intravenous or oral) is only recommended for those who are confirmed to have an identified tick that was estimated to have been attached for more than 36 hours, and when it is possible for treatment to be started within 72 hours (Franco & Ernest 2011). However, this detailed information is often not available, and because of the uncertainty in diagnosis, the American College of Obstetricians and Gynecologists recommends prophylaxis with oral antibiotics in areas where Lyme disease has a high prevalence (Lee 2008). In the UK the British Infection Association (BIA 2011) suggest this is not a general recommendation, for various reasons to do with the difference of the disease transmission. However in pregnancy, prophylaxis may be appropriate and urgent referral to a knowledgeable specialist should be made.

Early treatment normally clears the rash within several days and may prevent complications developing (HPA 2012). Treatment is much the same for pregnant women as for those who are not pregnant, apart from avoidance of some specific drugs (Stanek *et al.* 2012).

Careful observation of pregnant women, monitoring their skin appearance for presence of a rash and/or a pyrexia, is recommended following any contact with a tick, for Lyme disease as well as other tick-related illness (Franco & Ernest 2011). Women who develop Lyme disease during pregnancy should be followed for up to a year for late-stage disease symptoms, such as skin lesions or chronic Lyme arthritis of large joints.

POTENTIAL OUTCOMES

Identification of adverse pregnancy outcomes are difficult to assess, as the number of women diagnosed is small and there can be many causes resulting from combinations of several perinatal and neonatal indicators. However, one recently published piece of research (Lakos & Solymosi 2010) identified several suggested associations. They found that the interval when infection was diagnosed varied widely, from 0 to 280 days (average 33 days), but there was no clear relationship between the length of infection and adverse pregnancy outcome, although if the woman appeared to be infected long before conception and was untreated, there were no fetal or infant complications – suggesting an effective maternal antibody reaction. Pregnancy loss occurred most frequently when the infection was very early in pregnancy (Lakos & Solymosi 2010). Unlike other, earlier, reports, such as Strobino *et al.* (1999) they found no fetal cardiac abnormalities, but they did observe haemangioma in several of the infants.

In adults, acrodermatitis chronica atrophicans (ACA), a progressive fibrosing skin lesion, may be the most common outcome of chronic Lyme borreliosis in Europe, although it is rare (Brzonova *et al.* 2002). Chronic Lyme arthritis is seen most frequently in North America and usually affects the knee, although it can be present in any large joint (Bhate & Schwartz 2011b).

PREVENTION

A vaccine against Lyme disease has been developed, but it is not recommended during pregnancy. It also does not protect all recipients against *B. burgdorferi*, and there is no protection against other tick-borne diseases (Woensdregt *et al.* 2008). Potentially more effective vaccines are in development and there is a canine Lyme vaccine available in the United States (Schuijt *et al.* 2011).

BOX 13.4 AVOIDANCE OF TICK BITES

- Use of appropriate clothing: long-sleeved shirt and long trousers tucked into socks, and light coloured to show up ticks more easily
- Inspect skin frequently, especially in skin folds, and shower or bathe at the end of the day
- Check clothes and pets to ensure ticks are not brought home
- Consider using DEET insect repellent

(HPA 2012)

Advice is given to avoid areas where it is known the ticks are found or habitats that would support them (Franco & Ernest 2011). Ideally, actions should be taken to avoid being bitten by a tick (*see* Box 13.4), but if a tick is found it needs to be removed immediately and the Health Protection Agency (HPA 2012) suggests this should be done with tweezers, applied as close to the head area of the tick as possible to avoid compressing the abdomen, and pulling gently upwards away from the skin. Any substances such as alcohol or matches are not recommended (BIA 2011). Following removal, the area should be disinfected. Any rash or symptoms following this exposure should be reported.

ROLE OF THE MIDWIFE

- Appropriate advice to women on how to avoid exposure to ticks
- Recognition and referral when a vector-transmitted infection such as Lyme disease is suspected
- Support when women are undergoing treatment – in particular, encouragement of compliance to an antibiotic regimen

---

USEFUL RESOURCES

- British Infection Association (2011) The epidemiology, prevention, investigation and treatment of Lyme borreliosis in United Kingdom patients: A position statement by the British Infection Association. *Journal of Infection.* **62** pp. 329–38.
- Mygland A, Ljøstad U, Fingerle V, *et al.* European Federation of Neurological Societies (2010) EFNS guidelines on the diagnosis and management of European Lyme neuroborreliosis. *Eur J Neurol.* **17**(1): 8–16.
- The Health Protection Agency (now part of Public Health England) maintains a site that is a valuable resource for figures and updated general information (including leaflets that can be printed off for women). Available at: www.gov.uk/government/publications/lyme-disease
- NHS Choices has a publicly accessible website that also contains much relevant and up-to-date in formation. Available at: www.nhs.uk/Conditions/Lyme-disease/Pages/Introduction.aspx

CHAGAS' DISEASE

INTRODUCTION

Chagas' disease (also known as American trypanosomiasis) is the most important endemic parasitic infection in South and Central America and Mexico (Jannin & Salvatella 2006). The disease can become chronic, and midwives in the UK will usually see women in this stage of the infection. Although the woman may be asymptomatic, there is a high rate of vertical transmission, and an association with life-threatening diseases in later life.

Although Chagas' disease was initially restricted to South and Central America and Mexico, because of immigration there are now many known cases in North America, Europe, Japan and Australia (Jackson *et al.* 2009, Roca *et al.* 2011). Chagas' disease is considered a growing problem in Europe, especially in Spain, as migration from Latin America is common and chronic infection is asymptomatic (Roca *et al.* 2011).

Previously, Chagas' disease was endemic in Brazil, Uruguay, Chile and Argentina, but recent work has led to the Pan American Health Organization identifying these countries as being vector-transmission free (Moretti *et al.* 2005). However, these are recent developments and the woman may have been infected in her childhood before these measures took place, or even congenitally via her own mother: in countries such as Argentina it is now considered that congenital cases are at least 10 times more frequent than the acute cases by vector transmission (Gürtier *et al.* 2003). The risk of infected blood transfusion in endemic countries has also reduced, as screening of donations is in place in most countries (Castro 2009).

Work is being undertaken on the development of a vaccine; however, at present there is nothing available.

TRANSMISSION

Transmission of the flagellate protozoan, *Trypanosama cruzi*, responsible for Chagas' disease, can occur from mother to fetus or infant, from contaminated blood products or organ transplants, or through contaminated food or drink, although this is rare. However, the most common method of transmission is via an insect vector. At present in Europe, vertical, transfusional and transplantation routes have been responsible for all cases of transmission (Jackson *et al.* 2009).

Traditionally, transmission is usually via a bite from infected Triatomine bugs. These bugs breed and feed on many species of domestic and wild mammals, as well as humans (Morel & Lazdins 2003). Triatomines are commonly known as 'kissing bugs', as they tend to bite on the face, after falling from infested roofs (either thatched or containing cracks or crevices and usually in poor rural areas) onto exposed faces during the night. After the bugs bite and ingest blood, they defecate and the *T. cruzi* parasites are present in the insect faeces. As this is near the bite wound, the parasites can easily enter the bloodstream when scratched or itched. The parasites can also enter through intact mucous membranes, and this commonly occurs through the conjunctiva.

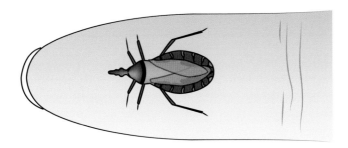

FIGURE 13.3 Triatomine bug

Little is known about the impact of Chagas' disease on pregnancy. Vertical transmission from mother to fetus will be the most relevant issue for most UK midwives, and this is thought to occur in 2%–20% of infected mothers. It is unknown if transmission takes place during pregnancy or at birth, although it is likely that both occur. It is also unknown what factors put the Chagas-positive woman at higher risk of transmitting the disease to her baby (Moretti *et al.* 2005); however, it is considered that the stage of the pregnancy, the stage of the disease (acute or later), her general health and the degree of parasitic load may all be possible contributors.

Most women seen in the UK maternity system will be in the chronic phase of the disease. However, one paper (Moretti *et al.* 2005) studied three pregnant women with acute chagasic infection (one of whom had become infected during a laboratory accident). The two women infected in the third trimester had uninfected children; however, the other woman who was infected earlier in pregnancy had an infected baby.

Maternal Chagas' disease has historically been considered an important cause of stillbirth.

CLINICAL FEATURES AND DIAGNOSIS

Acute Chagas' disease occurs immediately after the infection and if any symptoms (*see* Box 13.5) develop they usually disappear within about 3–8 weeks (Bern *et al.* 2007). The infection then becomes chronic, and about 20%–40% of these individuals will develop life-threatening digestive or cardiac conditions, usually very many years later. Symptomatic chronic disease is called 'determinate', and asymptomatic is called 'indeterminate' – midwives in the UK will usually only see those with indeterminate Chagas' disease.

Most commonly, signs and symptoms of acute Chagas' disease will be non-specific and mild; however, more severe symptomology is possible: one report of a laboratory worker infected during her work when 32 weeks pregnant described her needing intensive care admission (Moretti *et al.* 2005). More usually, the bite may go unnoticed, and after 4–6 weeks the chronic phase of Chagas' disease is entered. In

---

BOX 13.5 POSSIBLE SIGNS AND SYMPTOMS OF ACUTE CHAGAS' DISEASE

- Swelling around the bite (a chagoma)
- Pyrexia
- General malaise
- Diarrhoea and vomiting
- Swollen glands
- Hepatosplenomegaly (enlarged and tender liver and spleen)
- Schizotrypanids (a urticariform cutaneous rash, usually raised and red).
- Romaña's sign (swelling of eyelid near the bite wound)
- Ophthalmic ganglionar complex (inflammation of the ganglionar complex in the eye, usually causing visual disturbances and redness/swelling).

60%–80% of individuals they will remain asymptomatic for the rest of their life (Bern *et al.* 2007), although of course they can pass it on vertically, or through donation of blood or organs.

One distinguishing sign of the acute infection is Romaña's sign, which occurs if the bite is near an eye, and the parasitic faeces of the insect are rubbed into the eye. This involves swelling of the eyelid. Very rarely, vulnerable individuals (young children or those with weak immune systems) can develop myocarditis or meningoencephalitis in the acute stage.

At present Chagas' disease is rare in Europe, and since up to two-thirds of infected newborns are asymptomatic at birth, congenital infection may not be diagnosed. However, in a woman from an endemic area, examination of the placenta demonstrating liquid-filled cysts can lead to suspicion, and Chagas' can be diagnosed with histopathologic examination and serologic testing, congenital *T. cruzi* infection being confirmed by a positive blood microscopic finding in the infant and mother (Jackson *et al.* 2009). Screening with two sequential serologic tests is considered the most reliable (CDC 2010).

Babies are usually screened two to three times throughout their first year of life, and it is vital that the midwife emphasises to the woman the importance of these tests, and compliance with medication, even if – as is most likely – the baby appears well.

Healthcare professionals in Switzerland have implemented routine screening of pregnant women for Chagas' disease according to their place of origin (Jackson *et al.* 2009). However, in the UK, with limited resources and the probably small number involved, this has not been undertaken. However, the midwife needs to be aware of the risk groups and if, on questioning, she identifies increased risk (*see* Box 13.6) then referral for diagnosis may be appropriate. Early screening and effective treatment for the mother and infant would reduce vertical transmission in future pregnancies, as well as lowering the mother and child's risk of developing life-threatening cardiac and digestive complications in the future (Viotti *et al.* 2006).

BOX 13.6 INCREASED RISK OF CHAGAS' DISEASE

- Lived in rural areas of Mexico, Central America or South America – in particular, if in houses with walls having cracks or crevices
- Have seen a triatomine bug ('kissing bug')
- Previous stillbirth
- Blood transfusion in an endemic country before routine blood screening
- Previously tested positive
- Close relative who has tested positive (or who died from possible Chagas' related complications such as cardiac conditions)

TREATMENT

The drugs of choice for treatment are antiparasitic medication, and benznidazole or nifurtimox are commonly used. However, this is not given in pregnancy or when breastfeeding, and side effects are common, which can be serious and unpleasant (CDC 2010). Treatment will be given to the newborn, usually for an extended period of time, and is expected to be successful in clearing the parasites. The mother will also be similarly treated, but the cure rate for adults with chronic Chagas' disease is not usually as effective. However, treatment has been demonstrated to slow the onset of cardiac disease in adults with chronic Chagas' disease (Rassi *et al.* 2010).

ROLE OF THE MIDWIFE

- If a woman reveals she is from a high-risk area, the midwife should explore some of the other possible risk factors (*see* Box 13.6), which could then lead to a referral for a blood test to establish whether she is serum positive.
- If a woman reports any of the generally non-specific symptoms of Chagas' disease, the midwife should enquire as to her recent travel, keeping the possibility of Chagas' disease in her mind.
- If a woman is diagnosed with chronic Chagas' disease, the midwife must ensure the mother has all the information necessary to encourage compliance with treatment for herself and her baby.

USEFUL RESOURCE

- Centers for Disease Control and Prevention – up-to-date information and American guidelines available at: www.cdc.gov/parasites/chagas (click 'resources for health professionals').

REFERENCES

Adam I, Elhassan E, Mohmmed A, *et al.* (2011) Malaria and pre-eclampsia in an area with unstable malaria transmission in Central Sudan. *Malar J.* **10**: 258.

Akinleye S, Falade C, Ajayi O (2009) Knowledge and utilization of intermittent preventive treatment for malaria among pregnant women attending antenatal clinics in primary health care centers in rural southwest, Nigeria: a cross-sectional study. *BMC Pregnancy Childbirth.* **9**(28): 1–9.

Ansell, J, Hamilton K, Pinder M, *et al.* (2002) Short-range attractiveness of pregnant women to *Anopheles gambiae* mosquitoes. *Trans R Soc Trop Med Hyg.* **96**(2): 113–16.

Bader E, Alhaj A, Hussan A, *et al.* (2010) Malaria and stillbirth in Omdurman Maternity Hospital, Sudan. *Int J Gynecol Obstet.* **109**(2): 144–6.

Basurko C, Carles G, Youssef M *et al* (2009) Maternal and foetal consequences of dengue fever during pregnancy. European Journal of Obstetrics and Gynecology and Reproductive Biology 147(1): 29–32.

Bern C, Montgomery S, Herwaldt B, *et al.* (2007) Evaluation and treatment of Chagas disease in the United States: a systematic review. *JAMA.* **298**(18): 2171–81.

Bhate C, Schwartz R (2011a) Lyme disease: part I. Advances and perspectives. *J Am Acad Dermatol.* **64**(4): 619–36.

Bhate C, Schwartz R (2011b) Lyme disease: part II. Management and prevention. *J Am Acad Dermatol.* **64**(4): 639–53.

Bouwman H, Kylin H (2009) Malaria control insecticide residues in breast milk: the need to consider infant health risks. *Environ Health Perspect.* **117**(10): 1477–80.

Briand V, Bottero J, Noel H, *et al.* (2009) Intermittent treatment for the prevention of malaria during pregnancy in Benin: a randomized, open-label equivalence trial comparing sulfadoxine-pyrimethamine with mefloquine. *J Infect Dis.* **200**(6): 991–1001.

British Infection Association (BIA) (2011) The epidemiology, prevention, investigation and treatment of Lyme borreliosis in United Kingdom patients: a position statement by the British Infection Association. *J Infect.* **62**(5): 329–38.

Brzonova I, Wollenberg A, Prinz J (2002) Acrodermatitis chronica atrophicans affecting all four limbs in an 11-year-old girl. Br J Dermatol 147 (2): 375–8.

Castro E (2009) Chagas disease: lessons from routine donation testing. *Transfus Med.* **19**(1): 16–23.

Centers for Disease Control and Prevention (CDC) (2010) *Parasites – Amercian Trypanosomiasis (also known as Chagas Disease).* Available at: www.cdc.gov/parasites/chagas (accessed 11 June 2012).

Centers for Disease Control and Prevention (CDC) (2012a) *Outbreak Notice: Malaria in Greece.* 19 October 2012. Available at: www.cdc.gov/travel/notices/outbreak-notice/malaria-greece-sept-2012.htm (accessed 17 January 2013).

Centers for Disease Control and Prevention (CDC) (2012b) *Dengue.* Available at: www.cdc.gov/Dengue/faqFacts/index.html (accessed 20 September 2014).

Centers for Disease Control and Prevention (CDC) (2013) Ongoing dengue epidemic. *MMWR Weekly.* **62**(24): 504–7.

Chitra T, Panicker S (2011) Maternal and fetal outcome of dengue fever in pregnancy. *J Vector Borne Dis.* **48**(4): 210–13.

Chukwuocha U, Dozie I, Onwuliri C, *et al.* (2010) Perceptions on the use of insecticide treated nets in parts of the Imo River Basin, Nigeria: implications for preventing malaria in pregnancy. *Afr J Reprod Health.* **14**(1): 117–28.

Chye J, Lim C, Ng K, *et al.* (1997) Vertical transmission of dengue. *Clin Infect Dis.* **25**(6): 1374–77.

Clerk C, Bruce J, Greenwood B, *et al.* (2009) The epidemiology of malaria among pregnant women attending antenatal clinics in an area with intense and highly seasonal malaria transmission in northern Ghana. *Trop Med Int Health.* **14**(6): 688–95.

Daily J (2012) Malaria vaccine trials: beyond efficacy end points. *N Engl J Med.* **367**(24): 2349–51.

Desai M, ter Kuile R, Nosten F, *et al.* (2007) Epidemiology and burden of malaria in pregnancy. *Lancet Infect Dis.* **7**(2): 93–104.

Dorman E, Shulman C (2000) Malaria in pregnancy. *Curr Obstet Gynaecol.* **10**: 183–9.

Dorman E, Shulman C, Kingdom J, *et al.* (2000) Impaired utero-placental blood flow in pregnancies complicated by falciparum malaria. *J Obstet Gynaecol.* **20**(Suppl. 1): S15.

Franco A, Ernest J (2011) Parasitic infections. In: James D, Steer P, Winer C, *et al.* (editors). *High Risk Pregnancy: management options.* 4th ed. New York: Elsevier, Saunders. pp. 543–62.

Gamble C, Ekwaru J, ter Kuile I (2006) Insecticide-treated nets for preventing malaria in pregnancy. *Cochrane Database Syst Rev.* (2): CD003755.

Gould E, Solomon T (2008) Pathogenic flaviviruses. *Lancet.* **371**(9611): 500–9.

Gubler D (2010) Dengue viruses. In: Mahy B, Van Regenmortel M (editors). *Desk Encyclopedia of Human and Medical Virology.* Boston: Academic Press. pp. 372–3.

Gürtier R, Segura E, Cohen J (2003) Congenital transmission of *Trypanosoma cruzi* infection in Argentina. *Emerg Infect Dis.* **9**(1): 29–35.

Guzman M, Halstead S, Artsob H, *et al.* (2010) Dengue: a continuing global threat. *Nat Rev Microbiol.* **8**(12 Suppl.): S7–16.

Health Protection Agency (HPA) (2008) *Foreign Travel-Associated Illness: a focus on those visiting friends and relatives; 2008 Report.* London: HPA. Archived 13.4.13 and now can be viewed through www.nationalarchives.gov.uk/webarchive. (accessed 20 September 2014).

Health Protection Agency (HPA) (2012) *HPA Advises Public to be 'Tick Aware' to Reduce the Risk of Lyme Disease.* Available at: www.gov.uk/government/publications/tick-bite-risks-and-prevention-of-lyme-disease (accessed 20 September 2014).

Health Protection Agency (HPA) (2013) *Increase in Imported Dengue Fever: England Wales and Northern Ireland.* www.gov.uk/government/news/phe-publications-dengue-fever-chikungunya-annual-data (accessed 20 September 2014).

Ismail N, Kampan N, Mahdy Z, *et al.* (2006) Dengue in pregnancy. *Southeast Asian J Trop Med Public Health.* **37**(4): 681–3.

Jackson Y, Myers C, Diana A, *et al.* (2009) Congenital transmission of Chagas disease in Latin American immigrants in Switzerland. *Emerg Infect Dis.* **15**(4): 601–3.

Jannin J, Salvatella R (2006) *Quantitative Estimates of Chagas Disease in the Americas.* OPS/HDM/CD/425-06. Washington: Pan American Health Organization.

Kalilani L, Mofolo I, Chaponda M, *et al.* (2010) The effect of timing and frequency of *Plasmodium falciparum* infection during pregnancy on the risk of low birth weight and maternal anemia. *Trans R Soc Trop Med Hyg.* **104**(6): 416–22.

Knoop K, Stack L, Storrow A, *et al.* (editors) (2010) *Tropical Medicine: atlas of emergency medicine.* 3rd ed. New York: McGraw-Hill Professional.

Ladner J, Valériane L, Etienne K, *et al.* (2003) Malaria, HIV and pregnancy. *AIDS.* **17**(2): 275–6.

Lagerberg R (2008) Malaria in pregnancy: a literature review. *J Midwifery Womens Health.* **53**(3): 209–14.

Lakos A, Solymosi N (2010) Maternal Lyme borreliosis and pregnancy outcome. *Int J Infect Dis.* **14**(6): 494–8.

Lee R (2008) Vector-transmitted infections. In: Rosene-Montella K, Keely E, Barbour L, *et al.* (editors). *Medical Care of the Pregnant Patient.* 2nd ed. Philadelphia: ACP Press.

Lindsay S, Ansell J, Selman C, *et al.* (2000) Effect of pregnancy on exposure to malaria mosquitoes. *Lancet.* **355**(9219): 1972.

Mali S, Kachur S, Arguin P; Division of Parasitic Diseases and Malaria, Center for Global Health; Centers for Disease Control and Prevention (2012) Malaria surveillance: United States, 2010. *MMWR Surveill Summ.* **61**(2): 1–17. Available at: www.cdc.gov/mmwr/preview/mmwrhtml/ss6102a1.htm (accessed 13 January 2013).

Maroun S, Marliere R, Barcellus R, *et al.* (2008) Case report: vertical dengue infection [English, Portuguese]. *J Pediatr (Rio J).* **84**(6): 556–9.

Martina B, Koraka P, Osterhaus A (2009) Dengue virus pathogenesis: an integrated view. *Clin Microbiol Rev.* **22**(4): 564–81.

Mathew D, Loveridge R, Solomon A (2011) Anaesthetic management of caesarean delivery in a parturient with malaria. *Int J Obstet Anesth.* **20**(4): 341–4.

McGready R, Hamilton K, Simpson J, *et al.* (2001) Safety of the insect repellent N, N-diethyl-M-toluamide (DEET) in pregnancy. *Am J Trop Med Hyg.* **65**(4): 285–9.

Moore S, Davies C, Hill N, *et al.* (2007) Are mosquitoes diverted from repellent-using individuals to non-users? Results of a field study in Bolivia. *Trop Med Int Health.* **12**(4): 532–9.

Morel C, Lazdins J (2003) Chagas disease. *Nat Rev Microbiol.* **1**(1): 14–15.

Moretti E, Basso B, Castro I, *et al.* (2005) Chagas' disease: study of congenital transmission in cases of acute maternal infection. *Rev Soc Bras Med Trop.* **38**(1): 53–5.

Morgan M, Figueroa-Munoz J (2005) Barriers to uptake and adherence with malaria prophylaxis by the African community in London, England: focus group study. *Ethn Health.* **10**(4): 355–72.

Msamanga G, Taha T, Young A, *et al.* (2009) Placental malaria and mother-to-child transmission of human immunodeficiency virus-1. *Am J Trop Med Hyg.* **80**(4): 508–15.

National Travel Health Network and Centre (NaTHNaC) (2013) *Travellers: dengue fever reminder.* 15 May 2013. Available at: www.nathnac.org/travel/news/dengue_remind_150513.htm (accessed 1 February 2014).

Nelson-Piercy C (2006) *Handbook of Obstetric Medicine.* 3rd ed. Abingdon: Informa Healthcare.

NHS Choices (2013) www.nhs.uk/news/2013/08august/pages/new-malaria-vaccine-has-potential-to-save-millions.aspx

Pouliot S, Xiong X, Harville E, *et al.* (2010) Maternal dengue and pregnancy outcomes: a systematic review. *Obstet Gynecol Surv.* **65**(2): 107–18.

Procop G, Jessen R, Hyde S, *et al.* (2001) Persistence of *Plasmodium falciparum* in the placenta after apparently effective quinidine/clindamycin therapy. *J Perinatol.* **21**(2): 128–30.

Public Health England (PHE) (2014) PHE guidelines for malaria prevention in travellers from the UK 2014. Available at: www.gov.uk/phe (accessed 18 September 2014).

Ranjit S, Kissoon N (2011) Dengue hemorrhagic fever and shock syndromes. *Pediatr Crit Care Med.* **12**(1): 90–100.

Rassi A, Rassi A, Marin-Neto J (2010) Chagas disease. *Lancet.* **375**(9723): 1388–402.

Rijken M, Papageorghiou A, Thiptharakun S, *et al.* (2012) Ultrasound evidence of early fetal growth restriction after maternal malaria infection. *PLoS One.* **7**(2): e31411.

Roca C, Pinazo M, López-Chejade P, *et al.* (2011) Chagas disease among the Latin American adult population attending in a primary care center in Barcelona, Spain. *PLoS Negl Trop Dis.* **5**(4): e1135.

Royal College of Obstetricians and Gynaecologists (RCOG) (2010a) *The Diagnosis and Treatment of Malaria in Pregnancy.* Green-top Guideline 54B. London: RCOG.

Royal College of Obstetricians and Gynaecologists (RCOG) (2010b) *The Prevention of Malaria in Pregnancy.* Green-top Guideline 54A. London: RCOG.

Schuijt T, Hovius, van der Poll T, *et al.* (2011) Lyme borreliosis vaccination: the facts, the challenge, the future. *Trends Parasitol.* **27**(1): 40–7.

Shulman C, Marshall T, Dorman E, *et al.* (2001) Malaria in pregnancy: adverse effects on haemoglobin levels and birthweight in primigravidae and multigravidae. *Trop Med Int Health.* **6**(10): 770–8.

Smith A, Bradley D, Smith V, *et al.* (2008) Imported malaria and high risk groups: observational study using UK surveillance data 1987–2006. *BMJ.* **337**: a120.

Sotimehin S, Runsewe-Abiodun T, Oladapo O, *et al.* (2008) Possible risk factors for congenital malaria at a tertiary care hospital in Sagamu, Ogun State, South-West Nigeria. *J Trop Pediatr.* **54**(5): 313–20.

Srinivasan R, Kalyanasundaram M (2006) Ultra low volume aerosol application of deltacide (deltamethrin 0.5% w/v, S-bioallethrin 0.71% w/v & piperonyl butoxide 8.9% w/v) against mosquitoes. *Indian J Med Res.* **123**(1): 55–60.

Stanek G, Wormser G, Gray J, *et al.* (2012) Lyme borreliosis. *Lancet.* **379**(9814): 461–73.

Steketee R, Nahlen B, Parise M, *et al.* (2001) The burden of malaria in pregnancy in malaria-endemic areas. *Am J Trop Med Hyg.* **64**(1–2 Suppl.): 28–35.

Stramer S, Hollinger F, Katz L, *et al.* (2009) Emerging infectious disease agents and their potential threat to transfusion safety. *Transfusion.* **49**(Suppl. 2): S1–29.

Strobino B, Abid S, Gewitz M (1999) Maternal Lyme disease and congenital heart disease: a case-control study in an endemic area. *Am J Obstet Gynecol.* **180**(3 Pt. 1): 711–16.

Tagbor H, Bruce J, Browne E, *et al.* (2008) Malaria in pregnancy in an area of stable and intense transmission: is it asymptomatic? *Trop Med Int Health.* **13**(8): 1016–21.

Tan S, McGready R, Zwang J, *et al.* (2008) Thrombocytopaenia in pregnant women with malaria on the Thai-Burmese border. *Malar J.* **7**: 209.

Umbers A, Aitken E, Rogerson S (2011) Malaria in pregnancy: small babies, big problem. *Trends Parasitol.* **27**(4): 168–75.

Uneke C, Ogbonna A (2009) Malaria and HIV co-infection in pregnancy in sub-Saharan Africa: impact of treatment using antimalarial and antiretroviral agents. *Trans R Soc Trop Med Hyg.* **103**(8): 761–7.

Van Eijk A, Ayisi J, Kuile F, *et al.* (2003) HIV increases the risk of malaria in women of all gravidities in Kisumu, Kenya. *AIDS.* **17**(4): 595–603.

Van Eijk, Hill J, Alegana V, *et al.* (2011) Coverage of malaria protection in pregnant women in sub-Saharan Africa: a synthesis and analysis of national survey data. *Lancet Infect Dis.* **11**(3): 190–207.

Viotti R, Vigliano C, Lococo B, *et al.* (2006) Long-term cardiac outcomes of treating chronic Chagas disease with benznidazol versus no treatment. *Ann Intern Med.* **144**: 724–34.

White N (1998) Why is it that antimalarial drug treatments do not always work? *Ann Trop Med Parasitol.* **92**(4): 449–58.

Whitehorn J, Farrar J (2010) Dengue. *Br Med Bull.* **95**: 161–73.

WHO Expert Committee on Malaria (2000) *WHO Expert Committee on Malaria: twentieth report.* WHO Technical Report Series No. 892. Geneva: World Health Organization.

Wiwanitkit V (2010) Unusual mode of transmission of dengue. *J Infect Dev Ctries.* **4**(1): 51–4.

Woensdregt K, Lee H, Norwitz E (2008) Infectious diseases in pregnancy. In: Funai E, Evans M, Lockwood C (editors). *High Risk Obstetrics: the requisites in obstetrics and gynecology.* New York: Mosby, Elsevier. pp. 287–316.

World Health Organization (WHO) (2009) *Dengue: guidelines for diagnosis, treatment, prevention and control.* Available at: http://whqlibdoc.who.int/publications/2009/9789241547871_eng.pdf (accessed 2 February 2010).

World Health Organization (WHO) (2010) *World Malaria Report 2010.* Available at: www.who. int/malaria/world_malaria_report_2010/en/ (accessed 11 November 2014).

World Health Organization (WHO) (2014) *Malaria: Fact Sheet No. 94.* Available at: www.who. int/mediacentre/factsheets/fs094/en/index.html (accessed 20 September 2014).

Yap H, Lee Y, Zairi J, *et al.* (2001) Indoor thermal fogging application of pesguard FG 161, a mixture of d-tetramethrin and cyphenothrin, using portable sprayer against vector mosquitoes in the tropical environment. *J Am Mosq Control Assoc.* **17**(1): 28–32.

CHAPTER 14

Infection control issues

INTRODUCTION

'Infection control' addresses the spread of infections within a healthcare setting, including prevention, investigation and management. This includes not only the woman's health but also the midwives'. Infection control was historically a high-priority concern in midwifery practice. In the early part of the 1900s and before, when puerperal fever was a common killer of childbearing women (Loudon 2000), midwifery care firmly emphasised what they understood to be rigorous infection control procedures.

Infection has had a reduced profile in UK maternity care over the past several decades, not specifically because of low levels but largely because ease of access to – and efficiency of – antibiotics has resulted in very reduced morbidity and mortality levels. Overall better nutrition, housing and access to skilled care and blood transfusion have also improved outcomes. However, recently infection has again become the primary cause of maternal mortality in the UK (CMACE 2011).

Infection usually occurs when normally harmless organisms cause a pathological response. The risk of an infection occurring depends on the balance between the woman's immune system and the number and type of microorganisms she is exposed to. Childbearing women are very susceptible to compromised immune systems, as they are extremely likely to be sleep deprived, nutrient deficient and highly stressed.

Infection can only occur if there is a *source*, a *means of transmission* and a *means of entry* (Moore & Woodrow 2009), and the midwife can have a profound influence on all of these, as she could transport infection from one woman to another. The midwife also routinely carries out procedures including venepuncture, cannulation and catheterisation that breech the woman's normal defence barriers as well as providing a portal for entry of microorganisms.

Currently it is suggested that approximately one-third of hospital-acquired infections could be prevented by high-quality infection control practice (Wilson 2006).

Although this figure is not maternity specific, it does demonstrate that midwives may have lessons to learn from their nursing and medical colleagues in ensuring that women in their care receive the best standard of infection control practice, to confirm that midwives are not complicit in causing, or allowing, an infection to occur. Since women could be infectious before symptoms, or diagnosis, the midwife would not know their medical state. It is therefore important that the midwife incorporates practices into her care that will reduce the risk of transmission from one woman to another, and not just use 'infection control' when an infection is known. It is also important that the midwife employs best practices consistently, in order to protect herself (*see* Box 14.1 concerning 'universal precautions').

BOX 14.1 UNIVERSAL PRECAUTIONS AND STANDARD INFECTION CONTROL PRECAUTIONS

The idea of undertaking methods to protect against the spread of disease, largely through isolation techniques, began formally in the 1970s in the United States, although the practice had been widespread previously in the UK (e.g. tuberculosis hospitals). This approach only considered those ill with communicable diseases. This was then expanded to considering those undiagnosed, with no symptoms, following identification of HIV/AIDS in 1985, where the concept of applying 'universal precautions' (healthcare workers treating all patients/clients as if they were potentially infectious) was identified. In 1996, the Centers for Disease Control and Prevention in the United States replaced universal precautions with 'standard principles' (Garner & HICPAC 1996). In the UK the Department of Health has recently developed and accredited guidelines, the latest versions of which were published by the National Institute for Health and Care Excellence (NICE) (2012) and in 2014 by the *Journal of Hospital Infection* (Loveday *et al.* 2014).

'Isolation' (i.e. separating the woman – usually in a single room – from other women and casual caregivers) is sometimes a necessary technique to prevent the spread of a potentially dangerous infection, and midwives may occasionally be expected to undertake care of this woman, such as during the recent influenza epidemic. Different conditions will need different levels of isolation and use of equipment. Hospitals will have an identified team (e.g. 'the infection prevention and control team') who should be contacted at an early stage for guidance. The trust's infection control lead nurse should be accessed for advice concerning isolation whenever necessary. The local infection control nurse will be a valuable resource when information is needed for specific diseases, isolation precautions and indications for their use.

Precautions are usually divided into the following types.

- *Airborne*: transmitted by inhalation via tiny droplet nuclei from the respiratory tract. These may remain suspended in the air for some time. Examples include measles and tuberculosis.

- *Respiratory droplets*: transmitted via respiratory secretions, in particular sneezing, coughing or even talking. They will not remain airborne and so may not travel far. They may also be transmitted by contact. Examples include mumps, pertussis and some respiratory viruses.
- *Contact*: transmitted via contact with the patient ('direct') or the patient's environment ('indirect'). Some microorganisms can survive long periods to be transmitted by contact with equipment. Examples include *Clostridium difficile* and some antibiotic-resistant organisms such as methicillin-resistant *Staphylococcus aureus* (MRSA).

PERSONAL PROTECTION

All infection control practices benefit both the woman (to whom the midwife may transmit the infection) and the midwife (who is protecting herself, and her personal contacts such as her family).

Hand hygiene

The World Health Organization places hand hygiene as central to its global safety challenges, and it suggests that hand hygiene and cleaning equipment are the best ways to prevent cross-infection (WHO 2005). The hands are acknowledged to be the most common method of transmission of microorganisms between staff and those in their care (Weston 2008, Wilson 2006). Hands can be contaminated with transient skin flora and this has been identified following touching patients or after bed-making, etc. (Wilson 2006), but pathogens are usually found on the staff's skin in the largest number following contact with body fluids (Pittet 2008). Most transient microorganisms are acquired from obviously potentially contaminated contact, but many (e.g. methicillin-resistant *Staphylococcus aureus* or *C. difficile*) can also be acquired from contact with 'clean' surfaces – for example, bed curtains, bed linen and work surfaces (Weston 2008). As cleaning surfaces will only have a transient effect on numbers of microorganisms, there is never a guarantee of a pathogen-free environment, and therefore hand decontamination must always be undertaken before contact with the woman or baby (Loveday *et al.* 2014). It must be remembered that pathogens transferred by the midwife to non-vulnerable areas of the woman (or baby) can then cause colonisation and future infection (Loveday *et al.* 2014).

Although most midwives would agree as to the importance of hand hygiene, it is unlikely they are largely different from other healthcare workers, where it has been demonstrated that the actual amount of hand hygiene may be poorly – and infrequently – undertaken (Pittet 2008). Most transient microorganisms can be removed by even a brief wash with soap and water (Lucet *et al.* 2002), but obviously hands should be washed properly (*see* Box 14.2), applying soap to wet hands only, and following a systematic routine, allowing for all parts of the hands and wrists to be cleansed. The most common parts of the hands missed during washing are thumbs, in between fingers and fingertips. Microorganisms are also found frequently under nails, and this of course has the potential to be even more concentrated if the nails are long.

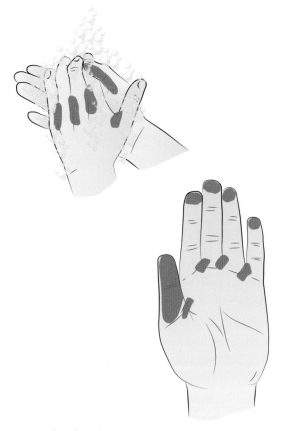

FIGURE 14.1 Areas commonly missed when cleansing hands

The drying of hands is also important, as moist hands can lead to dry and cracked skin, and damaged skin can easily be colonised with pathogens (Larson 2001). There is some research that suggests paper towels can remove some residual bacteria from the hands after washing, making this the preferred way of drying hands. It is also self-evident that paper towels do not have the potential to blow microorganisms from the hands, therefore making them less prone to possible cross-contamination than jet air or warm air hand dryers (Redway & Fawdar 2008).

The convenience and effectiveness of alcohol handrubs and gels have made them a routine part of clinical work. They have been shown to provide a higher reduction in bacterial counts on hands than either soap or antiseptic soap (Boyce & Pittet 2002), although to be effective it is necessary to rub hands together, covering all areas, until the alcohol has evaporated. It has been shown that this practice is often poorly performed, even when being observed (Laustsen *et al.* 2008). However, since handrubs cannot clean visibly soiled hands, soap and water washes continue to be necessary. Also, alcohol handrubs do not work on all pathogens (Hoffman *et al.* 2004) – *C. difficile* is the organism most common in midwifery practice where exclusive attention would need to be paid to soap and water washing.

Midwives need to care for the skin on their hands. A good emollient cream should be used regularly (Loveday *et al.* 2014). In one study almost one-third of healthcare workers reported contact dermatitis of the hands (Kampf & Loffler 2003). If there are any individual concerns with decontamination products damaging skin the occupational health provider should be contacted.

Long, artificial and/or polished nails can increase the number of bacteria on the skin (Jeanes & Green 2001). The 'Bare Below the Elbows' campaign (NICE 2012) is sensible, as some bacteria have been found to survive in the moist areas under rings (Hoffman *et al.* 1985). It is advised by NICE (2012) that before hand decontamination begins, all wrist and ideally hand jewellery should be removed.

The National Health Service has recently had a campaign based on a World Health Organization framework (WHO 2009), highlighting the basics of when to apply hand hygiene, identifying the '5 moments for hand hygiene at the point of care'.

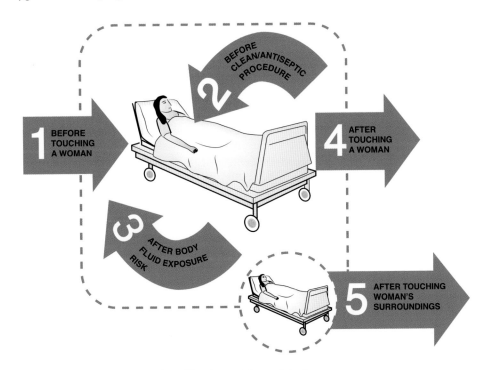

FIGURE 14.2 5 moments for hand hygiene at the point of care

BOX 14.2 HANDWASHING TECHNIQUE

1. Wet hands under tepid running water and then apply liquid soap.
2. Rub hands together vigorously for a minimum of 10–15 seconds, so all surfaces of the hand are covered: particular attention should be paid to the tips of fingers, the thumbs and between the fingers.
3. Hands should be rinsed thoroughly, using elbows to turn off the water, if possible, as taps might have been previously contaminated.

Hands need to be thoroughly dried, ideally with good-quality paper towels.

Use alcohol handrub to decontaminate physically clean hands (e.g. between dealing with different women, or women and their babies). To be effective, apply only to clean hands, and ensure that the handrub comes into contact with all surfaces of the hand, paying particular attention to the tips of fingers, the thumbs and between the fingers, rubbing until the solution has evaporated and the hands are dry.

Hands should be decontaminated:

- before and after contact with women or babies, and also during care if changing between 'clean' and 'dirty' procedures – general research has found that healthcare workers cleansed their hands between a dirty and clean body site on only 11% of occasions (Pittet *et al.* 1999)
- after gloves are removed
- after any contact with body fluid.

All products supplied for hand hygiene in the clinical area must comply with current British standards, and different preparations have different uses. As a general principle:

- use liquid soap – there is evidence microorganisms can grow on soap bars (Archibald *et al.* 1997) – for physically soiled hands
- use antiseptic soap solution before surgical or invasive procedures (e.g. suturing).

Gloves

The use of disposable gloves during midwifery care – when there is an inevitable risk of contact with body fluids – is vital. However, since gloves can be contaminated as they are put on, can contaminate the hands when they are removed, and may contain pinholes, they need to be seen as a way of reducing the risk of acquiring pathogens, not as an impermeable barrier. Gloves cannot be considered a substitute for hand hygiene (Loveday *et al.* 2014).

NICE (2012) recommends gloves be worn for all invasive procedures, contact with sterile sites and non-intact skin or mucous membranes, and all activities carrying a risk of exposure to blood, body fluids, secretions or excretions, or to sharp or contaminated instruments. To be effective gloves need to be changed between 'procedures' – for example, following delivery, where the midwife's gloves may be contaminated with faecal matter. Clean gloves should be used before active management of the third stage, when 'catching' the placenta may bring her contaminated gloves in contact with open areas of the perineum – and certainly should be changed before examination of the perineum for tears. For this reason many midwives 'double-glove' for delivery, removing the contaminated outer gloves after the birth of the baby. This is not an ideal practice, but it may be a compromise at a time when changing gloves with attendant handwashing may not be possible.

Linen, uniforms, scrubs, aprons, masks, eye protection

NICE (2012) and epic3 (Loveday *et al.* 2014) suggest that full-body fluid-repellent gowns must be worn where there is a risk of extensive splashing of blood, body fluids, secretions or excretions onto the skin or clothing of healthcare practitioners, and both use the example of 'assisting with childbirth' as an illustration. In many areas, midwives have abandoned the traditional 'gowning for delivery' as part of the drive to de-medicalise childbirth, but with the rise in the prevalence of infection it may be time to think again about protection of the women we care for, as well as for ourselves.

It has been demonstrated that used hospital linen, contaminated with microorganisms from body fluids, may not be decontaminated unless the wash is sufficient (71°C for 3 minutes or 65°C for 10 minutes is suggested) to kill these (Wilson 2006) – and scrubs or uniforms will need the same care. It is possible if midwives are laundering their own uniforms, or wearing their own clothes when giving clinical care, that they may not be adequately cleaning their workwear and therefore risk spreading infection – including to their own families.

Since the most obvious area susceptible to contamination besides hands is the front of the midwife's torso, plastic aprons should be worn when there is any risk of contaminating normal workwear, such as intimate care of the woman or stripping soiled beds. Bed linen should be disposed of in the appropriate bags (which have been taken to the bedside to avoid carrying soiled linen), and hands washed following any potential contamination.

Eye protection and a mask should be worn if there is a risk of body fluid splashing – caring for a woman in second stage with intact membranes is a common midwifery scenario. Splashes to mucous membranes within eyes and mouth make staff vulnerable to blood-borne viruses as well as other pathogens (Eaton 1996).

Care of sharps

Sharp instruments are a major cause of injury to healthcare workers and can cause transmission of blood-borne viruses (HPA 2008). The risk of transmission depends on many factors (*see* Box 14.3). It should be noted that although all midwives should be protected from hepatitis B, there is no vaccination for hepatitis C or HIV (*see* Chapters 7 and 8). In addition, it is known that the risk of acquiring HIV depends on the infectivity of the virus, and this is highest during seroconversion. Therefore, in a situation where HIV screening is undertaken only at booking, a subsequently infected woman may well be seroconverting at around the time of delivery. This is a timely reminder to always comply strictly with universal precautions and ensure sharps are handled with the maximum of care, irrespective of any known infection of the woman.

BOX 14.3 RISK OF DISEASE TRANSMISSION FOLLOWING NEEDLESTICK INJURY – POSSIBLE INFLUENCES

- The virus present: the risk is considered to be about 1:3 for hepatitis B, 1:30 for hepatitis C, and 1:300 for HIV (Loveday *et al.* 2014)
- Viral load*
- Depth of injury
- Bore of needle (wider, more blood present and increased risk)
- The presence of visible blood on apparatus causing injury
- Time elapsed since sharp was contaminated

* The highest risk of HIV is at the time of seroconversion.

It is unknown how many 'sharps' injuries occur, as it is highly likely many are not reported. However, a nursing survey found 48% of nurses had at least one needlestick injury during their career (Ball *et al.* 2008). It has been identified that commonly sharps injuries take place during venepuncture, and therefore particular care needs to be taken during this procedure. Vacuum blood collection systems are used widely and are considered to be safer than using a needle and syringe when taking blood. If the barrel is reusable (not advisable) then the needle should be removed with a re-sheathing device. NICE (2012) states that needle safety devices must be used where there are clear indications that they will provide safer systems of working for health-care personnel. It should be noted that the number of needlestick injuries reported by those not directly involved (e.g. from inappropriate disposal of contaminated sharps) has risen (HPA 2008) and midwives should take care to safely dispose of sharps used immediately. There have been many practices identified that should be adopted to help prevent sharps injuries (*see* Box 14.4).

BOX 14.4 PREVENTION OF SHARPS INJURIES

- Do not pass sharps directly hand to hand.
- Do not re-cap or re-sheath needles and do not disconnect syringes and needles.*
- Do not transport used sharps to the container; rather, portable 'sharps bins' should be taken to the woman's side or should be easily accessible from a delivery or suturing trolley.
- Sharps should be disposed of safely as soon as possible, and by the person using them.
- Equipment with safety devices should be used whenever possible.
- Sharps should only be discarded into a sharps container that conforms to current national and international standards.
- Sharps bins should only be filled to three-quarters full, or not above 'fill' line, and should then be sealed and replaced.
- Use safe handling and disposal procedures. In particular, ensure safe positioning of sharps bins – the danger of unsupervised toddlers on a postnatal ward is evident.
- Report potentially compromising exposures to body fluid.

* A particularly common risk situation occurs in midwifery when cord blood samples of the newborn are taken for blood gas analysis. After obtaining the sample, if conventional syringe/needles are used, either the needle and syringe need to be separated, and the needle discarded, or the needle needs to be re-sheathed, to enable the sample without an exposed needle to be carried to the blood gas analyser. If re-sheathing is to be done, the sheath should be placed, supported, on a flat surface and the needle inserted without holding the sheath (Wilson 2006), as most needlestick injuries during this procedure involve stabbing the hand holding the sheath. However, ideally a re-sheathing device should be used. In no circumstances should unsheathed needles be carried.

Suturing is a particularly high-risk activity, and many studies report high levels of needlestick injury during this procedure (Wilson 2006). However, none are specific for perineal suturing, and a focus on this area would be of great interest to midwives, especially as one dated study (Tokars *et al.* 1992) suggested that surgical suturing needlestick injuries were three times as common in vaginal hysterectomies (a procedure with some similarities to the suturing of the vaginal wall commonly done by midwives). In general studies it was shown the most common site for injury was the index finger of the non-dominant hand, as it was guiding the needle (Wilson 2006), and it is easy to visualise how this would be particularly so when suturing internal vaginal tears and the perineum. There are suggestions that blunt suture needles should be used to suture all tissues other than the skin, and that double-gloving can reduce the risk of the needle reaching the skin (Tanner & Parkinson 2006). However, the most effective strategy would probably be for the midwife to keep the risk of needlestick injury in the front of her mind, and take time when undertaking suturing – possibly a challenge on a busy labour ward. If exposure to body fluids occurs, the midwife must follow the accepted guidelines for her unit (*see* Table 14.1 for an example).

Occupational health regulations now require all midwives to be immunised against hepatitis B virus. Although some may maintain the benefit of immunisation, not all individuals do, and vaccine-induced antibodies to the hepatitis B virus can decline over time. Boosters may be necessary 5 years after the primary course. Around 10%–15% of adults fail to respond to the three doses of vaccine, and non-responders to the primary course are offered a repeat course and are retested in 1–4 months. Following exposure, hepatitis B immunoglobulin may be needed for additional protection. It is important that a midwife always ensures her immunisation is valid.

TABLE 14.1 Actions to be taken following exposure to body fluids

Needlestick injury	Mucus membrane exposure
Bleed wound under tepid running water. Wash with soap and water	Wash area with soap and water. In the case of a splash to the eyes, irrigate with eye wash solution (all hospital areas where births take place should have eye wash stations easily accessible).
Inform senior midwife, and attend occupational health, accident and emergency, or genitourinary medicine clinic (location depends on local arrangements and time of day) immediately. Counselling should then be received to establish level of risk and whether commencement of post-exposure prophylaxis to potentially prevent HIV is suggested. This medication should ideally be begun very quickly, so rapid action is necessary (as soon as possible and ideally within 1 hour of the exposure).	
Assessment should also be made of the woman's hepatitis C status, if this is not already known. Early antiviral treatment may prevent chronic infection (HPA 2008)	
Record accident – the local method of documentation should be known to the midwife	
It is a duty of employment to inform an employer of a sharps injury (HSE 2013)	

INTRAVENOUS SITES

Cannulation, and care of women with an intravenous (IV) cannula is a common part of midwifery care. However, an intravenous IV cannula can cause blood stream infection, and good care when inserting a cannula, while it is in situ, and on removal, can help prevent this. During general hospitalisation, it has been reported that 48% of bloodstream infections are caused by IV cannulae, and the risk of infection depends on the health of the patient, the type of cannula, how long it is in and how frequently it is manipulated (Coello *et al.* 2003).

The site of an IV cannula has been described as 'not unlike an open wound containing a foreign body' (Maki *et al.* 1973). Common use of IV cannulae may make health professionals lose sight of the vulnerability of these sites as a portal of entry for serious infection. Care of the IV site is therefore an area the midwife needs to pay particular attention to, as every time a cannula is inserted, lines are flushed or infusions started, there is the potential for microorganisms to enter the woman's bloodstream. Ensuring clean hands and taking care to avoid contaminating any area of the equipment that should remain sterile is vital. Insertion is a particularly high-risk time, as bacteria may be introduced into the bloodstream, either from the woman's own skin or from the midwife; therefore asepsis is important (O'Grady *et al.* 2011).

All IV sites should be 'sealed' and a sterile, transparent, semipermeable dressing is commonly used (Loveday *et al.* 2014). However, it is not unusual, especially during a hot and mobile labour, to see these dressings begin to lift – the midwife should ensure this area is kept sealed and that the IV lines are taped sufficiently to ensure the cannula cannot move, which besides perhaps causing the woman pain can also irritate the vein and lead to mechanical phlebitis and potentially infection. An inflammation of the vein at the cannula site (phlebitis) is said to develop in about one-third of general hospital patients with a peripheral IV (Wilson 2006), and this increases the risk of infection, as well as usually being very painful for the woman.

An IV cannula is often necessary for extended periods of time – for example, in a woman with major placenta previa in an antenatal ward. These cannulae should be inspected daily for any signs of inflammation. The use of a visual infusion phlebitis scale (Gallant & Schultz 2006) may provide an easy standardised assessment tool, and this is being introduced in many units. Studies have shown that the risk of colonisation and phlebitis (which increases the risk of blood-borne infection) in peripheral IV cannulae rises 72–96 hours after insertion (NICE 2012). However, a Cochrane review (Webster *et al.* 2013) found no evidence to support routinely changing cannulae in this time period, so individual assessment will be necessary and local guidelines should be available. Maternity units should ensure systems are in place that enable the date and time of IV insertion to be written on the covering dressing, and this information should be clearly documented in the woman's notes. All invasive devices should of course be removed as soon as possible when no longer required.

Microorganisms colonising the hub or access port are one of the most common causes of cannula-related bloodstream infection, and this contamination of the hub is increased by frequent manipulation (Mermel 2000). It is recommended that the hub or access port should be cleaned for a minimum of 15 seconds and allowed to dry before using (Loveday *et al.* 2014). Care also needs to be taken to ensure the connection from the fluid administration set remains sterile until it is attached – which can sometimes be a challenge when a busy midwife is quickly making up an infusion of IV antibiotics in a crowded drug preparation area – however, the importance of contamination or infection prevention should underlie all procedures.

URINARY CATHETERS

The presence of urinary catheters for women around the time of birth has grown extensively along with epidural use and the rise in caesarean sections. However, although common practice, it is still a procedure that carries risks to the woman, and all catheterisations should be carried out as an aseptic procedure (*see* Box 14.6). NICE (2012) suggests after training, healthcare personnel should be assessed for their competence to carry out catheterisation. Hospital-wide studies have demonstrated that urinary tract infections associated with catheterisation can lead to serious blood-borne bacteraemia (Coello *et al.* 2003). In addition, bacteria from a urinary tract infection can circulate around the body and cause secondary infection – for example, in wounds (Wilson 2006). It is considered that as well as enabling microorganisms to easily enter the bladder, the presence of the catheter (a foreign body) reduces the activity of white blood cells and damages the bladder mucosa (Wilson 2006).

Bacteria can enter the bladder:

- during insertion of the catheter
- by tracking up the interior of the tubing
- along the outside of the tube from the perineum.

Women with indwelling urinary catheters are very prone to infection, so good catheter care should be a midwife's priority. The midwife should ensure the catheter is removed as soon as possible and that she follows guidelines on catheter care (*see* Box 14.5) to reduce the risk of infection as far as possible. In addition, since bacteria cannot grow as well in dilute urine, encouraging the woman to drink, or ensuring she does not become dehydrated if not drinking, may be useful.

The use of a lubrication/anaesthetic gel when inserting a catheter is recommended practice (NICE 2012). In maternity care, catheters are most frequently inserted when the woman has an epidural or spinal anaesthesia. Since there is therefore usually minimum discomfort for women, the importance of gel may be overlooked, but the gel acts not only to improve comfort but also, and importantly, to protect the urethral mucosa, which is vulnerable to trauma during catheterisation.

Catheter tubing needs to be fixed to prevent movement of the device in the urethra, which can cause pain, irritation to the mucosa and potentially infection (Gould *et al.* 2010). It will also prevent pulling against vulnerable tissues if the urine collection bag is full and heavy, or if the tubing becomes caught. It is suggested from general research that the use of catheter fixation can reduce infection rates significantly (Freeman 2009). Commercially designed fixation devices include Velcro straps and adhesive swivel clips; however, it may not be possible to always provide these within the restricted budgets most maternity units operate, and with the lack of priority these devices may have when considering short-term use in healthy women. Although it may not be the ideal method, taping the tubing to the woman's inner thigh

---

BOX 14.5 CATHETER CARE GUIDELINES

- Avoid catheterisation if possible.
- Catheters should be inserted using aseptic technique, after cleaning of the vulval area according to local policies.
- Use topical anaesthetic/lubrication during catheterisation to minimise urethral trauma and infection.
- Fill the balloon with the specified amount of sterile water (usually 10 mL) – a partially filled balloon can become distorted and damage the bladder.
- Ensure the tubing is secured to the woman's thigh, to prevent unnecessary movement of the catheter in the urethra, causing trauma.
- Keep the catheter bag below the level of the bladder and off the floor.
- Ensure collection of specimens is done via the sampling port using aseptic technique.
- Maintain a closed sterile drainage system (i.e. only empty when three-quarters full, do not routinely change collection bags).
- Drainage bags should be emptied using clean gloves and collecting receptacle, and without allowing the drainage port to touch the receptacle.
- Keep indwelling catheters in for as short a time as possible.

---

is probably an adequate alternative, and will perform the function necessary in the short term.

Catheter drainage bags should be positioned below the level of the bladder, so that backflow is avoided. Backflow is associated with increased infection (Ward *et al.* 1997). If this cannot be maintained – for example, during a transfer of the woman – the tubing should be clamped for a short period, until the proper drainage position can be resumed (Wilson 2006).

An indwelling urinary catheter system is usually heavily contaminated with micro-organisms, which, after handling by staff, can be transferred to other women. Also pathogens carried on the hands of the midwife or other staff can be transferred to the drainage bag, therefore possibly entering the bladder and causing infection. If emptying drainage bags from more than one woman, gloves should be changed between each woman, as cross-infection has been identified in these circumstances (Wilson 2006). It has also been noted that staff do not regularly disinfect reusable containers effectively, so this is an area that requires particular attention (Wilson 2006).

To empty an indwelling catheter bag: wash hands, put on clean gloves and empty bag into a clean container, discard urine appropriately, disinfect or discard container, remove and discard gloves, wash hands.

Urinary tract infection usually has obvious symptoms (dysuria, frequency, urgency, pyrexia, loin or lower abdominal pain – *see* Chapter 2) but in pregnancy these may overlap with normal features of pregnancy, or at least have pregnancy-related causes. Diagnosis may become even more problematic in a catheterised woman, as many of the traditional symptoms will not be evident (Johnson *et al.* 2006). Therefore a urinary tract infection should be considered early in investigations for a catheterised woman who feels unwell and who may have a high temperature or abdominal pain. A catheter specimen of urine should be collected in an approved way from the sampling port – urine in the collecting bag will almost inevitably show some signs of 'infection', such as appearing cloudy. It should also be remembered that a 'sterile' catheter specimen would indicate infection at lower cell count levels than a normally voided specimen and it must be ensured that the laboratory request is accurately labelled as a 'CSU' (catheter specimen of urine) rather than the more normal 'MSU' (midstream specimen of urine).

WOUND CARE AND PREVENTION OF WOUND INFECTION

See Chapter 3, 'Wound infection'.

ASEPTIC TECHNIQUE

Aseptic technique is commonly used in midwifery practice. The Health and Social Care Act 2008 (DH 2008) requires that healthcare providers have to have a standardised aseptic technique in practice, where education and audit can be demonstrated.

Aseptic technique is a method of prevention of microorganisms entering a susceptible site. It will also prevent microorganisms from an infected site being transferred to the carer. The basic principles are that *sterile items do not come into contact with anything non-sterile* and *only sterile objects come into contact with the vulnerable site*. Any system that enables these principles to be followed can be used, and having a methodical and consistent routine will ensure it becomes second nature. Box 14.6 outlines an example of one method.

BOX 14.6 AN EXAMPLE OF ASEPTIC TECHNIQUE

- Discuss procedure and gain consent.
- Identify a clear, clean space to use, and collect all necessary equipment.
- Position the woman appropriately (although, if necessary, ensure her dignity is maintained by, for example, a draped sheet that she can remove herself when the midwife is ready).
- Wash hands or use alcohol handrub.
- Open sterile packs, cleaning/lubricating fluids as appropriate and gloves, carefully onto a 'sterile field', usually created from the main pack, ensuring nothing sterile touches a surface outside the sterile field.

- Decontaminate hands again (after touching non-sterile outer packs) and put on sterile gloves using an approved method.
- If, for example, cleaning the woman prior to urinary catheterisation, ensure a 'dirty' and 'clean' hand is identified to prevent touching non-sterile areas with the 'clean' hand, and transferring microorganisms onto sterile equipment.
- Use basic principles as already identified throughout the procedure.
- After completing the procedure, ensure all equipment, including any sharps, is appropriately discarded, gloves are removed, hands are washed again and the woman is made comfortable.
- All procedures need to be appropriately documented.

SUMMARY OF PROTECTION FOR THE MIDWIFE

- Cover cuts or grazes to the skin with waterproof dressing and replace as necessary.
- Wash hands with appropriate solution, dry hands properly and use hand cream as necessary to avoid contact dermatitis and other hand injury. Adhere to 'Bare Below the Elbows' to enable maximum cleanliness.
- After assessing risk of procedure, use appropriate protection (e.g. gloves, masks, eye protection, gowns) against direct contact with body fluid. It is common sense that the front of the midwife's body is the most vulnerable area to contamination; therefore, the use of disposable plastic aprons may be the easiest and most effective method of protection for most procedures. Eye protection and a mask should be worn if there is a risk of body fluid splashing.
- The protection emphasis in modern midwifery is against blood-borne viruses, but all body fluids may contain other pathogens. Blood-borne viruses tend to be fragile, but many other pathogens can live – and transfer to others – when dry and after some time has passed. When wet, cotton scrubs, which are commonly worn in delivery suites, allow microorganisms to easily pass through them. Therefore, there is a risk in, for example, not changing scrubs between caring for more than one woman giving birth, or in not washing hands (and showering if necessary) carefully after removing scrubs at the end of a shift.
- Wear gloves when undertaking venopuncture. It may be that when a needlestick injury does occur, the act of the needle going through the glove removes some of the pathogens.
- Ensure hepatitis B vaccination is up to date.
- It is estimated that many incidences of potentially harmful body fluid exposure is not reported. Although most studies are not done exclusively in maternity units, there is no evidence that midwives are any more conscientious, and certainly the scope for exposure to body fluid is greater in midwifery care than by most other

healthcare providers. However, it is only by reporting incidences, that areas of unsafe practice can be identified, and perhaps changes made to enable greater safety for all.

REFERENCES

Archibald L, Corl A, Shah B, *et al.* (1997) *Serratia marcescens* outbreak associated with extrinsic contamination of 1% chloroxylenol soap. *Infect Control Hosp Epidemiol.* **18**(10): 704–9.

Ball J, Pike G; Royal College of Nursing (RCN) (2008) *Needlestick Injury in 2008: results from a survey of RCN members.* London: RCN.

Boyce J, Pittet D (2002) Guideline for hand hygiene in health-care settings: recommendations of the Healthcare Infection Control Practices Advisory Committee and the HICPAC/SHEA/ APIC/IDSA Hand Hygiene Task Force. *Infect Control Hosp Epidemiol.* **23**(12): S1–40.

Centre for Maternal and Child Enquiries (CMACE) (2011) Saving Mothers' Lives: reviewing maternal deaths to make motherhood safer: 2006–2008. The Eighth Report of the Confidential Enquiries into Maternal Deaths in the United Kingdom. *Br J Obstet Gynaecol.* **118**(Suppl. 1): 1–203.

Coello R, Charlett A, Ward V, *et al.* (2003) Device-related sources of bacteraemia in English hospitals: opportunities for the prevention of hospital-acquired bacteraemia. *J Hosp Infect.* **53**(1): 46–57.

Department of Health (DH) (2008) *The Health and Social Care Act 2008: Code of Practice for the NHS on the prevention and control of healthcare associated infections and related guidance.* Available at: www.dh.gov.uk/en/Publicationsandstatistics/Publications/PublicationsPolicyAndGuidance/ DH 093762 (accessed 22 September 2014).

Eaton L (1996) Case notes – subject: Marilyn Smith [occupational risk of hepatitis A]. *Nurs Times.* **92**(24): 10.

Freeman C (2009) Why more attention must be given to catheter fixation. *Nurs Times.* **105**(29): 35–6.

Gallant P, Schultz A (2006) Evaluation of a visual infusion phlebitis scale for determining appropriate discontinuation of peripheral intravenous catheters. *J Infus Nurs.* **29**(6): 338–45.

Garner J; Hospital Infection Control Practices Advisory Committee (HICPAC) (1996) Guideline for isolation precautions in hospitals. *Infect Control Hosp Epidemiol.* **17**(1): 53–80.

Gould C, Umscheid C, Agarwal R, *et al.* (2010) Guideline for prevention of catheter-associated urinary tract infections 2009. *Infect Control Hosp Epidemiol.* **31**(4): 319–26.

Health and Safety Executive (HSE) (2013) *Health and Safety (Sharp Instruments in Healthcare) Regulations 2013: guidance for employers and employees.* Health Services Information Sheet 7. Available at: www.hse.gov.uk/pubns/hsis7.htm (accessed 21 August 2014).

Health Protection Agency (HPA) (2008) *Eye of the Needle: UK surveillance of significant occupational exposure to bloodborne viruses in healthcare workers.* London: HPA.

Hoffman P, Bradley C, Ayliffe G (2004) *Disinfection in Healthcare.* 3rd ed. Oxford: Blackwell Publishing.

Hoffman P, Cooke P, McCarville E, *et al.* (1985) Micro-organisms isolated from skin under wedding rings worn by hospital staff. *Br Med J (Clin Res Ed).* **290**(6463): 206–7.

Jeanes A, Green J (2001) Nail art: a review of current infection control issues. *J Hosp Infect.* **49**(2): 139–42.

Johnson J, Kuskowski M, Wilt T (2006) Systematic review: antimicrobial urinary catheters to prevent catheter-associated urinary tract infection in hospitalized patients. *Ann Intern Med.* **144**(2): 116–26.

Kampf G, Loffler H (2003) Dermatological aspects of a successful introduction and continuation of alcohol-based hand rubs for hygienic hand disinfection. *J Hosp Infect.* **55**(1): 1–7.

Larson E (2001) Hygiene of skin: when is clean too clean? *Emerg Infect Dis.* **7**(2): 225–9.

Laustsen S, Lunde, Bibby B, *et al.* (2008) The effect of correctly using alcohol-based handrub in a clinical setting. *Infect Control Hosp Epidemiol.* **29**(10): 954–6.

Loudon I (2000) *The Tragedy of Childbed Fever.* Oxford: Oxford University Press.

Loveday H, Wilson J, Pratt R, *et al.* (2014) epic3: national evidence-based guidelines for preventing healthcare-associated infection in NHS hospitals in England. *J Hosp Infect.* **86**(Suppl. 1): S1–70.

Lucet J, Rigaud M, Mentre F, *et al.* (2002) Hand contamination before and after different hand hygiene techniques: a randomized clinical trial. *J Hosp Infect.* **50**(4): 276–80.

Maki D, Goldman D, Rhame F (1973) Infection control in intravenous therapy. *Ann Intern Med.* **79**(6): 867–87.

Mermel L (2000) Prevention of intravascular catheter-related infections. *Ann Intern Med.* **132**(5): 391–402.

Moore T, Woodrow P (2009) *High Dependency Nursing Care: observation, intervention and support for level 2 patients.* 2nd ed. London: Routledge.

National Institute for Health and Care Excellence (NICE) (2012) *Infection Control: prevention of healthcare-associated infection in primary and community care.* Clinical Guideline 139. London: NICE.

O'Grady N, Alexander M, Burns L, *et al.* (2011) Guidelines for the prevention of intravascular catheter-related infections. *Clin Infect Dis.* **52**(9): e162–93.

Pittet D (2008) Hand hygiene: it's all about when and how. *Infect Control Hosp Epidemiol.* **29**(10): 957–9.

Pittet D, Mourouga P, Perneger T (1999) Compliance with handwashing in a teaching hospital. *Ann Intern Med.* **130**(2): 126–30.

Redway K, Fawdar S (2008) *A Comparative Study of Three Different Hand Drying Methods: paper towel, warm air dryer, jet air dryer.* European Tissue Symposium. Available at: www.europeantissue.com/pdfs/090402-2008%20WUS%20Westminster%20University%20hygiene%20study,%20nov2008.pdf (accessed 10 August 2010).

Tanner J, Parkinson H (2006) Double gloving to reduce surgical cross-infection. *Cochrane Database Syst Rev.* (3): CD003087.

Tokars J, Bell D, Culver D, *et al.* (1992) Percutaneous injuries during surgical procedures. *JAMA.* **267**(21): 2899–904.

Ward V, Wilson J, Taylor L, *et al.* (1997) *Preventing Hospital-Acquired Infection: clinical guidelines.* London: Public Health Laboratory Service.

Webster J, Osborne S, Rickard C, *et al.* (2013) Clinically-indicated replacement versus routine replacement of peripheral venous catheters. *Cochrane Database Syst Rev.* (4): CD007798.

Weston D (2008) *Infection Prevention and Control: theory and practice for healthcare professionals.* Chichester, West Sussex: John Wiley.

Wilson J (2006) *Infection Control in Clinical Practice.* 3rd ed. Edinburgh: Baillière Tindall, Elsevier.

World Health Organization (WHO) (2005) *Global Patient Safety Challenge: 2005–2006.* Geneva: WHO.

World Health Organization (WHO) (2009) *About SAVE LIVES: Clean Your Hands. My 5 moments for hand hygiene.* Geneva: WHO.

Glossary

abscess: A localised collection of pus.

acrodermatitis chronica atrophicans: A progressive fibrosing skin lesion.

active immunity: Protective immunity that develops after exposure to infection or vaccination.

acute: A short, sharp illness that may be severe but from which most people will recover in a few weeks without lasting effects.

aerobe: A microbe that grows in the presence of oxygen (*see* anaerobe).

alanine aminotransferase (ALT): A liver enzyme that enters the blood following liver damage.

albumin: The main protein in human blood, manufactured by the liver.

allergen: An antigen that causes an allergic reaction (either immediate or delayed).

anaerobe: A microbe that grows in the absence of oxygen (*see* aerobe).

anaphylaxis: A severe and rapid allergic reaction, causing constriction of the trachea (airway) and needing immediate and life-saving measures.

antibody: A protein produced by B-lymphocytes that appears in body fluids in response to contact with a foreign molecule (antigen) and which combines specifically with that antigen to destroy it.

antigen: A molecule (usually protein) on the surface of cells, viruses, fungi, bacteria and some non-living substances such as toxins, chemicals, drugs and foreign particles. The immune system recognises antigens and produces antibodies that destroy matter containing antigens.

antiseptic: A chemical used to kill microbes on body surfaces.

arthralgia: Joint pain.

ascites: Accumulation of fluid in the cavity that surrounds the bowel, leading to enlarged, swollen and painful abdomen.

asepsis: The complete absence of bacteria, fungi, viruses or other microorganisms that could cause disease.

aseptic non-touch technique (ANTT): Standardised aseptic technique, including identification and protection of the key parts of the procedure, performing effective hand hygiene, instituting a non-touch technique, wearing the appropriate personal protective equipment.

aseptic technique: Method developed to ensure only uncontaminated objects/fluids make contact with sterile or susceptible sites. It is the last line of defence for women from infection during any invasive clinical procedure.

aspartate aminotransferase (AST): A liver enzyme.

atopy: Genetic predisposition to allergy.

autogenous: From within the person.

autoimmune: A type of disease causing the body's immune system to attack another part of the body.

autologous: In blood transfusion, a situation in which the donor and recipient are the same person.

bacteraemia: The presence of bacteria in the blood, with clinical symptoms of infection.

bile: A yellow/green fluid made by the liver to help digest foods containing fat and cholesterol.

bilirubin: A product of the breakdown of haemoglobin.

cellulitis: A bacterial infection, usually involving the skin. It is commonly red, swollen and painful.

chemokines: 'Signalling proteins' that can attract cells to the site of the infection.

chemoprophylaxis: Administration of a drug to prevent disease or infection.

cholangiocarcinoma: Cancer of the bile ducts.

cholangitis: Inflammation of the bile ducts.

cholestasis: A condition where the flow of bile from the liver is reduced.

chronic: An illness that lasts a long time (>6 months), possibly for the rest of a person's life.

cirrhosis: Where inflammation and fibrosis have spread to disrupt the shape and function of the liver. Even with no signs or symptoms of liver disease, the working capacity of liver cells has been badly impaired and they are unable to repair the liver. This is permanent cell damage and can lead to liver failure or liver cancer.

coagulopathy: A condition where the blood's ability to clot is compromised.

co-infection: Being infected with more than one virus/bacteria at the same time.

colonisation: When bacteria live in the body without causing any harm or symptoms.

commensal: Naturally occurring bacteria, which cause no harm to the carrier.

compensated disease: Where medical treatment has counterbalanced damaged organ function. Decompensated disease is where treatment can no longer counterbalance severe organ damage.

complement: A cascade of serum enzymes activated by the presence of pathogens.

contamination: Soiling of inanimate objects or living material with potentially harmful infectious matter. Wounds can be contaminated by organisms on the surface of the wound bed when there is no replication or host response, and therefore no infection.

C-reactive protein (CRP): An acute-phase protein produced by the liver, with increases in serum and amniotic fluid, which can be used as a marker of inflammation and to monitor the inflammatory response.

cross-infection: Transmission of a pathogenic organism from one person to another.

cytokines: Soluble molecules used to transmit messages from cell to cell. Types of cytokine include interferons and chemokines.

decontamination: A process that removes hazardous substances, including chemicals or microorganisms.

disinfection: A process that reduces the number of microorganisms to a level where they should not be harmful. Bacterial spores and viruses may not be destroyed.

dyspnoea: Difficulty breathing.

dysuria: Pain on micturition (passing urine).

ELISA (enzyme-linked immunosorbent assay): A biochemical test used mainly in immunology to detect the presence of an antibody or an antigen in a sample.

encephalopathy: Disturbed brain function leading to mental confusion and memory loss.

endogenous: From within the body. Endogenous infection is caused by microbes that are carried by the woman in her own normal bacterial flora.

envelope: An outer membrane that surrounds the capsid of some viruses and may be derived partly or wholly from the host cell.

enzyme: A substance, usually a protein, produced by the body to help speed up a chemical reaction.

erythema (erythematous): Redness of the skin or mucous membrane, usually caused by injury, infection or inflammation.

exogenous: From outside the body.

fetal fibronectin (fFN) test: Assesses fFN in vaginal/cervical fluid, and is a good indicator of preterm birth in symptomatic women. If negative it can almost totally rule out preterm birth, although does not have a good positive predictive value in asymptomatic women.

fibroblasts: The most common cells of connective tissue, synthesising collagen and maintaining structural strength.

fibrosis: Where scar tissue is formed in an organ in response to ongoing inflammation.

focal infection: Infection of a small area of the body that causes subsequent infection elsewhere.

fulminant (or fulminating): Disease with rapid onset and following a short, severe course.

gastroenterologist: A doctor who specialises in treating digestive diseases.

glycogen: Glycogen is the way the body stores (in the liver and muscles) carbohydrates. It is easily changed back to glucose when the body needs energy quickly.

granuloma: Localised area of chronic inflammation, usually produced in response to a pathogen that is hard to clear.

haematopoiesis: The formation of blood cell components.

haemolysis: Destruction of the red blood cells.

HAV: Hepatitis A virus.

HBV: Hepatitis B virus.

HCC: Hepatocellular carcinoma, also called hepatoma. With biliary tree cancer, HCC is one of the two main types of primary liver cancer.

HCV: Hepatitis C virus.

hepatic: Anything relating to the liver.

hepatic artery: The artery that carries blood to the liver, pancreas, gall bladder, stomach and duodenal portion of the small intestine.

hepatocyte: A liver cell.

hepatologist: A doctor who specialises in liver diseases.

hepatomegaly: Enlarged and tender liver.

hepatosplenomegaly: Enlarged and tender liver and spleen.

hydrops fetalis: A condition of the fetus where there is an accumulation of fluid in fetal compartments.

hyperthermia: When the body's core temperature rises due to failed thermoregulation.

hypothermia: When the body's core temperature drops below that required for normal metabolism – usually <35°C.

hypovolaemia: Decreased blood volume.

iatrogenic: Resulting from healthcare treatment.

immunoglobulin: Found in the blood, other body fluids and in cell tissues. Proteins of animal origin, with known antibody activity, synthesised by lymphocyte and plasma. They bind to invading organisms to destroy them. Can be derived from pooled plasma originating from blood donations to use therapeutically.

incubation period: The interval between contact with the microbe and the development of the signs and symptoms of infection.

infection: Presence of a microorganism in the tissues that causes a host response.

inflammation: The first response of the immune system to microbes, commonly characterised by heat, swelling, pain and tenderness.

interferon: A cytokine with antiviral effects.

jaundice: A condition in which the whites of the eyes go yellow and in more severe cases the skin also turns yellow. This is caused by the build-up of bilirubin (containing yellow pigment), which is normally processed by the liver to be excreted.

latent infection: When the clinical signs of infection are absent and the causative organism may be temporarily undetectable, but under certain conditions the infection may again become obvious.

leucocytes: White blood cells, a vital part of the immune system.

macrophage: A type of long-lived phagocyte in the tissues.

myalgic encephalomyelitis (ME): Also known as chronic fatigue syndrome, a condition in which a person always feels tired without a clear-cut medical reason.

meningism: Neck stiffness.

meningitis: Inflammation of the membranes that cover the brain and spinal cord, usually a result of infection by any of several microorganisms.

monovalent: Single strain, as in vaccines.

myalgia: Pain in the muscles (common in many viral infections).

negative-pressure respiratory isolation: Where air is mechanically pulled into ducts from the room and moved to outside vents via a filter.

neutropenia: Reduction in the number of circulating white blood cells ($<1000\,mm^3$), which will compromise the immune response.

oncologist: A doctor who specialises in understanding and treating cancer.

ophthalmia neonatorum: Mucopurulent discharge, inflammation and possibly oedema of the eyelids in the newborn. Common causes are maternal chlamydia or gonorrhoea.

ophthalmic ganglionar complex: Inflammation of the ganglionar complex in the eye, usually causing visual disturbances and redness/swelling.

orthopnoea: Difficulty breathing when lying flat.

parametritis: Inflammation of the ligaments around the uterus.

parenteral: Administered via injection into the tissues (intravenously, intramuscularly, subcutaneously).

parenteral feeding: Administration of nutrients by an infusion into a vein.

paroxysmal nocturnal dyspnoea: A sensation of shortness of breath that wakes the woman up at night.

pathogen: A substance that can cause disease.

peritonitis: Inflammation of the peritoneum (the tissue that lines the inner wall of the abdomen, covering most of the abdominal organs).

phlebitis: Inflammation of a vein.

polymerase chain reaction (PCR): A laboratory technique used to make multiple copies of a segment of DNA from a sample.

post-exposure prophylaxis (PEP): Drug treatment administered as soon as possible after an exposure to reduce the risk of acquiring a blood-borne virus.

prophylaxis: Preventive medical treatment.

prothrombin time: A test measuring the clotting time of plasma.

pus: A fluid formed as a result of infection consisting of dead and living microbes, phagocytes and tissue cells.

resistance: The ability of an infectious organism to survive and multiply despite the administration and absorption of a medicine given in doses equal to or higher than those usually recommended.

salpingitis: Inflammation and infection of the fallopian tubes.

sensitivity: The susceptibility of certain organisms to specific agents.

sepsis: A complex syndrome that, as it progresses, can affect all body systems, eventually leading to multiple organ failure.

septicaemia: A rapid multiplication of bacteria, and the presence of bacterial toxins in the blood (also known as 'blood poisoning'). Accompanied by signs and symptoms of infection.

seroconversion: The production of specific antibodies in response to an antigen.

seroprevalence: The percentage of a population who have been previously exposed to the infection.

serotypes: Different types of capsular carbohydrates that identify a particular strain.

sharps: Instruments used in delivering healthcare that can inflict a penetrating injury.

shock: Physiological shock is a dangerous reduction of blood flow throughout the body that, if not treated, can lead to collapse, coma and death.

sterilisation: The removal or destruction of all living organisms including bacterial spores and viruses.

subclinical infection: Early stages, or a very mild form, of infection, which produce no signs or symptoms.

systemic: Involving the whole body.

thrombocytopenia: A reduction in the number of platelets (thrombocytes) in the blood. This may result in bleeding into the skin, spontaneous bruising or prolonged bleeding after injury.

topical: Usually referring to a drug that is applied to a body surface.

toxin: A poisonous substance produced by, usually, a microbe.

varices: Dilated (expanded) and protruding blood vessels.

viraemia: Presence of virus in the blood.

viral load: The amount of virus present in the blood.

vector: An animal (e.g. an insect or tick) that transfers an infectious microbe between hosts.

virulent: Extremely infectious, which commonly can overwhelm a person's immunity and can spread easily to others.

West Nile virus: A mosquito-borne arbovirus, usually involving birds as the prime reservoir, found in temperate and tropical regions of the world. Is often subclinical but can cause encephalitis.

Index

References in **bold** refer to figures, tables and boxes.

viral infections
    common childhood, 249, 252
    genital, 105
    and UTIs, 42
viral load
    in breast milk, 174–5
    at conception, 168
    in hepatitis A, 184
    in hepatitis B, 188
    in hepatitis C, 194
    and risk of transmission, 165, 172–3, 338
viral load assays, 171
viral pneumonia, 219
viral protease inhibitors, 169
viruses
    blood-borne, 345
    classification of, 5–7
    and immune system, 16–17
vitamin A deficiency, 67–8
vitamin B complex, and wound healing, 68
vitamin B$_6$, 227
vitamin C
    and smoking, 33–4
    and wound healing, 68
vitamin D
    deficiency of, 223
    supplements of, 33
vomiting
    and malaria, 305, 307–8
    and whooping cough, 240
vulval itching, 130, 137
VZIG (varicella zoster immunoglobulin), 269–71

Wakefield, Andrew, 259
warm shock, 84
water, contaminated, 10, 174, 184–5
WBCs (white blood cell) count
    in pregnancy, 86
    reference ranges for, **28**
    rising, 48, 76

WBCs (white blood cells)
    environment encouraging, 66
    in immune system, 15
weight loss
    and HIV, 163
    postnatal, 32
whooping cough
    2012 outbreak of, 3, 24, 239–41
    clinical features of, 239–40
    contact with cases of, 244–5, **246**
    transmission of, 240, 333
    vaccination for, 240, **241**, 242–6; *see also* diphtheria-pertussis-tetanus vaccination
woman-centred approach, 227
worms, 5, 8, 22
wound care, 72, 74, 78
wound cleaning, 72
wound healing
    environment for, 66–7
    and inflammatory response, 17, 26
    influences on, **67**, 68–71
    and midwifery, 72–4
    primary and secondary intention of, 65
    and sleep, 34
    and smoking, 33
    stages of, 61–4
    and stress, 35
wound infection, 61
    and GBS, 156
    increased risk of, **66**
    midwifery reducing, 72
    organisms causing, 9
    and pyrexia, 51
    and sepsis, 85
    signs and symptoms of, **76**, 77
    from surgical procedures, 70–1, 74

yeast infections, 105, 153
yellow fever, 24, 181

zinc, absorption of, 33
zinc deficiency, 67

CPD with Radcliffe

You can now use a selection of our books to achieve CPD (Continuing Professional Development) points through directed reading.

We provide a free online form and downloadable certificate for your appraisal portfolio. Look for the CPD logo and register with us at: www.radcliffehealth.com/cpd

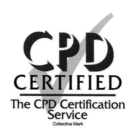